Bladder Cancer
Principles of Combination Therapy

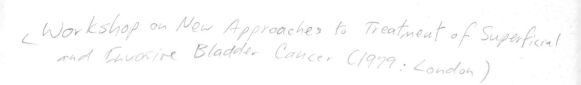
Bladder Cancer
Principles of Combination Therapy

R.T.D. Oliver, MD, MRCP

Senior Lecturer in Medical Oncology,
Institute of Urology, London

W.F. Hendry, ChM, FRCS

Consultant Urologist,
St Bartholomew's Hospital, London

H.J.G. Bloom, MD, FRCP, FRCR, FACR(Hon)

Consultant Radiotherapist and Oncologist,
Royal Marsden Hospital and Institute of Cancer Research, London

BUTTERWORTHS
London - Boston
Sydney-Wellington-Durban-Toronto

First published 1981

© Butterworth & Co (Publishers) Ltd, 1981

British Library Cataloguing in Publication Data

Workshop on New Approaches to Treatment of
    Superficial and Invasive Bladder Cancer,
    London, 1979.
    Bladder cancer.
    1. Bladder — Cancer — Congresses
    I. Title II. Oliver, R T D III. Hendry, W F
    IV. Bloom, H J G V. University of London.
    Institute of Urology
    616.9'94'62   RC280.B5   80-41725

ISBN 0-407-00187-5

Typeset by Scribe Design, Gillingham, Kent
Printed and bound by Mackays of Chatham

Acknowledgements

This book is derived from papers presented at the Institute of Urology Workshop on New Approaches to Treatment of Superficial and Invasive Bladder Cancer, held on 1st and 2nd July, 1979. We gratefully acknowledge the additional sponsorship of this workshop by the International Union Against Cancer (UICC) and the Imperial Cancer Research Fund Department of Medical Oncology, St Bartholomew's Hospital. We also acknowledge the support given by Lederle, ICI, Mead Johnson, Montedison, Ward Blenkinsop and Glaxo. Our thanks are due to Miss Anthea Minchom and Miss Linda Hayes of the Institute of Urology for editorial assistance and retyping of the edited manuscript, and to Miss Lindsey Pegus of the Department of Medical Arts, Royal Marsden Hospital and Institute of Cancer Research for the design of the motif on the spine of the cover.

Contributors

A. Akdas, MD
Clinical Research Fellow, Unit of Cancer Research, University of Leeds

†J.P. Blandy, DM, MCh, FRCS
Department of Urology, The London Hospital, London

*†H.J.G. Bloom, MD, FRCP, FRCR, FACR(Hon)
Consultant Radiotherapist and Oncologist, Royal Marsden Hospital and Institute of Cancer Research, London and St. Peters Group of Hospitals, London

Brigid Breckman, SRN
Department of Urology and Stomatherapy, Royal Marsden Hospital, London

L. Denis, MD
Dienst Urologie, A.Z. Middleheim, Antwerp, Belgium

John P. O'Donohue, MD
Professor and Chairman, Department of Urology, Indiana University Medical Center and Indianapolis Veteran's Administration Hospital, Indianapolis, USA

---

*These contributors are members of the London and Oxford Cooperative Urological Cancer Group which comprises Grant Williams (Chairman), Prof M. Alderson, H.J.G. Bloom, H.T. Ford, W.F. Hendry, R.J. Shearer, P.A. Trott (The Royal Marsden Hospital); J. Malpas, R. Sandland, H. Whitfield (St Bartholomew's Hospital); N. Howard, E. Newlands, P.F. Philip (Charing Cross Hospital); J. Boyd (St Helier Hospital); M. Snell (St Mary's Hospital); R. Durrant, G. Fellows, J.C. Smith (Oxford); R.T.D. Oliver, P.R. Riddle (St Peter's Hospitals); G.F. Abercrombie, I. Cade and J. Vinnicombe (Portsmouth)

†Participant in workshop

†F. Edsmyr, MD
WHO Collaborating Centre for Research and Treatment of Urinary Bladder Cancer, Radiumhemmet, Karolinska Sjukhuset, Stockholm, Sweden

†Lawrence E. Einhorn, MD
Associate Professor, Department of Medicine, Indiana University Medical Center and Indianapolis Veteran's Administration Hospital, Indianapolis, USA

†H.R. England, MB ChB(NZ), FRCS
Consultant Urologist, Department of Urology, The London Hospital, London

†P.-L. Esposti, MD
Radiumhemmet, Karolinska Sjukhuset, Stockholm, Sweden

†R.C.L. Feneley, MB, MChir, FRCS
Consultant Urologist, Department of Surgery, University of Bristol and Bristol and Weston Health District (Teaching), Bristol

V.C. Harral
District Administrator, District Headquarters, University of Bristol and Bristol and Weston Health District (Teaching), Bristol

*†W.F. Hendry, ChM, FRCS
Department of Urology, St. Bartholomew's Hospital, London

N.J. Hodson, BSc, MB ChB, FRCR
Department of Diagnostic Radiology and Radiotherapy, Royal Marsden Hospital and Institute of Cancer Research, Royal Marsden Hospital (Surrey Branch), Sutton

†H.F. Hope-Stone, MB BS, FRCR
Consultant Radiotherapist and Oncologist, Department of Radiotherapy and Oncology, The London Hospital, London

†Janet E. Husband, MB BS, MRCP, FRCR, DCH, DObstRCOG
Department of Diagnostic Radiology and Radiotherapy, Royal Marsden Hospital and Institute of Cancer Research, Royal Marsden Hospital (Surrey Branch), Sutton

†Günther H. Jacobi, MD
Department of Urology, University of Mainz Medical School, Mainz, West Germany

M.A. Jones, MB, FRCS
Department of Urology and Stomatherapy, Royal Marsden Hospital, London

*A. Lachand, MD
Service d'Urologie, Hôpital H. Mondor, Créteil, France

N. Manning, MB BS
Department of Urology, St. Bartholomew's Hospital, London

†C. Merrin
Urologic Oncologist, Cancer Treatment Center, Swedish Covenant Hospital, Chicago, USA; Associate Clinical Professor of Urology, Stritch Medical School, Chicago, USA

†E. Molland, MD, MRCPath
Department of Histopathology, The London Hospital, London

†Alvaro Morales, MD, FRCS(C), FACS
Department of Urology, Queen's University, Kingston, Canada

William M. Murphy, MD
Associate Professor, Department of Pathology, University of Tennesse Center for Health Science, Memphis, USA

*†R.T.D. Oliver, MD, MRCP
Senior Lecturer in Oncology, Institute of Urology, London

†Carol O'Toole, PhD
Department of Immunology, London Hospital Medical College, London

A.M.I. Paris, MB, FRCS, DObstRCOG
Department of Urology, The London Hospital, London

M. De Pauw
EORTC Data Center, Institut Jules Bordet, Brussels, Belgium

†M. Pavone-Macaluso, MD
Institute of Urology, University Polyclinic Hospital, Palermo, Italy

N.M. Perry, MB BS
Department of Urology, St. Bartholomew's Hospital, London

†J.P. Pryor, MS, FRCS
Dean, Institute of Urology, London

†R.C.B. Pugh, MD, MRCS, FRCPath
Consultant Pathologist, St. Peter's Hospitals and the Institute of Urology, London

†B. Richards, MD, FRCS
Department of Urology, York District Hospital, York

*†P.R. Riddle, MS, FRCS
St. Peter's Hospitals and the Institute of Urology, London

C.C. Rigby, MB ChB, FRCPath
Institute of Urology, London

M.R.G. Robinson, MB, FRCS(Eng.), FRCS(Ed.), DObstRCOG
Yorkshire Urological Cancer Research Group, The General Infirmary, Pontefract, Yorkshire

†C.C. Shulman, MD
Department of Urology, Erasme University Hospital, Brussels, Belgium

†P.H. Smith, MB, FRCS
*Head, Department of Urology, St. James's Hospital, Leeds
Chairman, EORTC Urological Group*

†Mark S. Soloway, MD
Associate Professor, Department of Urology, University of Tennessee Center for Health Science, Memphis, USA

M. Staquet
EORTC Data Center, Institut Jules Bordet, Laboratoire de Statistique Médicale, Université Libre de Bruxelles, Belgium

R. Sylvester
EORTC Data Center, Institut Jules Bordet, Brussels, Belgium

M.O. Symes, MD, MB ChB
Consultant Senior Lecturer in Immunology, Department of Surgery, University of Bristol and Bristol and Weston Health District (Teaching), Bristol

*P.A. Trott, MB BChir, MRCPath
Royal Marsden Hospital (Surrey Branch), Sutton

Alan G. Turner, MB BS, FRCS(Eng.), FRCS(Ed.)
Consultant Urologist, Peterborough District Hospital, Northamptonshire

*H.N. Whitefield, MA, MB BChir, MChir, FRCS
Department of Urology, St. Bartholomew's Hospital, London

†Willet F. Whitmore, Jr., MD
Urologic Service of the Department of Surgery, Memorial Sloan-Kettering Cancer Center, New York, USA

J.E.A. Wickham, BSc, MS, FRCS
Department of Urology, St. Bartholomew's Hospital, London

*†Grant B. Williams, MSc, MS, FRCS
Royal Marsden Hospital (Surrey Branch), Sutton

Stephen D. Williams, MD
Assistant Professor, Department of Medicine, Indiana University Medical Center and Indianapolis Veteran's Administration Hospital, Indianapolis, USA

†Alan Yagoda, MD
Associate Attending Physician, Solid Tumor Service, Memorial Sloan-Kettering Cancer Center, New York, USA

Contents

Part IV Immunotherapy

Introduction

W.F. Hendry, R.T.D. Oliver and H.J.G. Bloom

Bladder tumours are common: they comprise a significant part of the urologist's work and can confront him with many difficult problems. In some cases their management is quite straightforward — for example, many papillary tumours can be resected completely and seldom if ever recur; yet on other occasions, when apparently similar tumours are dealt with in an identical manner, the bladder produces a crop of recurrences which become increasingly difficult to manage at each cystoscopy. How can the urologist predict this behaviour? Should he persist with cystodiathermy; will radiotherapy help; what about intravesical chemotherapy; should cystectomy be considered — it would certainly solve the problem, but is it essential? The opportunity to eradicate the tumour must not be missed, thereby allowing possible progression and dissemination to occur by simple inactivity. Most superficial tumours are initially curable, but selection of the appropriate treatment and correct assessment of the therapeutic response is not easy, and with increasing experience the urologist recognizes these difficulties.

The situation should be more clear-cut with solid tumours. The tumour is infiltrating (it has declared its malignant character) and, with accurate assessment of the depth of invasion, an appropriately aggressive approach can be made with regard to its treatment. But the chance of successfully eradicating the disease has to be balanced against the morbidity produced by treatment, which may vary with the individual patient. The value of radiotherapy is universally recognized, but when should it be given, and how much, and by what technique? Should cystectomy be done as an early elective procedure, or should the bladder be saved for as long as possible and only removed when all other measures have failed? Chemotherapy has produced spectacular improvement in the results of treatment in other fields of oncology such as Hodgkin's disease, paediatric tumours and testicular teratomas. Some patients with advanced bladder cancer do show a transient response to cytotoxic drugs — would these agents prove more successful if given earlier in the course of the disease, especially when the metastases are microscopic?

These are questions that face the urologist daily, and should be discussed with colleagues who share in the management of the patient. Urologists have worked closely with radiotherapists for many years. This close collaboration has not only improved treatment results but has also reduced the incidence of complications as each specialist has become aware of the benefits and hazards associated with the other's specialty. The advent of the medical oncologist has brought expertise in the administration of drugs which, in view of the disseminated nature of malignant disease, holds the promise of systemic cancer therapy, but carry the added risk of potentially lethal side-effects. The successful combination of surgery, radiotherapy and chemotherapy in the treatment of bladder cancer forms the main substance of this book, which has developed from a meeting on this topic held by the Institute of Urology under the sponsorship of the International Union Against Cancer (UICC) in London in July 1979.

The first essential step in the treatment of bladder cancer is the recognition of the extent of the tumour and its degree of malignancy (stage and grade) in order to plan the appropriate treatment; hence the first part of this book is devoted to the pathological aspects of bladder tumours and their relationship to prognosis. Superficial tumours are most often papillary, and when these lesions escape from control by simple endoscopic methods, intravesical chemotherapy may not only help to control the tumour, but also to define, on the basis of non-response, patients for whom more radical therapy is necessary. Experience with various chemotherapeutic agents in treating recurrent superficial tumours, and interpretation of response, is the subject of Part IIA. In Part IIB special attention is given to flat in situ carcinoma, the incidence, the frequent widespread nature and the serious prognostic significance which has only been recognized in recent years. Of particular interest in this section is the new information or response of this condition to chemotherapy although, as with patients with extensive papillary non-invasive tumours, cystectomy is still occasionally required to forestall the progression of this condition to frank invasive tumours.

Deeply infiltrating bladder cancer is universally recognized as a threat to life, but there is much controversy concerning the best approach to its management. The case for radical radiotherapy is debated in Part IIIA, and is compared with the results obtained by pre-operative radiotherapy and elective cystectomy. Regardless of the method or treatment used, the need for effective systemic adjuvant therapy is obvious, since over half the patients die of cancer, often with distant metastases. The results obtained with chemotherapy in advanced disease are detailed in Part IIIB. Possible methods of integrating chemotherapy with radiotherapy and surgery are described in the context of the early experiences of some ongoing trials in Part IIIC. Finally, immunotherapy, a therapeutic enigma, is considered in Part IV.

The contents of this book are a record of work in progress. The results described with superficial tumours may help the urologist in the management of these tumours, which make up so much of his day-to-day work load. For invasive tumours, the controversy surrounding the test use of established treatment such as radiotherapy and cystectomy continues. However, until results from controlled trials in progress become available, the value of adjuvant systemic chemotherapy with respect to improved control of the primary tumour and its metastases has yet to be determined. Experience with paediatric tumours, lymphomas and testicular teratomas has shown the way for integrating chemotherapy into multidisciplinary treatment. Assuredly, it is only a question of time, with persistent trial and careful documentation of results, before such an approach will lead to improvement in survival of patients with bladder cancer.

I

Diagnosis, staging and experimental pathology

1

Histological Staging and Grading of Bladder Tumours

R.C.B. Pugh

Many different classifications of bladder tumours have evolved over the years, some based principally on tumour grading (Broders, 1922; Bergkvist *et al.,* 1965; Miller *et al.,* 1969) and others taking account of the clinical and pathological stage or depth of infiltration (Jewett and Strong, 1946; Dukes and Masina, 1949; Franksson, 1950). The TNM system for the classification of malignant tumours was developed by Denoix in France between 1943 and 1952 (UICC, 1978), and the International Union Against Cancer (UICC) TNM Classifications of Bladder Tumours produced in 1963 and 1974 are now widely used throughout the world (UICC, 1963; Wallace *et al.,* 1975). Before the 1963 publication a small subcommittee comprising six urologists and four pathologists from five European countries and the United States met to see how the clinical and pathological features and terms might be correlated: in 1973, the World Health Organization published a booklet, *'Histological Typing of Urinary Bladder Tumours'*, which contained a section on pathological staging, designating the PIS, P1, P2, P3 and P4 stages according to the depth of infiltration of the bladder wall. These stages corresponded exactly to the T stages of the UICC TNM scheme (Pugh, 1973). The 1963 TNM bladder tumour scheme permitted, for the very first time, the use of the results of a biopsy in the determination of the T status, thus clearly establishing the important role of the histopathologist in the assessment of the malignant potential of a patient's tumour. The 1963 and 1974 classifications were substantially the same and, in a paper to the British Association of Urological Surgeons in 1974, Wallace and his colleagues (Wallace *et al.,* 1975) emphasized the value of the TNM scheme as a descriptive shorthand method for recording factors which might be of importance in therapy and prognosis. However, they emphasized that the P staging was determined by examination of the operative specimen only and was not applicable to biopsy material.

Early in 1979, the third edition of the TNM Classifications became available (UICC, 1978), and it is now proposed that the 'clinical staging' be replaced by 'pre-treatment clinical staging', which is to be based on the same investigations as were mandatory in the 1974 scheme. 'Pathological staging' (or P stage) has been replaced by 'post-surgical histopathological classification', designated as pTNM. The document stresses that the TNM categories, once established, must remain unchanged. The booklet also states that the effective date for the introduction of the new classification was to be 1 January 1979 and, moreover, that all

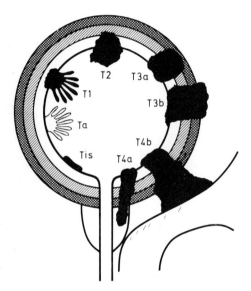

Figure 1.1 Diagrammatic representation of UICC 1978 classification

the classifications listed in the booklet should remain unchanged for at least 10 years. It stressed that, in order to develop and sustain a classification system acceptable to all, it is necessary to ensure the closest liaison by all national and international committees, thus permitting the use of a common language in comparing clinical material and assessing results. It would seem, though, that the new system for the bladder has so far been approved by only four of eight national and international bodies listed.

This paper will concentrate on pathological staging, but some aspects of grading will also be discussed very briefly. In the St Peter's Group of Hospitals and the Institute of Urology, the TNM schemes have been in use for many years and the only modification that has been introduced during this time has been the subdivision of the pathological P1 stage into P1a, where there is breakthrough of the basement membrane and infiltration of the stromal core of a papillary tumour, and P1b, where there is infiltration of the true lamina propria. In most instances this distinction is not difficult to make, particularly if attention is paid to the pattern of blood vessels, which tend to be fine in the core and are often of considerable size in the lamina propria. The justification for the subdivision has been shown by Pryor (1973) in his analysis of bladder cancer patients seen and treated at St Paul's between 1960 and 1969. In the non-invasive, in situ stage there was an 88% three-year survival rate which fell to 77% in the P1a, 64% in the P1b, 52% in the P2 and 24% in the P3 stages respectively.

Table 1.1

COMPARISON OF 1974 AND 1978 UICC TNM CLASSIFICATION WITH ST PETER'S PATHOLOGICAL CLASSIFICATION

St Peter's 1973 *Pathological* *stage*	*UICC 1974* *Histo-* *pathological* *category*	*Clinical* *stage*	*Tumour*	*UICC 1978* *Pre-treatment* *clinical stage*	*Post-* *surgical* *histo-* *pathological* *classification*
	PIS	TIS	Pre-invasive	Tis flat Ta papillary	pTis pTa
P1a cores P1b lamina propria	P1	T1	Lamina propria	T1	pT1
	P2	T2	Superficial muscle	T2	pT2
	P3	T3 a– b–	Deep muscle Through muscle	– a T3 – b	pT3
	P4	T4 a – b –	Fixed to or invading:- Prostate, uterus, vagina Pelvic/abdominal walls	– a T4 – b	pT4

Table 1.1 sets out the two UICC classifications and the St Peter's Hospitals modification and it will be seen that the only significant difference between UICC 1974 and UICC 1978 is the subdivision of the pre-invasive tumour (previously TIS PIS) into Tis, when the lesion is flat, and Ta when it is papillary, the corresponding post-surgical histopathological classifications being pTis and pTa. This is a very sound move as, hitherto, there has often been confusion in the use of the term 'in situ', which either described a pattern of tumour growth (e.g. flat carcinoma in situ) or indicated that a lesion, usually a papillary one, was not invasive. In both classifications there is an apparently clear-cut distinction between superficial and deep muscle invasion, the midpoint of the muscle being the line of demarcation between the two. In some instances it is a simple matter to see in the pathological specimen that only the superficial muscle is involved, or alternatively

that the tumour had grown right through into the perivesical tissues, but all too often the exact mid-point of the muscle cannot be determined with any certainty. A rigid separation of T2 and T3 tumours is therefore not always altogether justified, and this fact needs to be fully appreciated and reported when the results of a particular therapy are described: in those instances where there is this doubt, it would probably be more accurate to describe the tumour as being in the P2/P3 stage. Another area of potential confusion concerns the reporting of prostatic involvement. In the 1974 and 1978 UICC schemes, invasion of the prostate would be classified as P4 or pT4 respectively. A recent investigation of 33 cystectomy specimens examined in the St. Peter's Hospitals Group laboratory (R. Johri, 1979; personal communication) has shown that an important and practical distinction can be made between those tumours involving the prostatic ducts or acini, and those in which there is infiltration of the interstitial tissues of the gland. The former have been designated P4aa and the latter P4ab (*Table 1.2*).

Table 1.2
ST PETER'S GROUP PROPOSED HISTOPATHOLOGICAL CLASSIFICATION

ALL specimens to be staged

Stages:	Pis	Flat pre-invasive Ca: Ca in situ
	Pa	Papillary non-invasive
	P1a	Stromal cores
	P1b	Lamina propria
	P2	Superficial muscle
	P3a	Deep muscle
	P3b	Perivesical
	P4a	Prostate, uterus, vagina
	P4b	Pelvic or abdominal wall

P4a tumours involving prostate 4aa ducts and acini only
4ab intersitital tissue
Depth of tissue in specimen to be noted (symbol D) e.g. P1a/D2

There are 11 P4aa tumours and eight of these patients (72%) are still alive for periods of 2 months, 3, 4, 5, 5, 8, 9 and 9 years after examination. One patient died of a pulmonary embolism shortly after cystoprostatectomy: the other two died from unknown causes, 1 and 5 years after operation. Of the 22 patients with P4ab tumours only five (23%) are alive – three for periods of months and two each for 3 years. Twelve of the 17 deaths are known to be due to tumour.

On the basis of these findings, there is a good case for modifying the new UICC scheme by including the subdivisions of the earliest stages of invasion (i.e. 1a and 1b) and by being more precise with regard to prostatic involvement. *Table 1.2* details the staging scheme which has recently been put into use in our Group. In view of the fact that so many patients are now being continuously monitored by serial and/or multiple bladder biopsies in the follow-up of flat carcinoma in situ, or are being treated with intracavitary agents, or are having their bladders 'mapped' when a radical operation such as cystectomy is under consideration, it is believed that there is a case for the pathologist to stage *all* the specimens he receives and not merely to confine staging to the initial biopsy and post-surgical specimen, as UICC recommends. It is therefore logical to revert to P staging, rather than pT, to designate all biopsy and surgical specimen findings. The modified scheme nevertheless remains within the general UICC framework, although there is still no entirely satisfactory means of making a clear separation between the P2 and P3a tumours.

In order to further amplify the 'shorthand' description of a specimen, the depth of tissue present in it can be indicated by the pathologist by the use of the symbol D, so that, for example, a P1a/D2 tumour would be one in which there is invasion of the stromal cores in a specimen which contains some muscle on its deep aspect.

Tumour grading is, to some extent, a subjective exercise and it is not nearly so easy to be as consistent as it is with staging. The two ends of the spectrum (i.e. differentiated and anaplastic) are relatively easy to recognize, but it is the intervening grey area which often presents difficulty. Nevertheless, survival rate correlates with grade and it will be seen in *Table 1.3* that the rate falls as the tumours become less differentiated and more infiltrative.

Table 1.3
SURVIVAL BY GRADE AND STAGE

3-year survival rate (%)	Pattern and grade of tumour	Number of patients			
		Total	Pa	Stage P1	P2,3,4
81	Pap differentiated	102	58	42	2
62	Pap and solid differentiated	29	–	16	13
58	Pap and solid intermediate	31	–	14	17
44	Pap and solid anaplastic	41	–	9	32
22	Solid anaplastic	48	–	7	41

(Adapted from Pryor, 1973)

Grading and staging are essential pieces of information that the urologist must have if he is to evaluate and treat his patients in a rational manner: the pathologist has a duty to attempt to grade and stage all the material submitted to his laboratory.

REFERENCES

BERGKVIST, A., LJUNGQVIST, A. and MOBERGER, G. (1965). Classification of bladder tumours based on the cellular pattern. *Acta Chirurgica Scandinavica*, **130**, 371–378

BRODERS, A.C.(1922). Epithelioma of the genito-urinary organs. *Annals of Surgery*, **75**, 574–604

DUKES, C.E. and MASINA, F. (1949). Classification of epithelial tumours of the bladder. *British Journal of Urology*, **21**, 273–295

FRANKSSON, C. (1950). Tumours of the urinary bladder – a pathological and clinical study of 434 cases. *Acta Chirurgica Scandinavica*, 151 (Supplement)

JEWETT, H.J. and STRONG, G.H. (1946). Infiltrating carcinoma of the bladder. *Journal of Urology*, **55**, 365–372

MILLER, A., MITCHELL, J.P. and BROWN, N.J. (1969). The Bristol Bladder Tumour Registry. *British Journal of Urology*, **41** (Supplement)

PRYOR, J.P. (1973). Factors influencing the survival of patients with transitional cell tumours of the urinary bladder. *British Journal of Urology*, **45**, 586–592

PUGH, R.C.B. (1973). The pathology of cancer of the bladder: an editorial overview. *Cancer*, **32**, 1267–1274

UICC (INTERNATIONAL UNION AGAINST CANCER) (1963). *Malignant Tumours of the Urinary Bladder.* Research Committee on Clinical Stage Classification and Applied Statistics

UICC (INTERNATIONAL UNION AGAINST CANCER) (1978). *TNM Classification of Malignant Tumours,* 3rd Edition. Ed. by M.H. Harmer. Geneva; UICC

WALLACE, D.M., CHISHOLM, G.D. and HENDRY, W.F. (1975). TNM Classification for Urological Tumours (UICC) – 1974. *British Journal of Urology*, **47**, 1–12

WORLD HEALTH ORGANIZATION (1973). *Histological Typing of Urinary Bladder Tumours.* Ed. by F.K. Mostofi. Geneva; WHO

2

Urinary Cytology for Diagnosis, Grading and Monitoring Response to Treatment

P.-L. Esposti

The value of routine cytological examination of urine and bladder washings for diagnosis of urinary tract malignancy seems well established. After Papanicolaou and Marshall (1945) reported their results with urine sediment smears as a diagnostic procedure, numerous reports have been published introducing new techniques and discussing results. Books and atlases of urinary cytology for the education of pathologists and urologists are now available (Koss, 1968; De Voogt et al., 1977).

Exfoliative cytology from the urinary tract is at present accepted as a useful complement of other techniques in the early diagnosis of carcinoma of the bladder and lower urinary tract. Its significance in a more accurate grading of tumour malignancy and in monitoring response to treatment is being assessed.

PREPARATORY TECHNIQUES

Collection of samples

A preliminary cytological test, especially in outpatients, is easily performed on sediments of spontaneously voided urine. In the female, voided urine usually contains abundant squamous epithelial cells from vulva and vagina: to avoid contamination, examination of urine obtained by catheterization is advisable. Cells degenerate rather rapidly in urine: the first morning sample, consisting of urine that has gathered in the bladder during the night, is therefore discarded. The next sample (100 – 200 ml) is considered to be suitable for processing. Some kind of fixation (see below) is recommended if the sample of urine cannot be processed immediately. All patients with clinical suspicion of bladder tumour are submitted to cystoscopy: during this procedure it is usual to rinse the bladder with physiological saline. These wash-outs seem to provide better diagnostic material than urine (Esposti *et al.*, 1970; Harris *et al.*, 1971). Cells do not disintegrate as quickly in physiological saline, and immediate fixation is usually not necessary.

Cell concentration, preparation and staining of smears

At Karolinska Hospital, urine and bladder washings in volumes of up to 200 ml are sent to the cytological laboratory within 1–2 hours of collection. The specimens are centrifuged for 10 min at 35 g in 200 ml round-bottomed tubes. The supernatant is decanted and the sedimented cells resuspended in a few drops of the fluid left in the tube and fixed by the addition of 10 ml of methanol–acetic acid mixture (45 parts methanol, 10 parts glacial acetic acid and 45 parts distilled water). This resuspended material is decanted in 10 ml test tubes and again centrifuged for 10 minutes at 350 g, after which the supernatant is removed. The sediment is then transferred with a Pasteur pipette to a glass slide.

To the drop of sediment, a drop of an adhesive solution is added. This solution consists of 0.2 g pectin in 40 ml glycerine diluted with distilled water to 1000 ml, as recommended by Rofe (1955). The material is mixed well, spread over the slide and air-dried overnight. The dry slides are then stained according to the method of Papanicolaou. Different techniques of cell collection, cell concentration and smear preparation are recommended by different authors. For details, readers are referred to other sources (Koss, 1968; De Voogt *et al.*, 1977).

THE NORMAL URINARY SEDIMENT

The urinary tract is lined with transitional epithelium or urothelium. This is a pluristratified (3–7 layers of cells), non-keratinized epithelium. The urothelial cells vary in size and shape from the basal layer to the surface. The basal layer exhibits small, round cells with scant cytoplasm and dark, round nuclei. Intermediate cells show larger, often elongated, nuclei and a cytoplasmic tail reaching down to the basal layer. At the surface, large cells exhibit abundant cytoplasm and often more than one nucleus; they are commonly called 'umbrella' cells.

Urine or wash-out from a normal bladder are, as a rule, poor in cells. A great variety in cell shape and size characterizes the normal sediment. Large, often multinucleated umbrella cells, elongated cells from the intermediate layers and smaller cells from the deeper layers with a darker nucleus can be recognized. Occasionally a few columnar cells and squamous epithelial cells may be observed. It is a common mistake of the inexperienced cytologist to give a report of unsatis-factory material when examining the scant sediment of a normal bladder. The clean background, the absence of cell detritus and the presence of a few well-recognizable urothelial cells of the various layers should suffice for a benign cytological report.

CYTOLOGICAL FINDINGS IN BENIGN UROTHELIAL LESIONS

Inflammatory changes are usually attributable to bacterial infection (acute and chronic cystitis). The sediment will contain an increased number of urothelial cells as well as polymorphonuclear granulocytes, histiocytes and cellular debris. Nuclear atypia of the epithelial cells is usually slight and does not cause diagnostic problems. In cases of *lithiasis* the shedding of the urothelium is, as a rule, increased and cellular atypias, such as nuclear enlargement, slightly coarse chromatin and prominence of nucleoli, are more accentuated. These atypical cells can erroneously be interpreted as malignant (Beyer-Boon, 1977). As a result of chronic irritation of the mucosa, *squamous metaplasia* may be observed: squamous cells are predominant in the sediment, often exhibiting orange cytoplasm in the Papanicolaou stain, as a sign of keratinization. Anucleate squames may be present.

UROTHELIAL TUMOURS

Histopathological classification

Over 95% of the tumours of the bladder are of epithelial type, pre-dominantly originating from the transitional epithelium. When con-sidering the pattern of growth, four main types of urothelial tumours are recognized:
(1) papillary,
(2) solid;
(3) mixed papillary and solid;
(4) non-papillary or flat 'carcinoma in situ'.
  To evaluate the degree of anaplasia of these tumours, the WHO histological classification (1973) proposes three grades: grade 1 applies to carcinomas with the least degree of cellular anaplasia; grade 3 to carcinomas with marked cellular anaplasia, while grade 2 lies in between. If the tumour is covered by regular epithelium not more than six layers thick, the name 'papilloma' is used.

Cytological findings in urothelial tumours

Papillomas and low-grade papillary carcinomas cannot as a rule be diagnosed by examination of the cells exfoliated in the urine or bladder washings. Cell morphology is similar to that of benign conditions, but nuclear atypia is often greater than in non-neoplastic lesions *(Figure 2.1).* Papillary clusters or fronds of transitional cells in the sediment, as described by Allegra *et al.* (1966), are, in the experience of the author, not sufficiently frequent to be of practical importance. On the other hand, a repeated cytological report of benign urothelial cells in cases where papillary tumours have been cystoscopically detected, gives the urologist the important information that the lesions are not of the dangerous, aggressive type.

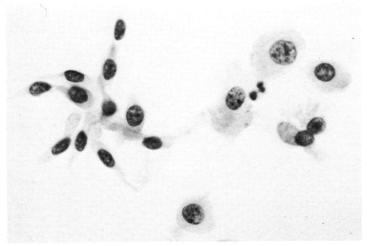

Figure 2.1 Urothelial cells from bladder washings of a patient with papillary carcinoma grade 1. The morphology is similar to that of cases without bladder tumour (× 800)

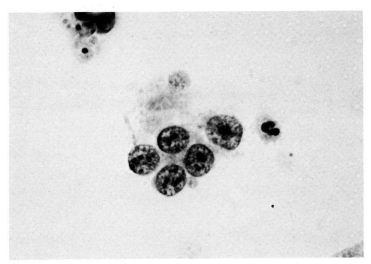

Figure 2.2 Carcinoma cells of low-grade anaplasia from bladder washings of a patient with tumour of histological grade 2 (× 800)

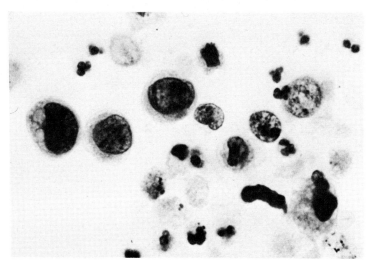

Figure 2.3 Carcinoma cells of high-grade anaplasia from bladder washings of a patient with tumour of histological grade 3 (× 800)

Urothelial carcinomas of higher-grade malignancy (grade 2 and 3) will, as a rule, shed abundant carcinoma cells, singly or in clusters. Nuclear abnormalities typical of malignancy are present and the cyto-pathologist will have no hesitation in reporting carcinoma.

By careful analysis of the exfoliated cells it is possible to assess a cytological grading of the malignancy of the tumour (Esposti and Zajicek, 1972). Urothelial tumours, histologically classified as grade 2, will as a rule shed malignant cells in small clusters, with enlarged nuclei exhibiting moderate anaplasia (*Figure 2.2*). On the other hand, malignant cells exfoliated from grade 3 tumours are mostly single and exhibit a high degree of nuclear pleomorphism. Degenerative changes such as cytoplasmic vacuolization and nuclear pyknosis are often present (*Figure 2.3*).

The cytological findings in 428 untreated bladder tumours, histo-logically diagnosed following the WHO classification, are summarized

Table 2.1
CYTOLOGICAL REPORTS IN 428 BLADDER TUMOURS

Cytological report	Histological diagnosis: carcinoma		
	Grade 1	*Grade 2*	*Grade 3*
Non-malignant	56	49	11
Suspicious	12	23	16
Malignant	2	80	179
Total	70	152	206

Table 2.2
CYTOLOGICAL DEGREE OF ANAPLASIA IN POSITIVE SMEARS OF 259 PATIENTS
WITH BLADDER CARCINOMA OF HISTOLOGICAL GRADE 2 AND 3

Cytological malignancy	*Histological grade*	
	2 (80 patients)	*3 (179 patients)*
Low-grade	80%	10%
High-grade	20%	90%

in *Table 2.1.* The degree of anaplasia in exfoliated carcinoma cells (cytological malignancy) is correlated with the histological grade in *Table 2.2.*

THE ROLE OF CYTOLOGY IN MONITORING RESPONSE TO TREATMENT

Surgical procedures

Papillary tumours of low grade and low stage are usually controlled by endoscopic resections or partial cystectomy. Clinical and cystoscopic examination at regular intervals is mandatory. Cytological examinations should be performed on these occasions and also at intermediate intervals, especially if suspicious changes in the mucosa have been observed. As shown in *Table 2.1,* the majority of grade 1 tumours do not shed malignant cells and a benign cytological report will be the rule over many years, even in patients with recurrence. The finding of carcinoma cells in the sediment must, however, be considered to be an alarm signal: it usually reveals a change in the biological behaviour of the tumour and, in general, of the urothelium, and is often followed by the appearance of a more aggressive, invasive type of neoplasm.

Radiotherapy

At Radiumhemmet, high-grade, high-stage bladder tumours are, as a rule, submitted to high-dose radiotherapy. Regular cytologic controls after irradiation give valuable information to the clinician (*see Table 2.3*). The disappearance of tumour after radiotherapy is usually accompanied by the disappearance of carcinoma cells in the sediment. The presence of cells with radiation changes does not, as a rule, constitute a major diagnostic problem, provided that the cytologist receives accurate

Table 2.3
CYTOLOGICAL MALIGNANCY AND CLINICAL FOLLOW-UP IN 226 PATIENTS AFTER
RADIOTHERAPY FOR BLADDER CARCINOMA

Clinical follow-up	Number of patients	Percentage of patients cytologically positive
Free from tumour	87	4
Suspected recurrence	31	45
Recurrence	68	90
No response to therapy	40	95

clinical information and has a basic knowledge of the morphology of irradiated cells. In patients free from tumour after radiotherapy, the persistence or the reappearance of malignant cells after a free interval will be followed, usually within one year, by a macroscopic recurrence in the bladder. However, in some cases, a positive cytology is observed for several years without any sign of exophytic tumour. This might be explained by the persistence of areas of 'carcinoma in situ', even if it has not been possible in all cases to verify histologically the 'in situ' lesions by repeated mucosal biopsies.

Chemotherapy

The effect of certain alkylating agents on the urothelium is well known (Forni *et al.*, 1964). Nuclear abnormalities are evident in exfoliated cells from the bladder of patients receiving parenteral cytotoxic chemotherapy. The question has been raised whether the atypical changes observed in the urothelial cells of these patients might, in some cases, progress to a frank malignancy. Clinical data confirming this suspicion have been gathered from the literature (Beyer-Boon, 1977).

Intravesical instillations of anticancer drugs have been used for treatment of superficial bladder tumours. There are many publications on the effect of *thiotepa,* demonstrating regression in about 50% of papillary neoplasms after intravesical instillation of this drug. More recently, *doxorubicin* has been found to be an active topical treatment of flat in situ (Tis) lesions of the bladder (Edsmyr *et al.*, 1978), and its effect on exfoliated cells has been described (Esposti *et al.*, 1978). Smears prepared from urinary sediments from patients with 'carcinoma in situ' usually contain abundant malignant cells, usually exhibiting high-grade anaplasia. A rapid reduction in the number of these cells is observed as a result of local doxorubicin treatment. Marked cellular alterations are seen in the remaining cells, including nuclear and cytoplasmic vacuolization, nuclear swelling or pyknosis, and other changes which suggest acute cellular injury. In the group of patients considered as 'responders', continued treatment will result in complete disappearance of carcinoma cells. In other cases, however, strongly atypical cells will persist, intermixed with degenerated cells. As a consequence it can become difficult to confirm or rule out malignancy: an inconclusive cytologic report is then given.

EXFOLIATED CELLS FROM THE BLADDER IN UROLOGICAL RESEARCH

Cells from bladder washings of patients with bladder tumours have been analyzed using a rapid-flow cytofluorometer in order to perform quantitative DNA measurements (Tribukait and Esposti, 1978; Tribukait *et al.*, 1979). The results indicate that there is a relation between the frequency of occurrence of aneuploidy, the histological grading of the tumour and the cytological findings in the bladder washings. In addition to aneuploidy as an important criterion for malignancy, the degree of proliferation appears to be of major biological significance. Similarly, quantitative DNA cytofluorometric studies have been performed on cells exfoliated from bladders with 'carcinoma in situ' lesions (Esposti *et al.*, 1978). Cytological findings and results of DNA analyses before and during treatment with doxorubicin are summarized in *Table 2.4*. A decrease in the number of

Table 2.4
CYTOLOGY AND PLOIDY IN PATIENTS WITH CARCINOMA IN SITU OF THE BLADDER

	Cytology positive	Aneuploidy
Before treatment	24/24 (100%)	16/19 (84%)
After treatment	11/24 (46%)	13/23 (57%)

positive cytological findings during treatment is paralleled by a decrease in the frequency of aneuploid cells. However, an increase in the number of aneuploid cells is observed when the therapy is discontinued. It would seem that these quantitative DNA aspects, together with the results of cytomorphological analysis, are of importance in the identification of the 'non-responders', for the early detection of drug resistance and in planning further therapy.

REFERENCES

ALLEGRA, S.R., FANNING, J.P., STREKER, J.F. and CORVESE, N.M. (1966). Cytologic diagnosis of occult and 'in situ' carcinoma of the urinary system. *Acta Cytologica*, **10**, 340–349

BEYER-BOON, M.E. (1977). *The Efficacy of Urinary Cytology*. Thesis, Delft; University of Leyden

DE VOOGT, H.J., RATHERT, P. and BEYER-BOON, M.E. (1977). *Urinary Cytology*. Berlin-Heidelberg-New York; Springer-Verlag

EDSMYR, F., BERLIN, T., BOMAN, J., DUCHEK, M., ESPOSTI, P. -L., GUSTAFSON, H. and WIKSTRÖM, H. (1978). Intravesical therapy with adriamycin in patients with superficial bladder tumours. In *Diagnostics and Treatment of Superficial Urinary Bladder Tumours*, p. 45. Proceedings of WHO Collaborating Centre Meeting at Radiumhemmet, Karolinska Hospital, Stockholm, September 15

ESPOSTI, P. -L and ZAJICEK, J. (1972). Grading of transitional cell neoplasms of the urinary bladder from smears of bladder washings. A critical review of 326 tumors. *Acta Cytologica*, **16**, 529–537

ESPOSTI, P. -L., MOBERGER, G. and ZAJICEK, J. (1970). The cytologic diagnosis of transitional cell tumors of the urinary bladder and its histologic basis. A study of 567 cases of urinary-tract disorders including 170 untreated and 182 irradiated bladder tumors. *Acta Cytologica*, **14**, 145–155

ESPOSTI, P. -L., TRIBUKAIT, B. and GUSTAFSON, H. (1978). Effects of local treatment with adriamycin in carcinoma in situ of the urinary bladder: cell morphology and DNA analysis for quantification of malignant cells. In *Diagnostics and Treatment of Superficial Urinary Bladder Tumors*, p. 71. Proceedings of WHO Collaborating Centre Meeting at Radiumhemmet, Karolinska Hospital, Stockholm, September 15

FORNI, A.M., KOSS, L.G. and GELLER, W. (1964). Cytological study of the effect of cyclophosphamide on the epithelium of the urinary bladder in man. *Cancer*, **17**, 1348–1355

HARRIS, M.J., SCHWINN, C.P., MORROW, I.W., GRAY, R.L. and BROWELL, B.M. (1971). Exfoliative cytology of the urinary bladder irrigation specimen. *Acta Cytologica*, **15**, 385–399

KOSS, L.G. (1968). *Diagnostic Cytology and its Histopathological Basis*. 2nd edition. Philadelphia; Lippincott

PAPANICOLAOU, G.N. and MARSHALL, V.F. (1945). Urine sediment smears as a diagnostic procedure in cancers of the urinary tract. *Science*, **101**, 519–520

ROFE, P. (1955). The cells of normal human urine. A quantitative and qualitative study using a new method of preparation. *Journal of Clinical Pathology*, **8**, 25–31

TRIBUKAIT, B. and ESPOSTI, P. -L.(1978). Quantitative flow-microfluorometric analysis of the DNA in cells from neoplasms of the urinary bladder: correlation of aneuploidy with histological grading and the cytological findings. *Urological Research*, **6**, 201–205

TRIBUKAIT, B., GUSTAFSON, H. and ESPOSTI, P. -L. (1979). Ploidy and proliferation in human bladder tumors as measured by flow-cytofluorometric DNA-analysis and its relation to histopathology and cytology. *Cancer*, **43**, 1742–1751

WORLD HEALTH ORGANIZATION (1973). Histological typing of urinary bladder tumours (1973). In *International Histological Classification of Tumours*. Geneva; WHO

3

The Effects of a Haematuria Service on the Early Diagnosis of Bladder Cancer

W.F. Hendry, N. Manning, N.M. Perry, H.N. Whitfield and
J.E.A. Wickham

Delay in the diagnosis of bladder tumours which are infiltrating muscle
has a serious effect on the prognosis. At the Royal Marsden Hospital,
Wallace and Harris (1965) showed that, for such cases, the crude three-
year survival rate when treatment was started within 1 month of the
onset of bleeding was 60%, whereas with a delay of 1–6 months, the
crude 3-year survival rate fell to 25%. A haematuria diagnostic service
was introduced at the Royal Marsden Hospital in 1973 so that patients
with haematuria could be seen immediately in the outpatient clinic and
return with the results of urinalysis, cytology and intravenous urogram
to the next clinic. The patient was admitted for cystoscopy without
delay under general anaesthetic (Turner *et al.*, 1977). Having shown
the effectiveness of the haematuria diagnostic service at the Royal
Marsden Hospital, a similar service was introduced at St Bartholomew's
Hospital, in February 1977. In this paper we describe our experiences,
with an analysis of the cases that have been seen, and of the effects of
the service on the distribution of the stage of bladder cancer patients at
diagnosis.

PATIENTS AND METHODS

At St Bartholomew's Hospital, computerization of records (Wickham
et al., 1975) was introduced in January 1973, and classification of
tumours was standardized using the TNM system (UICC, 1974) after
this date. Since then, 173 patients presenting with haematuria were
diagnosed as having carcinoma of the bladder. Between January 1973

and January 1977, 108 patients were diagnosed by the traditional methods of outpatient referral, intravenous urogram and subsequent cystoscopy (Group A). From February 1977 to July 1979, a further 65 patients were diagnosed through the 'emergency' haematuria service (Group B).

At the Royal Marsden Hospital, direct referral to the haematuria service was invited, but at St Bartholomew's Hospital all referrals were by letters from general practitioners, which were read on receipt by the chief assistant. Patients stated to have passed blood in the urine were automatically included in a clinic within a week. An intravenous urogram was performed, and patients were seen with the result within 2 weeks. The patients then underwent cystoscopy with general anaesthetic as inpatients or day cases.

Two studies have been done. First, an analysis was made of 127 patients seen in the haematuria service in the first year of its activity, to analyse the nature of cases referred and the malignancy pick-up rate. Subsequently, an analysis has been made of all the patients with bladder cancer seen since 1 January 1973, to study the distribution of the various stages of bladder cancer at diagnosis, before and after the introduction of the haematuria service.

RESULTS

Analysis of all Cases Seen in the First Year of Haematuria Service

The age distribution of the patients seen in the first year of the haematuria service is shown in *Table 3.1,* indicating a preponderance of patients aged more than 50 years. *Table 3.2* shows the duration of symptoms prior to referral. Most patients were referred within 4 weeks of the onset of the symptom. *Table 3.3* shows the interval between the doctor's letter and the first outpatient appointment, the majority being

Table 3.1
DISTRIBUTION OF AGE AND SEX OF 127 PATIENTS SEEN IN FIRST YEAR OF HAEMATURIA SERVICE (1977–78)

Age group (years)	Male	Female
< 20	1	2
20–29	10	8
30–39	9	3
40–49	11	4
50–59	19	11
60–69	19	8
70	20	2
Total (N = 127)	89	38

Table 3.2
DURATION OF SYMPTOMS IN 127 PATIENTS (1977—78)

Duration of symptoms (weeks)	Number of patients (N = 127)
≤ 1	51
1— 4	22
5—12	15
13—26	8
27—52	1
> 52	7
Unknown	12
Not haematuria	11

Table 3.3
TIME FROM RECEIPT OF DOCTOR'S LETTER TO FIRST OUT-PATIENT APPOINTMENT (1977—78)

Time in weeks	Number of patients
1	62
2	33
3	14
4+	3
Not known	15
Total	127

Table 3.4
TIME FROM FIRST TO SECOND OUTPATIENT APPOINTMENT (1977—78)

Time in weeks	Number of patients
1	37
2	21
3	9
4+	12
No 2nd appt.	33
Did not attend	7
Not haematuria	8
Total	127

seen within 2 weeks of the doctor's letter being written. The interval from the first to the second outpatient appointment is shown in *Table 3.4;* 33 patients were brought in directly, with no second outpatient visit. The interval from the outpatient appointment to cystoscopy (*Table 3.5*) was less than 4 weeks in most cases. The distribution of tumours related to stage and grade are shown in *Table 3.6:* patients

Table 3.5
TIME FROM OUTPATIENTS TO INPATIENT CYSTOSCOPY
(1977–78)

Interval	Time in weeks			
	2	2–4	5–8	8+
Outpatients to cysto-scopy (all cases)	12	25	13	8
Outpatients (2 visits) to cystoscopy (cases with tumours)	14	3		
Outpatients (no second visit) to cystoscopy (cases with tumours)		6		

Table 3.6
SITE OF PRIMARY TUMOUR, STAGE AND GRADE RELATED TO AVERAGE
DURATION OF SYMPTOMS IN 127 PATIENTS (1977–78)

Tumour site	Stage	Number	Grade			Average duration of symptoms (weeks)
			G1	G2	G3	
Bladder	T1	11	4	6	1	29.3
	T2	4		2	2	4.2
	T3	4		2	2	22.2
	T4	0				
	TX	2		1	1	20.5
Renal pelvis		2				
		23/127 (18%)				

with early stage (T2) invasive tumours had, on average, shorter duration of symptoms than those with more advanced disease. Overall, the malignancy pick-up rate was 18%.

Analysis of 173 Bladder Tumour Cases (Diagnosed 1973–79)

Forty-nine per cent of the patients diagnosed before the introduction of the haematuria service (Group A) had initial cytoscopy within 5 weeks of referral, compared to 74% of the patients diagnosed since then (Group B).

Table 3.7 shows the distribution of the bladder tumours that were diagnosed, analyzed by TNM classification (*Figure 3.1*). It may be seen that, after instituting the haematuria diagnostic service, the proportion of T1 (non-infiltrating) tumours stayed about the same. However, of the entire series the proportion of T2 tumours (into superficial muscle) increased by 6.1% while the proportion of T3 tumours (into deep muscle or perivesical fat) diminished by 5.6%. T4a tumours (infiltrating

Table 3.7

DISTRIBUTION OF T CLASSIFICATION OF BLADDER TUMOURS AT DIAGNOSIS
BEFORE AND AFTER INTRODUCTION OF HAEMATURIA SERVICE

Classification	(1973–76) – Routine service Group A		(1977–79) – Haematuria service Group B	
	Number (N = 108)	Percentage	Number (N = 65)	Percentage
T1	69	64	43	66
T2	10	9	10	15
T3	21	19	9	14
T4a	2	2	1	2
T4b	3	3	0	0
TX	3	3	2	3

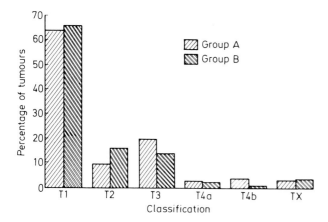

Figure 3.1 Distribution of T classification of 173 bladder tumours before and after introduction of haematuria diagnostic service

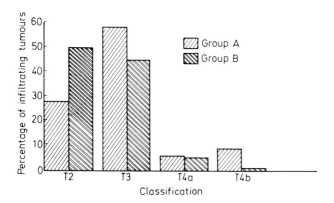

Figure 3.2 T classification of 56 infiltrating bladder tumours: note increase in proportion of early (T2) cases, reduction of more advanced (T3) lesions and elimination of fixed inoperable (T4b) tumours since the diagnosis of haematuria was accelerated.

prostate) continued to be seen. There were no T4b (fixed tumour) cases in Group B, but there were only 3 in Group A. A small proportion of tumours continued to present as TX (most commonly situated in a diverticulum). When infiltrating tumours alone were considered, the striking increase in early (T2) lesions from 28% to 50% became even more apparent (*Figure 3.2*), with a reduction in more advanced (T3) lesions from 58% to 45%.

DISCUSSION

We have found that it is possible to run an efficient 'emergency' haematuria service in a busy general hospital with minimal interference with other hospital procedures. It is simply necessary to recognize haematuria as demanding an accelerated service and to respond accordingly. Analysis of our data shows that the proportion of early, potentially curable (T2) tumours can be increased, and the proportion of probably incurable (T3) tumours decreased, in the population with infiltrating tumours. T1 tumours are mostly non-invasive and the proportion of these is likely to remain the same, irrespective of the degree of delay in diagnosis. However, infiltrating carcinoma invades the wall of the bladder progressively and the depth of invasion increases with time. It is for these patients (who comprise about one-third of all patients with bladder cancer) that early diagnosis is essential if conservative methods of treatment, sparing the bladder, are to have a reasonable chance of success. For example, 5-year survival rates of 50–60% can be achieved with T2 tumours using interstitial or external beam radiotherapy (Werf-Messing, 1965, Caldwell *et al.,* 1967), compared with 20–29% with T3 tumours treated by radiotherapy only (Wallace and Bloom, 1976; *see* Chapter 17. Although radiotherapy and cystectomy can improve the 5-year survival rate to 34–50% (for a review *see* Chapter 17) this improvement can be achieved only at greatly increased cost in terms of patient morbidity, time lost from work and use of hospital facilities. It is clear that early diagnosis of invasive bladder cancer is not only better for patients' survival, but is also cost-effective, because most early-stage cases can be treated by relatively conservative methods, often on an outpatient basis.

The malignancy pick-up rate of 18% in this series (1977–78) confirms the importance of providing an accurate diagnostic service for patients referred with haematuria, and almost certainly reflects a high degree of discrimination by doctors in selecting patients for hospital investigation. Our initial fears of a flood of young ladies with cystitis have not been realized (*see Table 3.1*). The value of a second outpatient visit is debatable; however, it did provide an opportunity to review the X-rays and urine results, and to channel the patients with tumours most expeditiously towards day-case cystoscopy, further investigation (*Table 3.5*), or inpatient treatment such as nephrectomy. In our series, 97.5% of patients with bladder tumours presented with haematuria — this symptom provides a golden opportunity to expedite their diagnosis and treatment.

REFERENCES

CALDWELL, W.L., BAGSHAW, M.A. and KAPLAN, H.S. (1967). Efficiency of linear acceleration X-ray therapy in cancer of the bladder. *Journal of Urology*, 97, 294—303

TURNER, A.G., HENDRY, W.F., WILLIAMS, G.B. and WALLACE, D.M. (1977). A haematuria diagnostic service. *British Medical Journal*, 2, 29—31

UICC (INTERNATIONAL UNION AGAINST CANCER) (1974) *TNM Classification of Malignant Tumours*. Geneva; UICC

WALLACE, D.M. and BLOOM, H.J.G. (1976). The management of deeply infiltrating (T3) bladder carcinoma: controlled trial of radical radiotherapy versus pre-operative and radical cystectomy (first report). *British Journal of Urology*, 48, 587—594

WALLACE, D.M. and HARRIS, D.L. (1965). Delay in treating bladder tumours. *Lancet*, 2, 332—334

WERF-MESSING, B. VAN DER (1965). Treatment of carcinoma of the bladder with radium. *Clinical Radiology*, 16, 16—26

WICKHAM, J.E.A., CHARLTON, C.A.C., RICHARDS, B., HENDRY, W.F., WARD, J.P., O'DONOGHUE, E.P.N., HAMSHERE, R.G. and FRANKLIN, D.A. (1975). A computer-based record and organisation system for a department of urology. *British Journal of Urology*, 47, 345—357

4

Computerized Axial Tomography for Staging and Assessing Response of Bladder Cancer to Treatment

Janet E. Husband and N.J. Hodson

Computed tomography (CT) has important implications for staging and monitoring therapeutic response in patients with bladder cancer, because both the intraluminal tumour and extravesical tumour spread can be demonstrated. Hitherto, the radiological techniques used to assess extravesical disease included fractionated cystography (Connolly *et al.,* 1966), arteriography (Lang *et al.,* 1966) and intravesical and perivesical gas insufflation (Gosalbez and Gil-Vernet, 1962), but these procedures have not found widespread acceptance, because of their invasive nature. In the majority of centres, clinical staging is therefore performed using urography, cystoscopy with biopsy and bimanual examination under general anaesthesia. The accuracy of bimanual examination is limited: the majority of errors occur in those patients with advanced disease, because of the difficulty of assessing the true extent of extravesical involvement (Werf-Messing, 1979). Ultrasound and computed tomography provide new techniques which are likely to complement and improve the conventional staging of these tumours. Ultrasound does, however, have the disadvantage that it is highly dependent upon the skill of the operator but, in those centres where adequate expertise is available, a high degree of accuracy can be obtained (Morley, 1978).

The purpose of this review is to discuss the value of computed tomography for assessing both the primary tumour (T stage) and spread to the regional lymph nodes (N stage). The technique of examination is described, guidelines for interpretation presented and the difficulties encountered emphasized. The accuracy of CT is discussed with reference to studies carried out at the Royal Marsden Hospital and to other reported series.

TECHNIQUE

Patients are referred to the CT scanning unit after clinical assessment according to the classification recommended by the International Union Against Cancer (UICC, 1978). TNM staging is performed using urography, cystoscopy, bimanual examination under general anaesthesia with biopsy and, in addition, lymphography is carried out in the majority of patients. CT examinations are performed using an EMI whole-body scanner (CT 5005) which has a scan time of 20 s and slice thickness of 13 mm. The physical principles of this system have previously been described (Hounsfield, 1973). The procedure is undertaken with the patient's bladder full in order to demonstrate the intraluminal tumour: in this way, that area of the bladder wall is located which must be scrutinized carefully for the presence of extravesical tumour spread. A full bladder also facilitates interpretation by displacing small bowel loops out of the pelvis into the abdomen. Urine has a significantly lower density than the soft-tissue tumour: the majority of lesions are therefore clearly seen without the need for intravenous iodinated contrast medium. It is, therefore, our practice to reserve contrast for those patients in whom the intraluminal tumour cannot be adequately demonstrated, or in whom a diverticulum causes difficulty in interpretation, or where accurate location of the ureters is required (*Figures 4.1, 4.2*). The patient is allowed to empty his bladder before the intravesical injection of contrast medium, in order to prevent layering of contrast in the posterior portion of the bladder. We use a relatively low dose (30 ml meglumine iothalamate 60% w/v) because higher doses produce dense opacification of the bladder which may obscure the intravesical tumour. Intravenous contrast medium is also occasionally required to distinguish vascular structures from suspected lymphadenopathy. In this situation, contrast medium is injected intravenously throughout the duration of the scan. We currently use 60 ml meglumine iothalamate 60% w/v.

Even with detailed knowledge of the pelvic anatomy, interpretation may be difficult. This is partly because small bowel loops (which have a similar density to other soft tissue structures) may lie alongside, or in front of, the bladder and can easily be mistaken for tumour; also because there may be little, if any, fat between such organs as the rectum, vagina and prostate and the posterior bladder wall. Several techniques have, therefore, been developed to identify as many anatomical structures as possible, in order to facilitate interpretation. Thus,

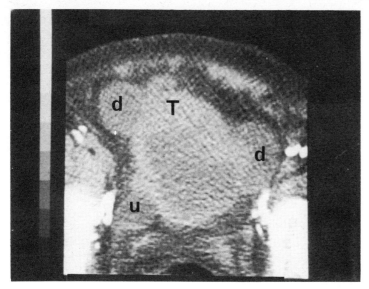

Figure 4.1 *CT scan without contrast medium showng tumour on anterior bladder wall (T). There are two diverticula (d). The right ureter (u) is dilated*

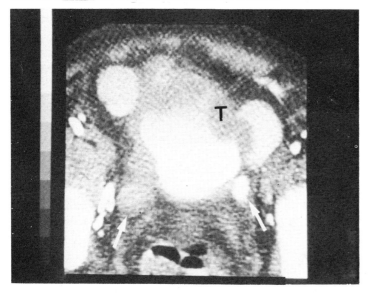

Figure 4.2 *CT scan in same patient after injection of intravenous contrast medium. Tumour (T) is seen extending into the diverticula. Both ureters are dilated (arrowed)*

all patients receive a dilute solution of oral contrast medium (300 ml 5% sodium/meglumine diatrizoate) 30 min before the examination, to outline as much of the small bowel as possible. The same solution is also given rectally immediately before the scan, to delineate the colon.

Female patients are asked to insert a vaginal tampon, which locates the position of the vaginal vault because air is entrapped between its fibres.

Streak artefacts from gas in a moving bowel degrade the CT image, but these can largely be eliminated by giving an intramuscular injection of an anticholinergic agent (hyoscine-N-butyl bromide 20 mg) just before the examination. This is not necessary with new machines which have scan times of 3–5 s.

The internal pelvic anatomy demonstrated on each CT image is related to the axial skeleton on a conventional radiograph which is taken using a slit beam of X-rays to overcome geometric distortion. A metal marker is placed over the symphysis pubis; each CT section is then related in centimetres to this metal marker on the patient's skin, and its position indicated on the radiograph. All patients are scanned in the supine position. CT sections are taken from the symphysis pubis to the sacral promontory at 1.5 cm intervals. Approximately 10–12 CT sections are required to cover the whole pelvis. After viewing the initial series of scans, the radiologist decides whether intravenous contrast medium is indicated, or whether scanning in the prone or lateral decubitus position is required to facilitate interpretation. For example, a tumour on the posterior bladder wall is often better assessed with the patient in the prone position.

Seidelmann *et al.* (1977) have routinely used negative contrast medium (carbon dioxide) introduced by urethral catheterization for staging bladder cancer. They consider that this is the best method for demonstrating the intravesical tumour and bladder wall. However, catheterization is unpleasant for the patient and there is also the risk of introducing infection, particularly in patients being treated with radiotherapy. For these reasons we have not adopted this procedure for the assessment of bladder tumours.

CT OBSERVATIONS AND CRITERIA FOR STAGING

T stage

Superficial tumours (UICC classification T1 and T2) cannot be distinguished with CT but, in our view, involvement of deep muscle (T3a) can be identified if there is appreciable thickening of the bladder wall in direct continuity with the intraluminal mass. However, this sign should be regarded with caution in those patients who have undergone recent endoscopic transurethral resection, when the resulting mural oedema and inflammation may produce similar appearances.

The most important feature of CT is the ability to demonstrate extravesical tumour spread (T3b). Perivesical fat has a low density and thus provides excellent tumour/background contrast, enabling soft tissue tumour extension to be recognized readily. Minimal growth through the bladder wall appears as a loss of definition of the extra-vesical fat margin in the region of the tumour, while more advanced tumour spread is easily recognized as a definite mass extending into the perivesical fat. T4b lesions extend laterally to involve the obturator internus muscle (*Figure 4.3*) or anteriorly to involve the rectus abdominus muscle. Spread of tumour into adjacent organs (T4a) is difficult to identify when there is no fat plane between them and the

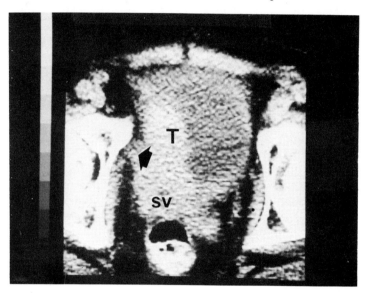

Figure 4.3 Carcinoma of the bladder involving the right lateral and posterior bladder walls. The tumour (T) extends to the right obturator internus muscle (arrowed) and also involves the right seminal vesicle, (sv)

bladder wall. This is a particular problem in attempting to assess involvement of the prostate by a tumour at the bladder base. However, involvement of the seminal vesicles is easily recognized because there is a well-defined fat angle between the posterior bladder wall and the seminal vesicles in the normal subject. Obliteration of this angle by soft tissue tumour indicates seminal vesicle involvement (*Figure 4.3*).

There are several pitfalls in attempting to interpret CT examinations in patients with bladder cancer. Normal structures lying in the peri-vesical fat may be misinterpreted as tumour extension if they lie adjacent to the bladder – for example, loops of small bowel which have not been opacified with contrast medium. The presence of bladder diverticula may also cause confusion in attempting to assess extra-vesical involvement. Following transurethral resection, blood clot and oedema of the bladder wall may be mistaken for tumour and, if all the intraluminal growth has been resected, then it is usually impossible to detect minimal extravesical extension. Similar problems may also occur in patients treated with radiotherapy, when the bladder capacity is markedly reduced and is accompanied by mural oedema.

N stage

Bladder neoplasms spread via the lymphatics to the external and internal iliac lymph node chains. Paravesical and obturator nodes may also be involved. Although enlarged pelvic lymph nodes can be identified with CT, they are more difficult to recognize than in other sites (such as para-aortic regions) because there is less adipose tissue surrounding them (Lee *et al.*, 1978). CT does not demonstrate the internal nodal architecture and enlargement is therefore the only criterion for diagnosing lymph node metastases. Lymph nodes equal to, or greater than, 1.5 cm in diameter are considered to be abnormal (Hodson *et al.*, 1979). If precise measurement is difficult, a useful sign is asymmetry of the soft tissues in the region of the external and internal iliac chains, comparing one side of the pelvis with the other. In general, enlarged external iliac lymph nodes are easier to recognize than those in the internal iliac chain, and it is only on rare occasions that abnormal lymph nodes in other sites such as the obturator group are recognized.

M stage

It is beyond the scope of this review to discuss the value of CT in assessing the tumour spread outside the pelvis. However, the technique is likely to have only a limited role in highly selected patients.

ACCURACY OF CT

The most critical information for assessing the accuracy of any staging technique is its correlation with histopathology. In patients with bladder cancer, this is difficult to achieve because few patients are treated by cystectomy alone. If radiotherapy is given before surgery, then the CT examination must be repeated in the immediate pre-operative period. For these reasons, there is insufficient correlative information at present to make conclusive statements, but the data which are available indicate a high degree of concordance between CT staging and pathological staging. Thus, Seidelmann *et al.* (1978) report an accuracy with CT of 81% in 21 patients in whom surgical confirmation was available. Kellett *et al.* (1980) compared CT findings with pathological staging in 15 patients. Agreement was found in 12 cases (80%); one patient was understaged by CT because invasion of the prostate was missed and two patients were overstaged, one because of observer error and one because of the difficulty in evaluating muscle wall thickening after endoscopy.

At the Royal Marsden Hospital we have demonstrated a similar accuracy, comparing CT with cystectomy specimens in 14 patients,

Table 4.1
COMPARISON OF CT FINDINGS WITH PATHOLOGICAL STAGING: CYSTECTOMY
FOLLOWING RADIOTHERAPY (14 PATIENTS)

| P stage | Number of patients | CT findings | | | |
		Thickened wall	T3a	T3b	T4a
pT0	4	3		1	
pT2	1	1			
pT3a	3	1		2	
pT3b	4		1	3	
pT4a	2		1		1
Total	14	5	2	6	1

following chemotherapy. The detailed results are shown in *Table 4.1*. The two major errors were due to failure to recognize the prostatic involvement in one patient and misinterpretation of a uterine fibroid which simulated tumour extension in another. In five patients, thickening of the bladder wall was the only abnormal CT finding after radiotherapy. None of these patients was found to have a mass at cystectomy, but two had microscopic evidence of tumour within the bladder wall. This emphasizes the inability of CT to exclude microscopic tumour which persists after therapy.

The results of these small series suggest that CT improves the accuracy of clinical staging. We have, therefore, compared CT staging with clinical staging in 75 patients (*Table 4.2*). These results show that 10 out of 13 patients with clinical T2 disease were upstaged by CT although seven of them showed evidence of intramural thickening only

Table 4.2
COMPARISON OF CT STAGING AND CLINICAL STAGING (75 PATIENTS)

| Clinical stage | Number of patients | CT stage | | | | |
		T2	T3a	T3b	T4a	T4b
T2	14	4	7	3		
T3	36		10	23	3	
T4a	12			8	3	1
T4b	13			6		7

(T3a). Distinction between T3a and T3b tumours by clinical examination may be difficult but with CT we were able to identify extravesical tumour spread in 23 out of 36 patients with clinical T3 category disease; organ involvement was detected in three patients. Twelve patients had clinical evidence of invasion of adjacent organs (T4a) but CT downstaged eight of these. It is also interesting that lower CT stage was demonstrated in half the patients who were assessed clinically as T4b. This finding may indicate that CT scanning is less accurate than clinical assessment for these stages, but histopathological correlation is required to confirm this.

The accuracy of CT in detecting lymph node metastases is even more difficult to determine than its accuracy for T staging. In our group of 14 patients who underwent cystectomy, all but one patient had negative lymph node biopsies. In this patient, a normal-sized node showed microscopic evidence of tumour. Lymphography and CT were negative in all 14 patients. We have compared CT findings with lymphography in 36 patients and have shown that CT is inferior to lymphography for demonstrating lymph node metastases in patients with bladder cancer. Out of 11 patients with positive lymphograms, CT was positive in only four (Hodson *et al.,* 1979). The main reason for this is that a lymph node metastasis frequently produces little, if any, enlargement of the node. It is therefore easily missed with CT, but can be clearly seen on the lymphogram film. These results support the study by Lee *et al.* (1978) in which CT was also found to be less accurate then lymphography for detecting lymph node metastases from a variety of primary pelvic cancers.

MONITORING THERAPEUTIC RESPONSE

The progress of patients being treated with radiotherapy or chemotherapy can be followed by sequential CT examinations on an outpatient basis. In a group of 20 unselected patients who were scanned both before and after varying doses of radiotherapy, we were able to demonstrate good tumour regression (greater than 25%) in half the patients, but only a poor response in the others. CT may have a useful role in assessing therapeutic response and may enable early modification of treatment policy without the need for repeated cystoscopies.

CONCLUSIONS

Computed tomography is a new technique which appears to be more accurate than the current methods available for the staging of bladder cancer. However, a thorough knowledge of anatomy and of the techniques used to facilitate interpretation is a prerequisite to obtaining highly accurate results. The additional information provided by CT is likely to be important for patient management. It is hoped that treatment can be tailored to the individual patient, precluding the need for surgery in those cases which are clearly inoperable and providing a more accurate selection of patients for radical cystectomy.

ACKNOWLEDGEMENTS

We gratefully acknowledge the help of Mrs D. Mears in scanning the patients, and Miss D. Harding, who prepared the manuscript. We would also like to thank our clinical colleagues for permission to report patients under their care.

REFERENCES

CONNOLLY, J.G., CHALLIS, T.W., WALLACE, D.M. and BRUCE, A.W. (1966). Use of the fractionated cystogram in the staging of bladder tumours. *Canadian Journal of Surgery*, **9**, 39–43

GOSALBEZ, R. and GIL-VERNET, J.M. (1962). Bladder tomography: the use of air intra- and peri-vesically in the radiologic study of bladder tumors. *Journal of Urology*, **88**, 312–317

HODSON, N.J., HUSBAND, J.E. and MACDONALD, J.S. (1979). The role of computed tomography in the staging of bladder cancer. *Clinical Radiology*, **30**, 389–395

HOUNSFIELD, G.N. (1973). Computerised transverse axial scanning (tomography); I. Description of system. *British Journal of Radiology*, **46**, 1016–1022

KELLETT, M.J., OLIVER, R.T.D., HUSBAND, J.E. and KELSEY FRY, I.(1980). CT scanning as an adjunct to bimanual examination for staging bladder tumours. *British Journal of Urology* **52**, 101–106

LANG, E.K., NOURSE, M.H., WISHARD, W.N., Jr., and MERTZ, J.H.O. (1966). The accuracy of pre-operative staging of bladder tumors by arteriography: a five year study. *Journal of Urology*, **95**, 363–367

LEE, J.K.T., STANLEY, R.J., SAGEL, S.S. and McCLENNAN, B.L. (1978). Accuracy of CT in detecting intra-abdominal and pelvic lymph node metastases from pelvic cancers. *American Journal of Roentgenology*, **131**, 675–681

MORLEY, P.(1978). Clinical staging of epithelial bladder tumours by echotomography. In *Ultrasound in Tumour Diagnosis*, pp. 145–161. Ed. by C.R. Hill, J.R. McCready and D.O. Cosgrove. London; Pitman Medical

SEIDELMANN, F.E., COHEN, W.N. and BRYAN, P.J. (1977). Computed tomographic staging of bladder neoplasms. *Radiologic Clinics of North America*, **15**, 419–440

SEIDELMANN, F.E., COHEN, W.N., BRYAN, P.J., TEMES, S.P., KRAUS, D. and SCHOENROCK, G. (1978). Accuracy of CT staging of bladder neoplasms using the gas-filled method: report of 21 patients with surgical confirmation. *American Journal of Roentgenology*, **130**, 735–739

UICC (INTERNATIONAL UNION AGAINST CANCER) (1978). *TNM Classification of Malignant Tumours,* 3rd Edition. Geneva; UICC

WERF-MESSING, VAN DER B. (1979). Pre-operative irradiation followed by cystectomy to treat carcinoma of the urinary bladder category T3 NX, 0–4, MO. *International Journal of Radiation, Oncology, Biology and Physics,* **5**, 394–401

5

Chemotherapy of Murine Bladder Cancer

Mark S. Soloway and William M. Murphy

Chemotherapy is increasingly being introduced into the treatment of both superficial and invasive bladder cancer. The demonstrated effectiveness of a few drugs and the limitations of surgery and radiotherapy are two major reasons for this interest. In dealing with superficial tumours the recurrence rate of 50–70% following local resection poses a major dilemma for the urologist (Nichols and Marshall, 1956; Williams *et al.*, 1977). Intensive intravesical chemotherapy has been shown to reduce the rate of tumour regrowth, but not of the number of patients who show a recurrence; however, only two drugs, thiotepa and ethoglucid, have had a significant clinical trial (Soloway, 1980). Numerous other antineoplastic agents with demonstrated effectiveness by the systemic route deserve evaluation for intravesical therapy. Patients with multifocal, superficial, tumours, who are not suited for long sessions of endoscopic resection or fulguration may also be excellent candidates for an effective intravesical drug programme.

At the other end of the spectrum are patients with tumours which have invaded the bladder muscle or spread to regional lymph nodes. Radiotherapy and/or radical surgery have not substantially improved the relatively poor survival in this group over the last few years. Improvement in the quantity and quality of survival in such cases may require systemic therapy.

Because only a few of the multitude of drugs exhibiting some antineoplastic activity in broad screening programmes can ever be evaluated clinically in bladder cancer, the availability of an animal model which closely simulates the disease in man has proved to be useful in evaluating potential intravesical or systemic agents and in determining which drugs should have priority for clinical trials. The animal model has also been useful in testing hypotheses which can be controlled only in a laboratory setting, such as the role of tumour cell implantation as a factor in high recurrence rates, or the antitumour synergism of radiation and chemotherapy.

This report will briefly describe a murine model for bladder cancer and enumerate some of the studies which have helped to guide and stimulate clinical chemotherapy trials.

THE ANIMAL MODEL

The transplantable and primary tumours used in our laboratory are induced by the carcinogen N-[4-(5-nitro-2-furyl)-2-thiazolyl] formamide (FANFT). FANFT is a nitrofuran which induces urothelial, primarily bladder, tumours in mice (Erturk *et al.*, 1970a; Soloway, 1975), rats (Erturk *et al.*, 1967, Erturk *et al.*, 1969), and dogs (Erturk *et al.*, 1970b) in an incidence approaching 100%. The histogenesis of the epithelial changes varies among species and with the concentration of carcinogen. By 38 weeks, almost all C3H/He mice ingesting 0.1% FANFT will have multifocal dysplasia. The tumours closely resemble

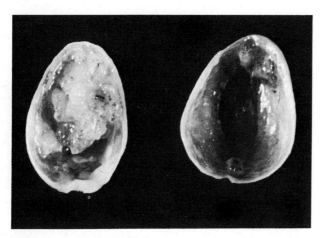

Figure 5.1 *Typical multifocal papillary tumours induced by FANFT*

those in man, both grossly (*Figure 5.1*) and histologically (*Figure 5.2*). Approximately 90% of the tumours are transitional cell; the remainder are squamous. They may be papillary or sessile. The lesions progress through the stages of hyperplasia, dysplasia and carcinoma in situ to frank malignancy (Tiltman and Friedell, 1971). Some of these tumours are immunogenic (Soloway *et al.*, 1978).

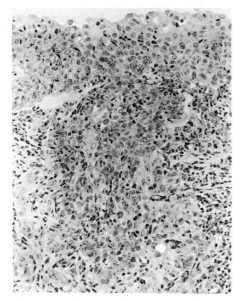

Figure 5.2 Histological appearance of typical transitional cell tumour induced by FANFT. Superficial normal-appearing urothelial cells are identified despite invasion of the carcinoma into the lamina propria (PAS × 250)

ROLE OF TUMOUR IMPLANTATION

The existence of multicentric foci of urothelial abnormalities (atypia, carcinoma in situ, and carcinoma) in patients with bladder cancer is well documented (Melamed *et al.*, 1964, Cooper *et al.*, 1973; Farrow *et al.*, 1976, Heney *et al.*, 1978; Murphy *et al.*, 1979) and the progression of these lesions is the probable aetiology for the majority of clinical 'recurrences' following initial resection or fulguration of a bladder tumour. Another hypothesis which might contribute to this high recurrence rate is the implantation or seeding of tumour cells on areas of traumatized urothelium. Although current methods of investigation probably are unable to provide proof that this phenomenon occurs clinically, there is strong circumstantial evidence that it is a factor. Franksson (1950) observed an apparent susceptibility of the bladder neck as a site of recurrent tumours. He suggested that trauma to this region during resection accounts for the predilection of this site to implantation. Boreham (1956), Hinman (1956), and Kiefer (1953) also emphasized the occurrence of implantation after urothelial trauma, citing their personal experience with vesical neck recurrences. Boyd and Burnand (1974) and more recently Page *et al.* (1978) observed that recurrent tumours were much more likely than initial tumours to be located on the dome or posterior wall. Both reports suggested that these were tumour implants, and implicated mechanical or thermal trauma to these regions during surgical resection as factors predisposing to implantation.

Initial laboratory experiments seeking to corroborate the clinical impressions that tumour cells were capable of implanting in the bladder, lacked a syngeneic transitional cell tumour model. Nevertheless, McDonald and Thorson (1956) evidently transplanted a β-naphthylamine-induced bladder tumour from one dog to a mucosal-lined pouch in another. Wallace and Hershfield (1958) injected rat sarcoma cells down the ureter or via the urethra into the bladder, and documented implantation of this anaplastic tumour. More recently,

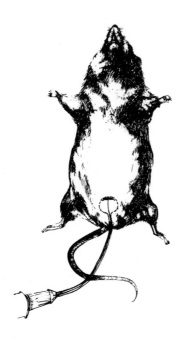

Figure 5.3 Technique for focal cautery of portion of murine bladder. Insulated electrode attached to electrocautery unit passed transurethrally

Weldon and Soloway (1975) demonstrated that syngeneic murine transitional tumour cells will implant and grow on a diffusely altered urothelium, but rarely in the normal bladder. A single installation of N-methyl-N-nitrosourea (NMU) was used to produce a chemical cystitis and alter the mucosal surface. This single instillation in itself does not cause tumours (Hicks and Wakefield, 1972). When tumour cells were instilled transurethrally into both normal and NMU-treated bladders, only 13% of normal bladders developed tumours, whereas 60% of mice exposed to a single instillation of NMU had tumours when they were killed ($P < 0.001$). Implantation was the only way that these tumours could have occurred.

In an effort better to simulate transurethral fulguration of a bladder tumour, a technique of injury, by electrocautery, of a portion of the murine bladder has been devised (Soloway and Masters, 1979). An insulated wire electrode was inserted transurethrally and the tip positioned against the posterior wall of the bladder (*Figure 5.3*). The wire was attached to a diathermy unit and a charge delivered for 5 s. One million cells from a transplantable transitional cell tumour designated MBT-683 were instilled transurethrally into 25 of 35 mice; 10 mice served as controls for the effect of cauterization alone. This group was compared with 25 mice receiving the same number of tumour cells but without alteration of the bladder. Four weeks later, all mice were killed and the incidence of tumour determined by gross and histological examination of the excised bladders.

Only 12% (3/25) of the mice which had the tumour cells instilled into a normal bladder (no cautery) developed tumours, in contrast to 54% (13/25) which had been given focal cautery, and which developed tumours ($P < 0.01$). Fulguration by itself did not cause tumours, as expected. Thus, transitional tumour cells preferentially implant on the cauterized urothelial surface.

INTRAVESICAL CHEMOTHERAPY

As prophylaxis against implantation tumours

The ability to fulgurate a portion of the murine bladder and to induce implantation of a transplantable transitional cell tumour provided a model for evaluation of the effectiveness of cytotoxic drugs in reducing the incidence of implantation. Earlier studies utilizing NMU to induce implantation demonstrated that intravesical ethoglucid and thiotepa would reduce the incidence of implantation (Soloway and Martino, 1976). As described above, bladders were cauterized with a transurethrally placed electrode and 1×10^6 MBT-2 or MBT-683 tumours cells were instilled via a PE-10 catheter. The initial experiment involved 65 female C3H/He mice. Twenty mice served as controls and received only sterile water. The treatment groups (15 each) received either thiotepa (5 mg/kg), cis-diamminedichloroplatinum (II) (DDP) (18 mg/kg), or mitomycin C (MMC) (6 mg/kg). All agents were diluted to instil the drug in a volume of 0.1 ml. Intravesical chemotherapy was started 24 h after placement of the tumour cells and continued weekly for 4 weeks. After 6 weeks all mice were killed and the bladders were distended with McDowell's solution for fixation, removed and examined macroscopically for the presence of tumour. The bladders were also sectioned at three levels so that the presence or absence of tumours could be confirmed by histological analysis.

Seventy-eight per cent of the mice receiving water irrigation alone (controls) developed tumours, confirming the high incidence of implantation following cauterization of a focal area of the bladder (*Table 5.1*). This also illustrated that water irrigation does not prevent implantation. DDP completely prevented tumour implantation; thiotepa and mitomycin C significantly reduced the incidence of tumours ($P < 0.02$).

Table 5.1
EFFECT OF INTRAVESICAL CHEMOTHERAPY ON INCIDENCE
OF LOCAL TUMOUR CELL IMPLANTATION

Therapy	Number of mice	Number of tumours	%	P
Control	18	14	78	---
Thiotepa	14	5	36	0.02
Mitomycin C	15	5	33	0.01
DDP	12	0	0	0.001

Day 0: cautery
Day 0: 1 X 10^6 MBT–683 cells intravesically
Days 1, 8, 15, 22: chemotherapy

This model will continue to be used to screen potential drugs for their use in intravesical chemotherapy. A recent clinical study by Burnand *et al.* (1976) reported a significant reduction in the recurrence rate of superficial bladder cancer when intravesical chemotherapy was started immediately after endoscopic resection. This clinical report appears to substantiate the hypothesis that implantation contributes to the high rate of subsequent tumours. Drugs effective in the animal model, such as thiotepa or MMC, (Crooke *et al.*, 1978) are among those which are effective clinically.

As treatment of carcinoma in situ and prophylaxis against tumour progression

The FANFT-induced transitional cell carcinoma (TCC) murine model has also provided a system to study the effect of chemotherapy on multifocal pre-neoplastic and neoplastic urothelial abnormalities, such as dysplasia and carcinoma in situ (Tis), as well as cancer. Patients with multifocal superficial bladder cancer or Tis pose a therapeutic dilemma because the natural history of the disease is quite variable from patient to patient. The high incidence of subsequent tumours following initial endoscopic resection has already been cited and the multifocal pre-neoplastic urothelial abnormalities probably provide the starting point in most cases. Cystectomy is curative but carries a high morbidity for this non-invasive lesion. Radiation is ineffective for Tis and, when used for superficial tumours, does not significantly reduce the incidence of subsequent tumours and often retards their diagnosis. Intravesical chemotherapy is an attractive option as it is relatively non-toxic, bathes almost the entire bladder and is amenable to an outpatient setting. Despite these advantages, only three agents have had any significant clinical evaluation: these are thiotepa (USA), ethoglucid (UK), and MMC (Japan and USA). Unfortunately, they have never been compared in a controlled, randomized trial. Because mice ingesting FANFT developed atypia, Tis and papillary tumours identical to those in man, the murine model seems ideal to investigate the comparative virtues of these and other drugs and to help select agents for clinical trials. To date, only one drug has been thoroughly evaluated in this system, but the methodology has now been established and comparative studies are in progress.

Thiotepa was the first drug selected to determine its effect on normal and abnormal urothelium. The dose of thiotepa was 5 mg/kg (515 mosmol/l) which is the LD_{10} when given weekly for a month. The control group in each study received intravesical saline.

Before evaluating the effect of thiotepa on the abnormal urothelium, the initial experiment analyzed possible alterations to the normal urothelium induced by a single instillation of thiotepa (day 0) compared with the effect of saline. Voided urine was obtained on days 1, 3, 7, and 22 following thiotepa instillation, and the bladder was removed and analyzed by light and electron microscopy. The urine was passed through a Millipore filter and stained with a modified Papanicolaou technique. There were no consistent morphological differences between treated and control groups, either cytologically or histologically. There were no cells with large, bizarre nuclei or hyperchromasia, such as those that have been described following radiation or cyclophosphamide. The same experiment was repeated after three weekly thiotepa instillations, with identical results. Thus, thiotepa induced few morphological alterations in the exfoliated cells or epithelium of normal bladders. This has clinical implications because it casts doubt on the so-called 'thiotepa effect' of exfoliated cells from bladders receiving this alkylating agent. Abnormal cells seen on cytological examination are likely to represent dysplasia or malignancy.

A similar investigation was then conducted to study the effect of thiotepa or saline on the abnormal urothelium (Murphy *et al.*, 1978). Intravesical therapy was started after the mice had ingested FANFT for 38 weeks and had atypia or Tis. Therapy was given weekly for 3 weeks, and the exfoliated cells as well as the bladders examined after various periods of treatment. Although cellular degeneration and vacuolization were prominent, nuclear changes were sparse. Multinucleated cells occurred infrequently in both thiotepa and saline groups. It was concluded that these alterations were primarily due to a toxic effect on the bladder epithelium rather than a metabolic effect. The incidence of tumours was similar in both groups, although the numbers were not sufficient to provide significant data. Another experiment was therefore designed to evaluate this critical factor.

Two groups of C3H/He mice ingesting FANFT were randomly divided into two groups (A and B) and each of these further divided into a treatment (thiotepa) and control (saline) group. Group A mice had either thiotepa or saline instilled weekly before the expected onset of tumour; in group B, intravesical therapy was started after tumours were evident on cytological analysis. Thus, the effectiveness of this alkylating agent on both developing (atypia, Tis) and established tumours could be evaluated. Upon removal of the bladders and histological analysis by serial sections of each bladder, no significant difference was found in overall tumour incidence between the treated and control mice in either group A or B. The administration of thiotepa, however, before tumour development (group A), resulted in significantly more low-grade, low-stage tumours than in the control mice, suggesting that thiotepa inhibited the progression of some tumours into high-grade, invasive lesions.

Thiotepa may be useful in the therapy of superficial bladder cancer by more than one mechanism. The toxic effect of thiotepa indicated in the initial studies may kill potentially implanting cells when these are introduced after local resection. This action may also alter the endoscopic appearance of papillary, low-grade lesions by denuding many of the cells from the fibrovascular stalk, and may thereby decrease the frequency of visible recurrences. The ability of thiotepa to prevent the progression of some tumours from low- to high-grade lesions, as indicated in the last experiment, suggests a metabolic action on rapidly dividing cells and has obvious therapeutic implications. This series of experiments is a prototype by which a number of other drugs are currently being analyzed.

SYSTEMIC CHEMOTHERAPY

Experiments using passaged tumour MBT-2 or MBT-683

A major step in the screening of drugs for use in bladder cancer is the selection of agents for clinical trials in patients with advanced disease. A systematic approach is used. The maximum tolerated dose (LD_{10}) of promising drugs is first determined. The mouse strains used in our studies are C3H/He or $B6C3F_1$. Initial antitumour studies are performed using a transplantable transitional cell tumour, usually MBT-2 or MBT-683. These tumours arose as invasive FANFT-induced

TCC in female C3H/He mice and have been serially transplanted sub-cutaneously. The transplanted-tumour studies allow relatively rapid evaluation of a number of agents. Tumour inhibition, assessed by comparison of the mean tumour diameter in treated mice as compared with controls at a specific time (usually when the tumours in the controls are about 11–12 mm in diameter), and prolongation of the median survival time (MST), are used as indicators of drug activity. The percentage increase in lifespan (% ILS) is calculated (MST of treated mice, minus MST of controls, divided by MST of control mice × 100). Mice actually cured by chemotherapy are not included in these cal-culations. Tumour growth delay is also calculated and used as an indicator of antitumour effect. This is the time (in days) required for the tumours in the treated group to reach a given size, usually 11 mm, minus the time for the controls to reach this size (T − C value). This value is similar to the duration of remission, used clinically.

In the first series of experiments, single-agent therapy was started 7 days after injection of 1 × 10^4 MBT-2 cells (Soloway *et al.*, 1973b). Doxorubicin and actinomycin D inhibited tumour growth and produced an ILS of 117% and 124% respectively. Cis-diaminedichloro-platinum (II) (DDP) yielded a dramatic ILS of 170%. This study was conducted in 1973, and stimulated a clinical trial in patients with recurrent transitional cell carcinoma of the bladder. The pronounced activity in man paralleled the murine data: DDP is currently the most active single agent against bladder cancer (Yagoda *et al.*, 1976; Soloway, 1978). Cyclophosphamide was highly active against this early generation MBT-2 tumour, curing all mice in the first major study. Although this drug possesses some activity in human bladder cancer, the response rates with cyclophosphamide do not approach those achieved with DDP.

A recent study evaluated two newly developed drugs, 4'-(9-acridinyl-amine) methanesulphon-m-anisidine (AMSA) and maytansine. Fifty-five C3H/He mice received 7.5 × 10^4 MBT-2 cells in their right hind limbs on day 0. Mice were randomly allocated on day 9 to a control

Table 5.2
EFFECTS OF AMSA AND MAYTANSINE ON MURINE BLADDER CANCER

Therapy	*Dose (mg/kg)*	*Number of mice*	*Mean tumour diameter (mm)*	*P*	*T−C value (days)*	*% ILS*
Control		23	11.7	− − −	− − −	100
AMSA	10	15	10.4	0.025	6.0	126
Maytansine	0.25	15	9.9	0.005	3.4	93

Day 0: 7.5 × 10^4 MBT−2 cells
Days 9, 16, 23: chemotherapy
Day 27: results
T − C: see text

(25) and two treatment groups (15). Therapy consisted of AMSA (10 mg/kg) or maytansine (0.25 mg/kg), and continued weekly for 3 weeks. The results (*Table 5.2*) indicated significant tumour inhibition by both agents on day 27. The controls reached MST on day 55. AMSA produced an ILS of 126%, while regrowth of tumour was more rapid in the maytansine group and no improvement in MST was achieved. Continuation of therapy might have produced a better response to maytansine.

A subsequent study evaluated four single agents: AMSA (10 mg/kg), methyl-GAG (100 mg/kg), DDP (6 mg/kg), and epipodophyllotoxin (VP16) (50 mg/kg). Therapy was started on day 7 and continued weekly for 2 additional weeks. Each agent effected a significant inhibition of tumour, as indicated in *Table 5.3*. Impressive improvements in the ILS were achieved by both DDP and VP16. On the basis of these results, VP16 appears to merit investigation in TCC in man.

Table 5.3
EFFECTS OF VP16, AMSA, METHYL–GAG, and DDP ON MURINE BLADDER CANCER

Therapy	*Dose (mg/kg)*	*Number of mice*	*Mean tumour diameter (mm)*	*P*	*T–C value (days)*	*% ILS*
Control		12	14.6	–––	–––	100
AMSA	10	13	12.5	0.025	6.3	104
Methyl-GAG	100	13	12.4	0.001	7.1	111
DDP	6	13	11.3	0.001	11.0	121
VP16	50	13	11.0	0.001	8.0	143

Day 0: 7.5×10^4 MBT-2 cells
Days 7, 14, 21: chemotherapy
Day 26: results
T – C: see text

Despite our earlier experience (Soloway, 1977) that methotrexate had little activity against any early generation of MBT-2, the clinical reports (Altman *et al.,* 1972; Turner *et al.,* 1977) that methotrexate is effective in bladder cancer, prompted us to re-investigate this agent. The current experiment used the MBT-683 tumour, which is a more rapid-growing, poorly differentiated transitional cell carcinoma. Two dose levels of methotrexate were compared with DDP. The rapid growth of the tumour is illustrated by the mean tumour diameter of 17.7 mm in the control group on day 23 (*Table 5.4*). Once again, the benefit of methotrexate was only modest, as indicated by the tumour diameter and T – C values: however, the higher dose did provide a significant improvement in the ILS. Mice receiving DDP once again experienced significant tumour inhibition ($P < 0.001$), with an ILS of 152%.

Combination chemotherapy offers the theoretical advantages of utilizing drugs which inhibit cell metabolism or replication by different

Table 5.4
EFFECT OF METHOTREXATE AND DDP ON MURINE BLADDER CANCER

Therapy	Dose (mg/kg)	Number of mice	Mean tumour diameter (mm)	P	T–C value (days)	% ILS
Control		18	17.7	———	———	100
Methotrexate	20	13	17.2	NS	1.3	111
Methotrexate	40	10	16.8	NS	1.6	133
DDP	6	15	7.9	0.001	†	152

† Reached MST before achieving mean tumour diameter of 17.7 mm
Day 0: 7.5×10^4 MBT–683 cells
Days 7, 14, 21: chemotherapy
Day 23: results
T – C: see text

mechanisms, but which have less than additive toxicity (Capizzi *et al.*, 1977). One such study used an early generation of the MBT-2. Chemotherapy was not started until the average tumour diameter had reached 8 mm (Soloway, 1977). Cyclophosphamide and DDP, when used alone in mice bearing these established tumours, produced similar tumour inhibition. The combination regimen produced a greater inhibition of tumour growth when measured on day 43, although the ILS was not improved, as a result of regrowth after therapy was discontinued. This animal study stimulated the use of this combination in man, with some prolongation in response duration, although the response rate was similar to that with DDP used alone (Yagoda, 1977; 1978).

An analogue of the transition state for the aspartate transcarbamylase reaction, N-phosphonacetyl-L-aspartate (PALA), has been synthesized and has shown some promise as an antitumour agent in initial screening tests (Johnson *et al.*, 1976). Theoretically, PALA should inhibit *de novo* pyrimidine nucleotide biosynthesis. Tumours with a low level of aspartate transcarbamylase have responded to PALA (Johnson *et al.*, 1978). In the initial study evaluating PALA in murine TCC, three dose levels were evaluated (200, 350 and 500 mg/kg) and

Table 5.5
EFFECT OF DDP AND/OR PALA ON MURINE TCC

Treatment	Dose (mg/kg)	Number	Tumour incidence	Mean tumour diameter (mm)	P	% ILS
Control		25	19 (76%)	9.07		100
DDP	6	15	11 (73%)	6.00	0.005	104
PALA	500	15	8 (53%)	6.30	0.05	114
DDP + PALA	6 + 250	15	8 (53%)	4.77	0.005	116

Day 0: 5.4×10^4 MBT–2 cells
Day 7, 14, 21: chemotherapy
Day 31: results

compared with DDP. The highest PALA dose and DDP produced both significant tumour inhibition and a significant prolongation of the ILS.

A subsequent study examined the combination of DDP and PALA. Seventy-six per cent (19/25) of controls developed tumours (*Table 5.5*). PALA and the PALA-DDP combination reduced the incidence of tumours to 53%. Each regimen produced a significant reduction in the average tumour diameter. This figure does not include the cures. The ILS of the combination was 116%, varying little from the groups receiving single-agent therapy. Phase I clinical trials with PALA have been started and are not conclusive, suggesting that the activity observed in murine models may not be as marked in humans.

Chemotherapy of primary unpassaged tumours

The selection of single or combination regimens for evaluation of efficacy in primary (autochthonous) murine bladder cancer is based on results in the transplanted tumour system (*see previous section*). The duration of each experiment is approximately 1 year, because therapy is not begun in most instances until a majority of the mice show severe dysplasia, Tis, or cancer, on cytological examination of the urine (Soloway, *et al.*, 1973a; Jacobs *et al.*, 1976). Chemotherapy was started after 40 weeks' ingestion of 0.1% FANFT. Chemotherapy was continued for 3 weeks; 2 weeks after completion of therapy, all mice were killed and the bladders removed, distended with formalin, and weighed. Serial histological sections of each bladder were made to determine the stage and grade of each tumour. An analysis of the difference between the weights of the bladders in each group was performed by taking the logarithm of each bladder weight to normalize the distribution before statistical analysis using Student's t test. The x^2 test was used to evaluate the significance of differences between the number of bladders bearing various stages of tumour.

In our first long-term study (Soloway, 1977) untreated mice (FANFT only) had a tumour incidence of 91.3% (31/34) with an additional three mice exhibiting Tis. Each chemotherapeutic agent significantly reduced tumour volume (reflected by the bladder weight) compared with the controls (108 mg) as follows: cyclophosphamide (42.9 mg), actinomycin D (49.6 mg); DDP (56.4 mg); and doxorubicin (69.5 mg). The combination of cyclophosphamide with doxorubicin (37.3 mg) or 5-fluorouracil (38.3 mg) was superior to cyclophosphamide alone. Despite the short duration of therapy (3 weeks) several regimes reduced the incidence of tumours invading the entire bladder wall (T3b). Nevertheless, despite this impressive reduction in tumour weight after 3 weeks' treatment, no regime reduced tumour incidence compared with that in the control group. However, there was a signficant reduction in incidence of deeply invasive lesions.

After the activity of PALA had been identified in the transplantable experimental model, this agent was evaluated with DDP in the primary tumour model. Therapy was started after 47 weeks on FANFT and consisted of a control (25) and four treatment groups (19). The treatment regimes and results are indicated in *Tables 5.6 and 5.7.* Each drug produced a significant reduction in the mean bladder weight, confirming activity in murine TCC. The combination of PALA and

Table 5.6
CHEMOTHERAPY OF PRIMARY FANFT-INDUCED BLADDER TUMOURS

Therapy (mg/kg)	*Number*	*Mean bladder wt. (mg)*	*Mean log bladder wt.*	*P*
Control (FANFT only)	25	56.9	3.94	---
PALA 400	18	46.2	3.62	0.05
PALA 250 + DDP 6	16	36.2	3.47	0.005
DDP 6	17	34.6	3.39	0.001
DDP 6 + CYCLO 50	19	29.6	3.36	0.001

Week 47: therapy started
Drugs given weekly ($\times$ 4)
Week 53: bladders removed

Table 5.7
CHEMOTHERAPY OF PRIMARY FANFT-INDUCED BLADDER TUMOURS

Therapy	*Number of bladders with tumour*	*Total number of mice*	*%*	*P*
Control (FANFT only)	18	25	72	---
DDP	10	17	59	NS
PALA	7	18	39	0.03
PALA + DDP	4	16	26	0.005
DDP + CYCLO	4	19	21	0.001

Week 47: therapy started
Drugs given weekly ($\times$ 4)
Week 53: bladders removed

DDP was superior to either agent alone in reducing tumour incidence, although the size of resulting tumours was not diminished by the addition of PALA to DDP. Although DDP used alone did not significantly reduce tumour incidence, the size of these tumours was significantly reduced. In addition, these experiments confirmed results of earlier studies, in that the addition of cyclophosphamide to DDP provided greater tumour inhibition than that achieved by DDP alone.

The benefit produced by the combination of cyclophosphamide and DDP in some studies has suggested that the three-drug combination of cyclophosphamide-DDP-doxorubicin might be more lethal to tumour cells than the single drugs alone, without a concomitant increase in toxicity. A series of experiments using the transplantable tumours varied the day of doxorubicin administration. The optimal antineoplastic effect was achieved when doxorubicin was administered 3 days after DDP and cyclophosphamide. This set the stage for a study using primary tumours. Therapy was started after 47 weeks on FANFT, and consisted of either cyclophosphamide, or DDP, or cyclophosphamide + DDP, or cyclophosphamide + DDP on day 0 with doxorubicin on day 3. Therapy was given every 10 days for 4-day cycles. Bladders were removed during week 53. The control group had a mean bladder weight of 43.2 mg with 14/19 bladders (74%) containing tumour (*Tables 5.8*

Table 5.8
CHEMOTHERAPY OF PRIMARY FANFT-INDUCED BLADDER CANCER

Therapy (mg/kg)	Number	Mean bladder wt. (mg)	SD	Mean log. bladder wt.	P
Control (FANFT only)	19	43.2	27.88	3.60	---
CYCLO 50	15	78.2	121.44	3.78	NS
DDP 5 + CYCLO 50	15	34.4	25.08	3.36	NS
DDP 5	15	31.2	30.25	3.19	NS
DDP 5 + CYCLO 50 + DOX 3†	14	27.9	20.50	3.19	0.05

†Doxorubicin given on Day 3 following each administration of DDP-CYCLO combination
Week 47: therapy started
Drug cycles every 10 days (× 4)
Week 53: bladders removed
SD: standard deviation

Table 5.9
CHEMOTHERAPY OF PRIMARY FANFT-INDUCED BLADDER CANCER

Therapy	Number of bladders with tumour	Total number of mice	%
Control	14	19	74
CYCLO	14	15	93
DDP + CYCLO	13	15	87
DDP	10	15	67
DDP + CYCLO + DOX	8	14	57

Week 47: therapy started
Drug cycles every 10 days (× 4)
Week 53: bladders removed

and 5.9). Cyclophosphamide failed to provide any tumour inhibition. The combination of DDP and cyclophosphamide was not superior to DDP alone. Because of large standard deviations in most groups, the only regime providing a significant reduction in the mean log bladder weight was the three-drug regime ($P < 0.05$). Mice in this group also had the lowest tumour incidence (57%). This study confirmed the suggested additional antineoplastic effect of this three-drug regime observed in the transplanted model. Clinical trials are in progress to determine whether response rates are higher or response duration longer with this three-drug regime than with DDP alone.

RADIATION THERAPY

The exact indications and schedules of radiation therapy in the treatment of bladder cancer are still under considerable discussion. There is suggestive evidence that pre-operative radiotherapy is capable of improving the survival achieved by surgery alone (Wallace and Bloom, 1976; Whitmore *et al.*, 1977) (*see* Chapters 17,18). Because further improvements in survival for patients with advanced disease will require systemic therapy, such as chemotherapy, a most useful drug would be one exhibiting not only a systemic effect but an additive or synergistic effect with radiotherapy against local disease. Such a drug given during pre-operative radiation and continued post-operatively, might lead to a long-term improvement in results.

The synergism between radiation and DDP in P-338 leukaemia (Wodinsky *et al.*, 1974) and the impressive activity of DDP in both murine and human transitional cell carcinoma, prompted us to investigate and combination of radiation and DDP. One hundred C3H/He mice had 5×10^4 MBT-2 cells (generation 43) placed in their hind limbs and they were then randomly allocated to one control (20) and eight treatment groups (10). The latter were given the following alternative regimes: cyclophosphamide; DDP; 1500 rad (250 rad twice weekly for 3 weeks); 1500 rad + cyclophosphamide; 1500 rad + DDP; 3600 rad + cyclophosphamide; and 3600 rad + DDP. Chemotherapy

Table 5.10

EFFECT OF CHEMOTHERAPY AND/OR RADIATION THERAPY ON TRANSPLANTED MURINE BLADDER CANCER

Therapy	Number of mice	Number of tumours	%	Median survival time (days)	% ILS
Control	19	17	(89)	56	– – –
DDP	10	9	(90)	60	107
CYCLO	10	10	(100)	60	107
1500 rad	9	8	(89)	67	120
3600 rad	10	4	(40)*	>180	>100
1500 rad + CYCLO	9	9	(100)	67	120
1500 rad + DDP	9	7	(78)	77	138
3600 rad + CYCLO	8	7	(88)	71	127
3600 rad + DDP	9	2	(22)*	>180	>100

* $P < 0.01$

Day 0: 5×10^4 MBT$-$2 cells

Days 7, 14, 21: therapy

was given on days 7, 14 and 21. Radiation was also started on day 7, using an AEC Theraton 80 ^{60}Co unit. Lead shielding assured that only the tumour-bearing limb received radiation.

In this high-generation, fast-growing tumour, DDP and cyclophosphamide produced little improvement in either cures or ILS (*Table 5.10*). In this study, calculations of MST and ILS include all mice beginning therapy. Radiation therapy was capable of curing some mice, particularly at the higher dose. The addition of cyclophosphamide to the radiation provided no additional benefit; however, the DDP-3600 rad regime resulted in 7/9 cures, as well as a significant inhibition of growth of those tumours that did grow, compared with either method used alone.

SUMMARY

To date there has been a relatively close correlation between agents found to be effective in the murine model and in clinical studies (*Table 5.11*). The efficacy of DDP in the FANFT model encouraged trials in

Table 5.11
SYSTEMIC CHEMOTHERAPY FOR BLADDER CANCER

Agent	Mouse	Man
DDP	+++	+++
Cyclophosphamide	++	+
VP16	++	?
PALA	++	?
AMSA	+	?
Methyl-GAG	+	?
Actinomycin D	+	?
Methotrexate	±	+
Maytansine	±	?
Doxorubicin	±	±
Hexamethylmelamine	−	?
Hydroxyurea	−	?
5–fluorouracil	−	±

human TCC: currently it is the most effective single agent for this tumour. It is hoped that this approach can continue to provide data which correlate with that in man. The increasing number of natural products and synthesized compounds with potential antitumour action, as well as the production of analogues of effective drugs, demand a reliable, systematic approach to the selection of drugs for clinical trial. The evaluation of combination chemotherapy, chemotherapy and radiation, and immunotherapy further magnify the task.

REFERENCES

ALTMAN, C.C., McCAGUE, N.J., RIPEPI, A.C. and CARDOZO, M.(1972). The use of methotrexate in advanced carcinoma of the bladder. *Journal of Urology*, **108**, 271–273

BOREHAM, P. (1956). The surgical spread of cancer in urology. *British Journal of Urology*, **28**, 163–175

BOYD, P.J.R. and BURNAND, K.G. (1974). Site of bladder-tumour recurrence. *Lancet*, **2**, 1290–1292

BURNAND, K.G., BOYD, P.J.R., MAYO, M.E., SHUTTLEWORTH, K.E.D. and LLOYD–DAVIES, R.W. (1976). Single dose intravesical thiotepa as adjuvant to cysto-diathermy in the treatment of transitional cell bladder carcinoma. *British Journal of Urology*, **48**, 55–59

CAPIZZI, R.L., KEISER, L.W. and SARTORELLI, A.C.(1977). Combination chemo-therapy – theory and practice. *Seminars in Oncology*, **4**, 227–253

COOPER, P.H., WAISMAN, J., JOHNSTON, W.H. and SKINNER, D.G.(1973). Severe atypia of transitional epithelium and carcinoma of the urinary bladder. *Cancer*, **31**, 1055–1060

CROOKE, S.T., JOHNSON, D.E. and BRACKEN, R.B. (1978). A phase I-II study of mitomycin C topical therapy in early transitional cell carcinoma of the bladder. *Proceedings of the American Association for Cancer Research*, **19**, 321

ERTURK, E., COHEN, W.M. and BRYAN, G.T. (1970a). Urinary bladder carcino-genicity of N-[4-(5-nitro-2-furyl)-2-thiazolyl] formamide in female Swiss mice. *Cancer Research*, **30**, 1309–1311

ERTURK, E., COHEN, S.M., PRICE, J.M. and BRYAN, G.T. (1969). Pathogenesis, histology, and transplantability of urinary bladder carcinomas induced in albino rats by oral administration of N-[4-(5-nitro-2-furyl)-2-thiazolyl] formamide. *Cancer Research*, **29**, 2219–2228

ERTURK, E., ATASSI, S.A., YOSHIDA, O., COHEN, S.M., PRICE, J.M. and BRYAN, G.T. (1970b). Comparative urinary and gall bladder carcinogenicity of N-[4-(5-nitro-2-furyl)-2-thiazolyl] formamide and N-[4-(5-nitro-2-furyl)-2-thiazolyl] acetamide in the dog. *Journal of the National Cancer Institute*, **45**, 535–542

ERTURK, E., PRICE, J.M., MORRIS, J.E., COHEN, S., LEITH, R.S., VON ESH, A.M. and CORVETTI, A.J. (1967). The production of carcinomas of the urinary bladder in rats by feeding N-[4-(5-nitro-2-furyl)-2-thiazolyl] formamide. *Cancer Research*, **27**, 1998–2002

FARROW, G.M., UTZ, D.C. and RIFE, C.C. (1976). Morphological and clinical obser-vations of patients with early bladder cancer treated with total cystectomy. *Cancer Research*, **36**, 2495–2501

FRANKSSON, C. (1950). Tumours of the urinary bladder: A pathological and clinical study of 434 cases. *Acta Chirurgica Scandinavica*, **100**, 664–667

HENEY, N.M., DALY, J., PROUT, G.R., JR., NEIH, P.T., HEANEY, J.A. and TREBECK, N.E. (1978). Biopsy of apparently normal urothelium in patients with bladder carcinoma. *Journal of Urology*, **120**, 559–560

HICKS, R.M. and WAKEFIELD, J.S.T.J.(1972). Rapid induction of bladder cancer in rats with N-methyl-N-nitrosourea. I. Histology. *Chemico-Biological Inter-actions*, **5**, 139–152

HINMAN, F., Jr. (1956). Recurrence of bladder tumours by surgical implanation. *Journal of Urology*, **75**, 695–696

JACOBS, J.B., ARAI, M., COHEN, S.M. and FRIEDELL, G.H. (1976). Light and scanning electron microscopy of exfoliated bladder epithelial cells in rats fed N-[4-(5-nitro-2-furyl)-2-thiazolyl] formamide. *Journal of the National Cancer Institute,* **57**, 63–66

JOHNSON, R.K., INOUYE, T., GOLDIN, A. and STARK, G.R. (1976). Antitumour activity of N-(phosphonacetyl)-L-aspartic acid, a transition-state inhibitor of aspartic transcarbamylase. *Cancer Research,* **36**, 2720–2725

JOHNSON, R.K., SWYRYD, E.A. and STARK, G.R. (1978). Effects of N-(phosphonacetyl)-L-(aspartate) on murine tumors and normal tissues in vivo and in vitro in the relationship of sensitivity to rate of proliferation and level of asparate transcarbamylase. *Cancer Research,* **38**, 371–378

KIEFER, J.H. (1953). Bladder tumor recurrence in the urethra: A warning. *Journal of Urology,* **69**, 652–656

McDONALD, D.F. and THORSON, T. (1956). Clinical implications of transplantability of induced bladder tumors to intact transitional epithelium in dogs. *Journal of Urology,* **75**, 690–694

MELAMED, M.R., VOUTSA, N.G. and GRABSTALD, H. (1964). Natural history and clinical behavior of in situ carcinoma of the human urinary bladder. *Cancer,* **17**, 1533–1545

MURPHY, W.M., SOLOWAY, M.S. and LIN, C.J. (1978). Morphological effects of thiotepa in mammalian urothelium: Changes in abnormal cells. *Acta cytologica,* **22**, 550–554

MURPHY, W.M., NAGY, G.K., RAO, M.K., SOLOWAY, M.S., PARIJA, G.C., COX, C.E. and FRIEDELL, G.H. (1979). 'Normal' urothelium in patients with bladder cancer: A preliminary report from the National Bladder Cancer Collaborative Group-A. *Cancer,* **44**, 1050–1058

NICHOLS, J.A. and MARSHALL, V.F. (1956). Treatment of histologically benign papilloma of the urinary bladder by local excision and fulguration. *Cancer,* **9**, 566–567

PAGE, B.H., LEVISON, V.B. and CURWEN, M.P. (1978). The site of recurrence of non-infiltrating bladder tumours. *British Journal of Urology,* **50**, 237–242

SOLOWAY, M.S. (1975). Animal models used for experimental chemotherapy of genitourinary tract tumors. In *Chemotherapy of Urogenital Tumors.* Ed. by G.P. Murphy and A. Mittleman, Springfield; Charles C. Thomas

SOLOWAY, M.S. (1977). Intravesical and systemic chemotherapy of murine bladder cancer. *Cancer Research,* **37**, 2918–2929

SOLOWAY, M.S. (1978). Cis-diamminedichloroplatinum (II) in advanced urothelial cancer. *Journal of Urology,* **120**, 716–719

SOLOWAY, M.S. (1980). The management of superficial bladder cancer. *Cancer,* **45**, 1856–1865

SOLOWAY, M.S. and MARTINO, C. (1976). Prophylaxis of bladder tumor implantation – Intravesical and systemic chemotherapy. *Urology,* **7**, 29–34

SOLOWAY, M.S. and MASTERS, S. (1979). Implantation of transitional tumor cells on the cauterized murine urothelial surface. *Proceedings of the American Association for Cancer Research,* **20**, 256

SOLOWAY, M.S., DE KERNION, J.B., ROSE, D. and PERSKY, L. (1973b). Effect of chemotherapeutic agents on bladder cancer. A new animal model. *Surgical Forum,* **24**, 542–544

SOLOWAY, M.S., MARTINO, C., HYATT, C. and MARRONE, J.C. (1978). Immuno-genicity of FANFT-induced bladder cancer. *Workshop in Genito-Urinary Cancer Immunology, National Cancer Institute Monograph,* **49**, 293–299

SOLOWAY, M.S., MYERS, G.H., Jr., MARRONE, J.C., DEL VECCHIO, P.R. and MALM-GREN, R.A. (1973a). Evaluation of urinary cytology as an indicator of bladder neoplasia in mice. *Journal of Urology,* **109**, 249–252

TILTMAN, A.J. and FRIEDELL, G.H. (1971). The histogenesis of experimental bladder cancer. *Investigative Urology,* **9**, 218–226

TURNER, A.G., HENDRY, W.F., WILLIAMS, G.B. and BLOOM, H.J.G. (1977). The treatment of advanced bladder cancer with methotrexate. *British Journal of Urology,* **49**, 673–678

WALLACE, A.C. and HERSHFIELD, E.S. (1958). The experimental implantation of tumour cells in the urinary tract. *British Journal of Cancer,* **12**, 622–630

WALLACE, D.M. and BLOOM, H.J.G. (1976). The management of deeply infiltrating bladder carcinoma: Controlled trial of radical radiotherapy versus preoperative radiotherapy and radical cystectomy (first report). *British Journal of Urology,* **48**, 587–594

WELDON, T.E. and SOLOWAY, M.S. (1975). Susceptibility of urothelium to neo-plastic cellular implantation. *Urology,* **5**, 824–827

WHITMORE, W.F., Jr., BATATA, M.A., GHONEIM, J.A., GRABSTALD, H. and UNAL, A. (1977). Radical cystectomy with or without prior irradiation in the treatment of bladder cancer. *Journal of Urology,* **118**, 184–187

WILLIAMS, J.L., HAMMONDS, J.C. and SAUNDERS, N. (1977). T1 bladder tumours. *British Journal of Urology,* **49**, 663–668

WODINSKY, I., SWINIARSKI, J., KENSLER, C.J. and VENDITTI, J.M. (1974). Com-bination radiotherapy and chemotherapy for P388 lymphocytic leukemia in vivo. *Cancer Chemotherapy Reports,* (Suppl.) **4**, 73–97

YAGODA, A. (1977). Future implications of phase II chemotherapy trials in ninety-five patients with measurable advanced bladder cancer. *Cancer Research,* **37**, 2775–2780

YAGODA, A., WATSON, R.C., GONZALEZ-VITALE, J.C., GRABSTALD, H. and WHIT-MORE, W.F., Jr. (1976). Cis-dichlorodiammineplatinum (II) in advanced bladder cancer. *Cancer Treatment Reports,* **60**, 917–923

IIA

Treatment of superficial disease: papillary
tumours

6

Introduction to the Management of Superficial Bladder Tumours

J.P. Pryor

In order to have a rational approach to the management of any tumour it is necessary to have a firm understanding of the 'natural' history of the disease. The malignant potential of superficial bladder tumours is low; other diseases which occur in the elderly patients who develop these tumours are often of equal or greater importance (30% of patients presenting with bladder cancer are over the age of 70 years and 10% over the age of 80). The mortality and morbidity of the treatment is therefore of importance, particularly when considering the role of a cystectomy in elderly patients with uncontrollable superficial tumours, and especially in the absence of precise information on the risks of leaving the condition untreated.

Reports on the survival of patients with superficial tumours (T1, NX, MX according to the UICC classification) show quite marked variation from series to series (*Figure 6.1*). This is hardly surprising, as it will be affected by the ages of patients being studied and the number of deaths from other causes. An additional factor is the proportion of patients whose tumours show evidence of early invasion. Pugh (1973) was the first to suggest that superficial T1 tumours could be separated into those where invasion had only just broken through the basement membrane (P1a) and those with invasion of the submucosa (P1b). Pryor (1973) demonstrated a higher death rate from bladder tumours in P1b (24% at 3 years) tumours compared with P1a (10% at 3 years), and patients in both these categories of T1 tumour did worse than patients whose tumours showed no evidence of invasion of basement membrane (Pa: 3% died from bladder tumours after 3 years' follow-up) (*Figure 6.2*). In this series, the extent of early invasion was

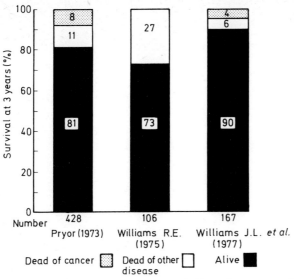

Figure 6.1 Superficial tumours of the bladder – 3-year survival in different series

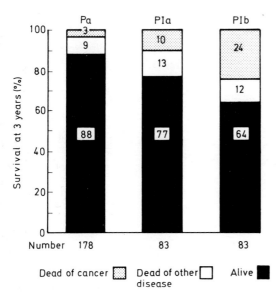

Figure 6.2 Superficial tumours of the bladder – 3-year survival based on histological evidence of invasion (data from Pryor, 1973)

found to be as important a prognostic factor as tumour grade when they were assessed in a series of 251 patients with P1–P3 tumours. All of the moderately (G2) or poorly differentiated lesions (G3) were found to be invasive, and 3-year survival rates based on grades alone were 76% (G1), 52% (G2) and 32% (G3) respectively.

The depth of invasion and grade of the tumour are clearly of importance in discussing the management of superficial bladder tumours. Most tumours are well controlled by endoscopic resection or fulguration and, as yet, there is no clear evidence that resection increases the risk of submucosal invasion. External beam radiotherapy has little to offer in the management of superficial well-differentiated non-invasive bladder tumours, but it is of value in the higher-grade tumours (G2 or G3), or where there is evidence of submucosal invasion.

Although the non-invasive superficial papillary tumour, Pa, rarely leads to death from tumour, at least 60% of patients develop recurrence and 5–10% develop such widespread growth over the whole bladder that cystectomy has to be considered. It is in these patients that the advent of intravesical chemotherapy has made such an impact; the next four chapters review the results achieved.

REFERENCES

PRYOR, J.P. (1973). Factors influencing the survival of patients with transitional cell tumours of the urinary bladder. *British Journal of Urology,* **45**, 586–592

PUGH, R.C.B. (1973). The pathology of cancer of the bladder: an editorial overview. *Cancer,* **32**, 1267–1274

WILLIAMS, J.L., HAMMONDS, J.C. and SAUNDERS, N.(1977). T1 bladder tumours. *British Journal of Urology,* **49**, 663–668

WILLIAMS, R.E. (1975). Strategy of treatment in transitional cell carcinoma of the bladder. In *The Biology and Management of Bladder Cancer.* Ed. by E.H. Cooper and R.E. Williams, Chap 8, pp. 163–192. Oxford; Blackwell

7

The Use of Intravesical Ethoglucid* in the Management of Superficial Bladder Tumours

P.R. Riddle

Fortunately the majority of bladder tumours are of the superficial variety, that is, without invasion of the muscle of the bladder wall. These tumours, although often associated with multiple recurrences, are thought to carry a good prognosis and are usually treated entirely by endoscopic means, either with resection or diathermy coagulation, or a combination of both these techniques. Occasionally it may be necessary to open the bladder in order to remove very large tumours, but the indications for this have become less over the years, largely because of the great improvement in endoscopic instruments and also in the expertise of their users.

Now that the concept of closed bladder treatment is firmly established, one has to have alternatives when endoscopic treatment no longer seems to be keeping up with the rate of growth and recurrence of these tumours. Where the growth is very bulky, so that large masses of tumour are recurring each time, or tumours are recurring in the urethra, it is probably wiser and certainly safer, not to procrastinate but to submit the patient to a radical cysto-urethrectomy and urinary diversion. However, if the tumours are small (less than 0.5 cm across), albeit numerous, and confined to the bladder, it seems unjustifiable to perform such a radical surgical procedure unless more conservative treatment has failed.

Although many alternative approaches to multiple superficial tumours have been used, the majority have failed in the long term. The instillation of alkylating agents into the bladder has probably been the most successful procedure. The two drugs in current use for this purpose are thiotepa, introduced by Jones and Swinney (1962) and

*Epodyl

63

ethoglucid. The latter, (triethyleneglycol diglycidyl ether) was first introduced by Abbassian and Wallace (1966). It was more extensively evaluated in 1971 by Riddle and Wallace, and in 1973 an analysis of the results of 64 patients treated with this drug was published (Riddle, 1973). The patients were reviewed after 3 months' treatment and 59% were found to be free of cystoscopically detectable tumours; 38% had improved but not cleared and in only 3% had the drug completely failed. At 1 year, 64% remained clear, 23% had failed and 14% were classed as partial responders. By 3 years, the patients appeared to fall equally into those who responded completely and those who failed.

It was apparent from these early results that the pattern is set, after the initial treatment, into either fully responsive or resistant cases. Those who initially respond fully have a good chance of remaining clear, while the partial responders are ultimately failures.

One of the problems of most published data on the use of intra-vesical chemotherapy is that long-term follow-up is often not reported. For this reason, it was decided to update this early series so that, not only would the ultimate fate of these patients be known, but also any factors influencing treatment or results could be ascertained. This long-term follow-up has been published in detail elsewhere (Fitzpatrick *et al.*, 1979) but the major findings will now be discussed.

The treatment regime has been previously described (Riddle, 1973): briefly, 100 ml of a 1% solution of ethoglucid in sterile distilled water at room temperature is introduced into the bladder and the catheter removed. The patients are then instructed to go about their daily routine and void the bladder contents after 1 hour. This is repeated weekly for the initial 3 months' treatment, and then monthly indefinitely, if indicated.

Sixty-three of the original 64 patients whose treatment started before 1972 are available for review at this time (1979). They fall into three groups:

(1)   complete response which is maintained (19 patients);
(2)   complete initial response, but relapse on treatment (20 patients);
(3)   failures from the start (24 patients).

There are, therefore, three roughly equal groups, all showing very different responses at the time of review. The mortality at the end of the review period is shown in *Table 7.1*. The eight deaths in Group 1 were all unrelated to their bladder tumours, whereas seven of the eight in Group 2 died of bladder cancer. In Group 3, 13 of the 17 deaths were due to bladder cancer; in this group, 19 needed subsequent radical treatment (13 cysto-urethrectomy and six radical radiotherapy).

In order to find any differences between the three groups, the initial histological stage based on the biopsy specimens was ascertained

Table 7.1
CURRENT STATUS OF 64 PATIENTS TREATED WITH INTRAVESICAL ETHOGLUCID,
BY TREATMENT RESPONSE

Status	Group 1	Group 2	Group 3	Total
Alive	11	11	6	28
Dead	8	8	17	33
Lost to follow-up	–	1	1	2

(*Table 7.2*). Superficial tumours are staged into three categories, Pa, P1a and P1b (*see* Chapter 1 and Pugh (1973)). Pa is where the basement membrane is intact throughout. P1a shows early invasion of the fronds of the tumour only, whereas in P1b there is breakthrough of the lamina propria at the base of the tumour.

Table 7.2
INFLUENCE OF INITIAL PATHOLOGICAL STAGING ON TREATMENT RESPONSE

Pathological stage	Group 1	Group 2	Group 3	Total
Pa	14	14	9	37
P1a	–	2	3	5
P1b	–	2	5	7
Px	5	2	7	14

Px represents unstaged tumours

All patients in Group 1, where the patients have all been complete and continued responders, were in the Pa histological category; in other words, there were no cases with any basement membrane breakthrough. In Group 3 approximately half the patients showed breakthrough, the majority being P1b, and in Group 2 the incidence of breakthrough was intermediate between those in Group 1 and Group 3. It would therefore appear that the initial pathological staging has a profound bearing on the response to ethoglucid and on the eventual outcome.

The overall survival rate at 5 years was 60%. The initial response to treatment was an important determinant of long-term survival. The

Table 7.3
CRUDE SURVIVAL RATE BY TREATMENT RESPONSE

Group	Number of patients	*Survival in years*				
		1	*2*	*3*	*4*	*5*
Group 1	19	18 (95%)	16 (84%)	13 (68%)	13 (68%)	12 (63%)
Group 2	19	19 (100%)	18 (95%)	18 (95%)	18 (95%)	18 (95%)
Group 3	23	21 (91%)	19 (82%)	16 (70%)	11 (48%)	10 (43%)
Total	61	58 (95%)	54 (86%)	47 (77%)	42 (69%)	40 (60%)

survival figures of the three groups at one year were similar (*Table 7.3*), although later there was a fall in Group 1 patients attributable to deaths from causes other than cancer. The worst survival rate was in Group 3, with death due mainly to invasive or metastatic tumour, although at 5 years 43% were still alive, most of whom had undergone radical surgery clearance of their disease.

The conclusions that can be drawn from this review are three-fold and must influence treatment:

(1) the histological stage of the tumour is clearly very important and, in general, intravesical ethoglucid is unsuitable for patients with P1b pathologically staged tumours;
(2) even with a favourable pathological stage, if the bladder cannot be cleared of tumour by ethoglucid within 1 year, radical surgery should be recommended;
(3) if the bladder is initially cleared of tumour which later recurs, then treatment has failed and cystectomy should be seriously contemplated.

The disturbing feature is the eventual invasive nature of tumours in many of these cases. It is by persisting with conservative treatment, when clearly it is not affecting tumour recurrence, that the chance for cure by radical surgery may be lost.

REFERENCES

ABBASSIAN, A. and WALLACE, D.M. (1966). Intracavitary chemotherapy of diffuse and non-infiltrating papillary carcinoma of the bladder. *Journal of Urology,* **96**, 461–465

FITZPATRICK, J.M., KHAN, O., OLIVER, R.T.D. and RIDDLE, P.R. (1979) Long-term follow-up in patients with superficial bladder tumours treated with intravesical Epodyl. *British Journal of Urology,* **51**, 545

JONES, H.C. and SWINNEY, J. (1962). The treatment of tumours of the bladder by transurethral resection. *British Journal of Urology,* **34**, 215–220.

PUGH, R.C.B. (1973). The pathology of cancer of the bladder. *Cancer,* **32**, 1267–1274

RIDDLE, P.R. and WALLACE, D.M. (1971). Intracavitary chemotherapy for multiple non-invasive bladder tumours. *Journal of Urology,* **43**, 181–184

RIDDLE, P.R. (1973). The management of superficial bladder tumours with intravesical Epodyl. *British Journal of Urology,* **45**, 84–87

8

Intravesical Thiotepa as Adjuvant to Cystodiathermy in Multiple Recurrent Superficial Bladder Tumours

H.R. England, A.M.I. Paris and J.P. Blandy

Intravesical thiotepa was first used to treat bladder tumours in the early 1960s (Jones and Swinney, 1961; Veenema *et al.*, 1962). When used alone as therapy in patients with multiple recurrent T1, low- or medium-grade tumours, it was successful in clearing the bladder in a third of the cases: however, it did not lead to indefinite control of recurrent tumours and, today, the main indication for its use is as an adjunct to cysto-diathermy to reduce or eliminate new tumour growth (Westcott, 1966; Veenema *et al.*, 1969; Burnand *et al.*, 1976). Used thus, thiotepa is thought to act in one of two ways: (1) it may destroy tumour cells left lying free within the bladder after endoscopic resection and prevent implantation tumours; (2) it may eliminate microscopic foci of tumour remaining after all visible tumour has been resected.

Several dosage schedules have been used but there are few compa-rative data. Most authors have used a single dose repeated at regular intervals. However, as a result of encouraging results reported when three doses were given in 5 days, repeated 3-monthly (Oravisto, 1972), we embarked on a study of this schedule.

To date, 40 patients have been treated (28 men and 12 women) whose ages at presentation ranged from 37 to 78 years with a mean of 62 years. The clinical problem in each was one of unstable epithelium, leading to multiple new tumours at every cystoscopy (*Figure 8.1*). The length of documented tumour history before starting thiotepa was less than 2 years in six patients, 2–5 years in 24 patients and more than 5 years in 10 patients (average 4.5 years). Twenty-seven patients had tumours of pathological grade G1 and of these, 13 showed no evidence of invasion (pTa). There were 13 patients with tumours in the G2 category, all with lamina propria involvement. Duration of follow-up ranged from 1.5 to 4 years.

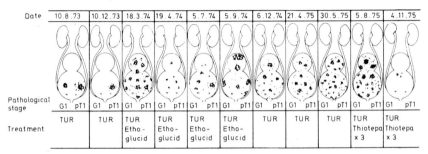

Date	10.8.73	10.12.73	18.3.74	19.4.74	5.7.74	5.9.74	6.12.74	21.4.75	30.5.75	5.8.75	4.11.75
Pathological stage	G1 pT1	G1 pT1	G1 pT1	G1 pT1	G1 pT1	G1 pT1	G1 pT1	G1 pT1	G1 pT1	G1 pT1	G1 pT1
Treatment	TUR	TUR	TUR Etho-glucid	TUR Etho-glucid	TUR Etho-glucid	TUR Etho-glucid	TUR	TUR	TUR	TUR Thiotepa x 3	TUR Thiotepa x 3

Figure 8.1 Pattern of bladder tumour recurrence in patient who subsequently responded completely on thiotepa

All tumours were meticulously resected and, using the regime suggested by Oravisto (1972), 30 mg of thiotepa in 50 ml of saline was instilled into the bladder for 2 h on post-operative days 1, 3 and 5. If pre-treatment blood counts showed evidence of marrow depression the dose was reduced to 15 mg.

Cystoscopy was repeated 3-monthly initially when any new tumours were resected, and further thiotepa was given. When the patient responded, the plan was to give one further course and then subsequently to reduce thiotepa instillations to individual minimum requirements, rather than to continue with a set routine. In this way, inconvenience for the patient was kept to a minimum. Sometimes thiotepa was reduced somewhat too enthusiastically, but that has helped rather than hindered the assessment of its value.

As this study was not a randomized trial, there were no controls, but with each case history known and the established pattern accurately documented for significant periods before starting thiotepa, these patients could reasonably be accepted as acting as their own controls.

RESULTS

A patient was considered to have responded to thiotepa if the bladder became clear of tumour or if the number of new tumours was reduced to a small fraction of the established pattern. In virtually all patients there were 20 or more tumours at cystoscopy before treatment and, accordingly, three tumours or less were considered to be a satisfactory response. According to this criterion, 31 (78%) of the treated patients responded, 26 became tumour-free after one to three courses of thiotepa and for the remaining five the number of new recurrences was limited to three or less. One of the latter patients died from lung metastases 20 years after original diagnosis, within 1 year of commencing thiotepa therapy: histology of the metastases was identical to that of the tumours in the bladder (pTa G1). Of the nine patients failing to respond (22%), two subsequently died from tumour (*Table 8.1*).

Table 8.1
RESPONSE TO THIOTEPA

Responders			
Becoming tumour-free			
After 1 course	11		
After 2 courses	10 } 26 (65%)		
After 3 courses	5		
		31 (78%)	40 (100%)
New tumours reduced to 3 or fewer	5 (1 death)		
Non-responders	9 (22% – 2 deaths)		

Patients with tumours of histological grades G1 and G2 both responded well. In the G1 group the response was better when the lamina propria was not invaded. However, in G2 tumours, despite involvement of the lamina propria, only two of 13 failed to respond (*Table 8.2*).

Table 8.2
HISTOLOGY AND RESPONSE

Histology	Responders	Non-Responders
G1.pTa	12	1
G1.pT1	8	6
G2.pT1	11	2

Eight (26%) of 31 responders have remained tumour-free without maintenance on thiotepa: of these eight patients, three had received one course of thiotepa, two had been given two courses and three had received three courses. One patient died after 6 months from myocardial infarction, bringing the total deaths in the series to four, the other three being from tumour. The remaining seven complete responders have been clear for 1–3 years since stopping thiotepa and their histology has followed the pattern of the series as a whole (*Table 8.3*).

Table 8.3
PATIENTS TUMOUR-FREE WITHOUT MAINTENANCE THIOTEPA

Tumour-free and remaining so	
After 1 course	3 (2, 1.5, 1 years)
After 2 courses	2 (3, 3 years)
After 3 courses	3 (2, 1, 0.5)
	—
	8 (26% of responders)
	—
Histology	
G1.pTa	3
G1.pT1	2
G2.pT1	3
	—
	8
	—

Twenty-two other responders have needed maintenance therapy. Seventeen are continuing to receive thiotepa (nine receiving one instillation, seven patients receiving two instillations and one patient receiving three instillations at 3-monthly intervals). Five other patients are now on 6-monthly review and have needed one or two instillations. The remaining responder was returned tumour-free to his local referring hospital 3 years ago (*Table 8.4*).

Table 8.4
MAINTENANCE THIOTEPA REQUIREMENTS IN RESPONDERS WHO CONTINUED ON TREATMENT

3-monthly	× 1	9	} 17	
	× 2	7		} 23 (74% of responders)
	× 3	1		
6-monthly	× 1	2	} 5	
	× 2	3		
Moved away		1		

Patients who responded, usually showed clear evidence of response after the first course of chemotherapy and always after the second. The commonest pattern was a dramatic drop in the number of new tumours after the first course (*Figure 8.1*), followed by clearance, both at cystoscopy and field biopsies, after the second course.

If responders grew new tumours after therapy had been stopped or reduced, they always responded again when thiotepa was restarted or increased to an effective level again (*Figure 8.2*).

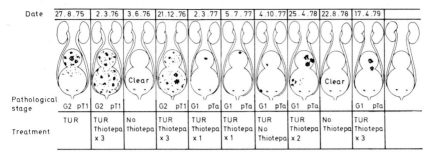

Date	27.8.75	2.3.76	3.6.76	21.12.76	2.3.77	5.7.77	4.10.77	25.4.78	22.8.78	17.4.79	
Pathological stage	G2 pT1	G2 pT1			G2 pT1	G1 pTa	G1 pTa	G1 pTa	G1 pTa		G1 pTa
Treatment	TUR	TUR Thiotepa x 3	No Thiotepa	TUR Thiotepa x 3	TUR Thiotepa x 1	TUR Thiotepa x 1	TUR No Thiotepa	TUR Thiotepa x 2	No Thiotepa	TUR Thiotepa x 3	

Figure 8.2 Titration of thiotepa dosage against recurrence rate in the bladder

Of the nine non-responders, four underwent tumour progression which involved muscle invasion or grade change to G3, or both (*Table 8.5*). The time intervals between presentation and progression were 9 months (patient died) and 1 year (patient died), 3 years (cystectomy) and 6 years (still alive)! Two of this group presented with single tumours of a type in which a good result usually can be expected with some confidence, long-fronded G1.pTa and G1.pT1 respectively.

Table 8.5
SUBSEQUENT COURSE OF NINE NON-RESPONDERS

	Initial stage	Current status
Tumour progression (n = 4)	G1.pTa G2.pT1	G3.pT2. m1 – died G3.pT4. m1 – died G2.pT3b – cystectomy G3.pT1 – alive
Upper tract urothelial tumour (n = 2)	G1.pT1	L. pelvis + R. ureter L. pelvis
Status unchanged (n = 3)	G1.pT1 G2.pT1	alive at 1½–2 years

Within 9 months the former had progressed despite thiotepa, to wide-spread G3 flat in situ carcinoma with multiple G3.pT1 tumours and widespread metastases. The second patient had a much slower progression but, when he eventually had a cystectomy after an initial refusal, tumour had spread to the perivesical tissues (*Figure 8.3*).

Two other non-responders, although not showing tumour progression within the bladder despite multiple recurrences, developed tumours of the upper urinary tract. The remaining three non-responders have so far shown no change in disease status, 1.5–2 years after thiotepa was given and 4, 5 and 10 years after initial presentation.

There were no complications of treatment. In particular, irritative bladder symptoms did not occur, treatment did not ever have to be

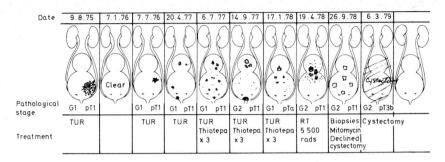

Date	9.8.75	7.1.76	7.7.76	20.4.77	6.7.77	14.9.77	17.1.78	19.4.78	26.9.78	6.3.79
Pathological stage	G1 pT1		G1 pT1	G1 pT1	G1 pT1	G2 pT1	G1 pTa	G2 pT1	G2 pT1	G2 pT3b
Treatment	TUR		TUR	TUR	TUR Thiotepa x 3	TUR Thiotepa x 3	TUR Thiotepa x 3	RT 5 500 rads	Biopsies Mitomycin Declined cystectomy	Cystectomy

Figure 8.3 Recurrence pattern in patient who progressed to T3 tumour on thiotepa

stopped because of bone marrow depression, and in only a few cases was thiotepa dosage reduced to 15 mg.

It is of interest that seven patients in the series had previously not responded to ethoglucid instillations, while one other was unable to tolerate that agent. Only two of these ethoglucid non-responders failed to benefit from thiotepa.

DISCUSSION

If it is accepted that the two main causes of new tumour growth, in patients with superficial bladder tumour, are implantation of tumour cells after endoscopy and microscopic tumour foci remaining after all visible tumour has been dealt with, then it makes sense to give thiotepa at endoscopy, or immediately afterwards, when these potential tumours are at their smallest and therefore their most vulnerable.

Thiotepa exerts its effect on actively dividing cells, interfering with nucleic acid synthesis: instillations given in quick succession may put the maximum number of dividing cells at risk. Indeed, a study by Nieh *et al.* (1980), in which H-thymidine uptake in rats was measured, has shown that intravesical thiotepa itself leads to peaks of mitotic activity in both tumour and normal urothelium 3 and 9 days later, a finding which supports the use of a regime similar to that suggested by Oravisto (1972). It is probable that much of the conflict apparent in the various reports on the efficacy of thiotepa is explicable in terms of the timing of administration.

In every series of low- or medium-grade T1 tumours there are patients who have a higher than average malignant potential and who, sooner or later, undergo tumour progression. The incidence of tumour progression is greater in patients who have multiple recurrences than in those who have only an occasional tumour. It is clear from our experience with thiotepa that demonstration of non-response in a patient is an important clinical sign, as it indicates patients with greater than average malignant potential, who ought to be considered for more radical treatment at an early stage.

SUMMARY

When using thiotepa in the regime described as an adjunct to cysto-diathermy, new tumour growth has been prevented or radically reduced in 31 of 40 patients with well-established and consistently high rates of tumour recurrence.

The procedure has been safe, causing little extra discomfort, and is less time-consuming and inconvenient than programmes employing more frequent instillations.

Lack of response to thiotepa probably indicates that the patient has tumours of higher than average malignant potential: as well as its thera-peutic value, therefore, this agent may help to identify at an early date those patients in need of more radical therapy.

REFERENCES

BURNAND, K.G., BOYD, P.J.R., MAYO, M.E., SHUTTLEWORTH, K.E.D. and LLOYD-DAVIES, R.W. (1976). Single dose intravesical Thiotepa as an adjuvant to cysto-diathermy in the treatment of transitional cell bladder carcinoma. *British Journal of Urology*, **48**, 55–59

JONES, H.B. and SWINNEY, J. (1961). Thiotepa in the treatment of tumours of the bladder. *Lancet*, **2**, 615–618

NIEH, P.T., DALY, J.J., IRWIN, R.J. and PROUT, G.R. Jr. (1980) Intravesical Thiotepa: a study of H-thymidine uptake in normal urothelium and FANFT-induced tumours in rats. Submitted to Grayson Carroll Essay Contest, American Urological Association

ORAVISTO, K.J. (1972). Optimal intravesical dosage of Thiotepa in the prophy-laxis of recurrent bladder papillomatosis. *Scandinavian Journal of Urology and Nephrology*, **6**, 26–28

VEENEMA, R.J., DEAN, A.L., Jr, ROBERTS, M., FINGERHUT, B., CHOWHURY, B.K. and TARASSOLY, H. (1962). Bladder carcinoma treated by direct instillation of Thiotepa. *Journal of Urology*, **88**, 60–63

VEENEMA, R.J., DEAN, A.L., Jr, USON, A.C., ROBERTS, M. and LARGO, F. (1969). Thiotepa bladder instillations: therapy and prophylaxis for superficial bladder tumors. *Journal of Urology*, **101**, 711–715

WESTCOTT, J.W. (1966). The prophylactic use of Thiotepa in transitional cell carcinoma of the bladder. *Journal of Urology*, **96**, 913–918

9

Preliminary Results from EORTC (European Organisation for Research and Treatment of Cancer) Studies on Chemotherapy for Superficial Bladder Tumours

C.C. Schulman, R. Sylvester, M. Robinson, P. Smith, A. Lachand, L. Denis, M. Pavone-Macaluso, M. De Pauw and M. Staquet

Additional participants:
J. Auvert (Hôpital H. Mondor, Créteil, France)
C. Bollack (Hospices Civils, Strasbourg, France)
C. Bouffioux (Hôpital de Bavière, Liège, Belgium)
G. Declercq (A.Z. Middelheim, Antwerpen, Belgium)
L. Denis (A.Z. Middelheim, Antwerpen, Belgium)
R. Glashan (Royal Infirmary, Huddersfield, England)
A. Lachand (Hôpital Henri-Mondor, Créteil, France)
Lardennois (CHU, Reims, France)
Lemaire (CHU, Reims, France)
D. Newling (Royal Infirmary, Hull, England)
M. Pavone-Macaluso (University Polyclinic Hospital, Palermo, Italy)
W. Reinhardt (Hospices Civils, Strasbourg, France)
B. Richards (York District Hospital, York, England)
M. Robinson (Castleford Normanton and District Hospital, Castleford, England)
S. Fantoni (University Hospital, Pavia, Italy)
C. Schulman (Hôpital Universitaire Erasme, Bruxelles, Belgium)
P. Smith, (St. James Hospital, Leeds, England)
M. Vandendris (Hôpital Universitaire Brugmann, Bruxelles, Belgium)
G. Viggiano (Ospedale Civile, Mestre, Italy)

INTRODUCTION

Superficial bladder tumours (T1, pT1 of the TNM classification (UICC, 1974) or Jewett Stage O and A) are usually treated by transurethral resection (TUR). However, recurrence of the tumour after complete resection occurs in about 60% of the patients (Marshall, 1956; Maltry, 1971) with a significant percentage of these recurrences showing a higher degree of malignancy (Marshall, 1956). In 10% of the cases the tumour progresses to invasive carcinoma (Greene *et al.,* 1973) and the 5-year survival rate following TUR is about 62% (O'Flynn *et al.,* 1975).

   Several adjuvant treatments to TUR have been advocated in an attempt to increase the survival rate, the disease-free interval and to reduce the recurrence rate. Periodic instillation of thiotepa, a cytotoxic alkylating agent, has been used for more than 15 years, both for pro-phylaxis and for the treatment of recurrent T1 bladder tumours, but controversy still continues regarding the precise indications for its use (Jones and Swinney, 1961; Veenema *et al.,* 1962; Esquivel *et al.,* 1965; Westcott, 1966; Veenema *et al.,* 1969; Mitchell, 1971). Staquet (1976) has reviewed nine non-randomized studies with intravesical thiotepa and found a success rate ranging from 24% to 100% (Abbassian and Wallace, 1966; Drew and Marshall, 1968; Edsmyr and Boman, 1971; EORTC, 1972; Byar and Blackard, 1977).

Objectives of the Study

This randomized clinical trial was designed by the EORTC Genito-Urinary Tract Cancer Cooperative Group to compare: (1) the disease-free interval; (2) the recurrence rate; (3) the number of patients with an increase in the T or G classification, in category T1 carcinoma of the bladder after TUR alone or TUR followed by bladder instillations of thiotepa or VM 26, a new epidophyllotoxin derivative reported to show some activity against bladder tumours (Pavone-Macaluso *et al.,* 1975; Schulman *et al.,* 1976).

SELECTION OF PATIENTS

Criteria for Admission

All patients shown on biopsy to have a primary or recurrent T1 papil-lary carcinoma of the bladder which was resectable transurethrally were considered to be eligible for the trial. T1 lesions were defined according to the 1974 TNM UICC classification, and represented tumours with no microscopic infiltration beyond the lamina propria. All visible lesions were completely resected and there was neither induration nor a mass palpable on bimanual examination under anaesthesia after TUR. In the case of urinary infection, the start of the trial was delayed until the urine was sterile.

Criteria for Exclusion

(1) Presence of another cancer or previous local or systemic cancer chemotherapy.
(2) Bladder lesions other than papillary lesions.
(3) General condition such that survival for the duration of the study was unlikely.
(4) Expected difficulties of follow-up related to overt psychosis, marked senility or too great a distance between patient's home and investigator's centre.
(5) White blood cell count (WBC) below $4500/mm^3$.
(6) Bladder papillomatosis not resectable by TUR.

DESIGN OF THE TRIAL

Three weeks after TUR, the following treatments were randomly allocated to eligible patients after stratification for primary or recurrent cases. Treatment group 1: intravesical thiotepa; treatment group 2: intravesical VM 26; treatment group 3: no treatment.

Thiotepa and VM 26 were administered for 1 year starting 1 month after TUR. All patients entering the trial were followed for 5 years or until death, whichever came first.

THERAPEUTIC REGIMES

The drugs (30 mg of thiotepa in 30 ml sterile water or 50 mg of VM 26 in 30 ml normal saline) were instilled into the bladder and retained for 1 hour. The drug instillation was started one month after TUR, given every week for 4 weeks, and then once every 4 weeks for 11 months (a total of 15 instillations) unless a recurrence occurred. If a recurrence was observed during the instillation treatment, a new complete schedule with the same regimen was repeated after TUR. Thus, one month after TUR, the drug instillation was started again every week for four instillations and then once every 4 weeks. The total duration of treatment was limited to 12 months beginning after the first TUR. Nitrofurantoin was given after each instillation at 3×100 mg/day for 3 days.

WBC and platelet counts were obtained before each chemotherapy administration. If haematological toxicity was suspected, drug administration was delayed until the WBC count was $\geqslant 4000/mm^3$ and the platelet count was $\geqslant$ 150 000/mm^3. Chemotherapy was also delayed whenever cystitis was present at the time of instillation. If severe drug-induced cystitis occurred, the drug was given in a total solution volume of 60 ml for the subsequent administrations. If severe drug-induced cystitis occurred again, no further instillations were given. Urinalysis was also performed before each drug instillation. Treatment was temporarily suspended in the case of urinary infection until control of the infection was achieved.

EVALUATION OF THERAPY

Cystoscopy was repeated every 12 weeks during the first year, every 16 weeks during the second year and then every 26 weeks during the following 3 years. All visible lesions seen on cystoscopy were biopsied, with recurrence being established only by histological examination of the biopsy material. The free interval was defined as the time interval between TUR and the date of the first positive biopsy.

RESULTS

Three hundred and forty patients from 20 participating institutions in six different countries have been admitted to this protocol from November 1975 to April 1978. While the analysis which is presented here is based on the 215 patients for whom follow-up is available, a similar analysis yielding essentially the same results was made, eliminating 16 ineligible or non-evaluable patients from the calculations. Kaplan–Meier curves were used to estimate the time until the first recurrence as shown by biopsy, and differences between the curves were tested using the Logrank and Gehan generalized Wilcoxon test procedures (Peto *et al.,* 1977). Two-tailed significance levels are reported in the text. A comparison of the recurrence rates (number of recurrences per patient months of observation) were performed using a χ^2 test (Potthoff and Whittinghill, 1966).

   The primary aim of the study was to discover if thiotepa or VM 26, when compared with no treatment, significantly increased the duration of the disease-free interval. Hence, Kaplan–Meier curves giving the time until first recurrence have been calculated for each treatment group. The median time to first recurrence was approximately 45 weeks for primary patients and 23 weeks for recurrent patients ($P = 0.01$). Comparison of the three treatment groups, with respect to the time until first recurrence and the percentage of patients developing one or more recurrences, showed no significant differences between thiotepa, VM 26 or no treatment, either in the whole patient population (*Figure*

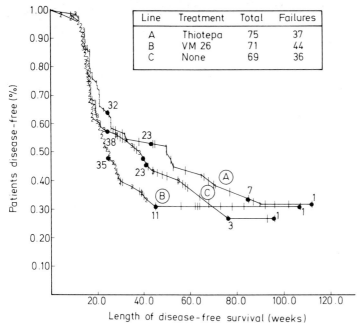

Figure 9.1 Disease-free survival of all patients according to treatment protocol

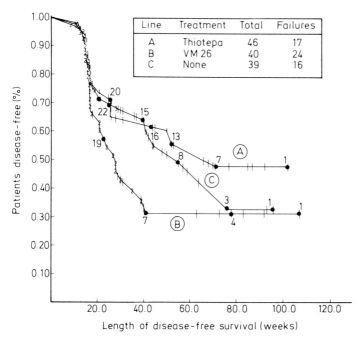

Figure 9.2 Disease-free survival of primary tumour patients according to treatment protocol

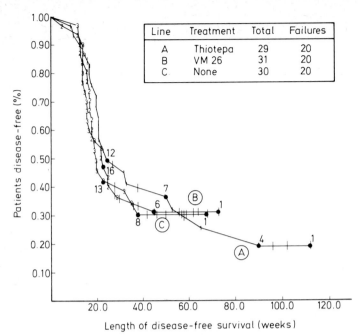

Line	Treatment	Total	Failures
A	Thiotepa	29	20
B	VM 26	31	20
C	None	30	20

Figure 9.3 Disease-free survival of recurrent tumour patients according to treatment protocol

Table 9.1
RECURRENCES BY TREATMENT (ALL PATIENTS)

Patient variables	Thiotepa	VM 26	No treatment	Total
Number of patients randomized	115	116	109	340
Number of patients with follow-up	75	71	69	215
Number of patients with recurrences	37	44	36	117
Percentage with recurrences	49.3	62.0	52.2	54.4
Total number of recurrences	58	69	68	195
Total months of follow-up	837	682	682	2201
Recurrence rate/100 patient-months	6.93	10.12	9.97	8.86

Table 9.2
RECURRENCES BY TREATMENT (PRIMARY PATIENTS)

Patient variables	Thiotepa	VM 26	No treatment	Total
Number of patients randomized	71	70	69	210
Number of patients with follow-up	46	40	39	125
Number of patients with recurrences	17	24	16	57
Percentage with recurrences	37.0	60.0	41.0	45.6
Total number of recurrences	23	36	26	85
Total months of follow-up	462	417	386	1265
Recurrence rate/100 patient-months	4.98	8.63	6.74	6.72

Table 9.3
RECURRENCES BY TREATMENT (RECURRENT PATIENTS)

Patient variables	Thiotepa	VM 26	No treatment	Total
Number of patients randomized	44	46	40	130
Number of patients with follow-up	29	31	30	90
Number of patients with recurrences	20	20	20	60
Percentage with recurrences	69.0	64.5	66.7	66.7
Total number of recurrences	35	33	42	110
Total months of follow-up	375	265	296	935
Recurrence rate/100 patient months	9.33	12.45	14.19	11.75

9.1, Table 9.1) or when the primary and recurrent patients were analyzed separately (*Figures 9.2, 9.3; Tables 9.2, 9.3*).

However, when the recurrence rates are determined for each treatment by dividing the total number of visits at which recurrence was present by the total patient-months of follow-up for all patients in a treatment group (average 10 months per patient), there were significant differences between thiotepa and either VM 26 ($P = 0.03$) or no treatment ($P = 0.04$) but not between VM 26 and no treatment. The recurrence rates per 100 months of follow-up were 6.93 for thiotepa, 10.12 for VM 26 and 9.97 for no treatment. *Tables 9.2 and 9.3* repeat these analyses for primary patients and recurrent patients separately. In each case, the recurrence rate for thiotepa was lower than that for no treatment or for VM 26, but overall the differences were not statistically significant ($P = 0.11$ for primary patients and $P = 0.17$ for recurrent patients).

Table 9.4 presents the number of patients with recurrences showing a higher histological grade (G category), while *Table 9.5* presents the

Table 9.4
PATIENTS WITH RECURRENCES SHOWING A HIGHER DEGREE OF MALIGNANCY

Patients	Thiotepa	VM 26	No treatment	Total
Primary	2/46	4/40	0/39	6/125
Recurrent	3/29	2/31	5/30	10/90
Total	5/75	6/71	5/69	16/215

Table 9.5
PATIENTS WITH RECURRENCES SHOWING AN INCREASE IN THE T CATEGORY

Patients	Thiotepa	VM 26	No treatment	Total
Primary	0/46	4/40	0/39	4/125
Recurrent	3/29	3/31	4/30	10/90
Total	3/75	7/71	4/69	14/215

number of patients with recurrences for which there has been an increase in the T stage when compared with pre-treatment histology. For the total patient population there were no significant differences between the three treatment groups with respect to changes in the G and/or T classifications. However, among primary patients there were more recurrences which had a higher G category and T stage in patients treated with VM 26 (x^2 = 4.3; P = 0.05).

DISCUSSION

Although thiotepa has been used for more than 15 years in the management of patients with recurrent superficial bladder tumours, its value is still uncertain. Used as therapy against actual tumour masses it undoubtedly does cause regression, although the incidence is low. The most encouraging results have followed its use as adjuvant therapy after cystodiathermy in patients who have had multiple recurrences uncontrollable by the latter procedure. The dose in these studies has varied, but the results reported have been better with 50 mg and 90 mg than those achieved after 30 mg, as used in this study. However, with the higher doses there have been problems of severe bone marrow suppression and, in one study, there were two deaths from marrow aplasia following 90 mg (Abbassian and Wallace, 1966).

In this study, rather than treat patients with multiple recurrences uncontrollable by cystodiathermy, we set out to investigate whether there was any justification for using thiotepa at an early stage, such as after primary transurethral resection or after the development of a single recurrence, in an attempt to reduce the known incidence (60%) of recurrence. As there were patients with a good prognosis, it was important that there should be no risk attached to the treatment, so that the lowest dose known to have activity was selected and started 1 month after transurethral resection, to be sure that there was minimal risk of chemical cystitis.

It is clear from the results reported, that thiotepa at this dosage is of little value in terms of disease-free intervals. However, the results do suggest that, used even at these low dosages and despite the month's delay in starting treatment, the rate of recurrence is less than that seen in a control group. In addition, this study has established that thiotepa is better than VM 26, which may in fact have been deleterious as there was a higher incidence of progression to more invasive tumours in patients receiving the latter drug.

Future studies planned by the EORTC Genito-Urinary Group aim to compare thiotepa with two of the newer agents recently reported to be active intravesically (doxorubicin and cis-platinum). However, before these studies can be started it is important to establish the most appropriate dosage and frequency of administration, in particular the extent of delay necessary after cystodiathermy, before treatment is begun.

ACKNOWLEDGEMENTS

This investigation was supported by Grant Number 5R10 CA11488–09, awarded by the National Cancer Institute, DHEW, Bethesda, Maryland, USA.

EORTC Genito-Urinary Tract Cancer Cooperative Group Protocol 30751.

REFERENCES

ABBASSIAN, A. and WALLACE, D.M. (1966). Intracavitary chemotherapy of diffuse noninfiltrating papillary carcinoma of the bladder. *Journal of Urology*, **96**, 461–465

BYAR, D. and BLACKARD, C. (1977). Comparisons of placebo, pyridoxine, and topical thiotepa in preventing recurrence of stage I bladder cancer. *Urology*, **10**, 556–561

DREW, J.E. and MARSHALL, V.F. (1968). Effect of topical thiotepa on the recurrence rate of superficial bladder cancers. *Journal of Urology*, **99**, 740–743 (1968)

EDSMYR, F. and BOMAN, J., (1971) Instillation of thiotepa (Tifosyl) in vesical papillomatosis. *Acta Radiologica; Therapy, Physics, Biology*, **9**, 395–400

EORTC COOPERATIVE GROUP FOR LEUKAEMIAS AND HAEMATOSARCOMAS (1972) Clinical screening of epipodophyllotoxin VM 26 in malignant lymphomas and solid tumours. *British Medical Journal*, **2**, 744–748

ESQUIVEL, E.L., MACKENZIE, A.R. and WHITMORE, W.F. Jr. (1965). Treatment of bladder tumours by instillation of thiotepa, actinomycin D, or 5-fluorouracil. *Investigative Urology*, **2**, 381–386

GREENE, L.F., HANASH, K.A. and FARROW, G.M. (1973). Benign papilloma or papillary carcinoma of the bladder? *Journal of Urology*, **110**, 205–207

JONES, H.C. and SWINNEY, J. (1961). Thiotepa in the treatment of tumours of the bladder. *Lancet*, **2**, 615–618

MALTRY, E. (1971). *Benign and Malignant Tumors of the Urinary Bladder.* New York; Medical Examination Publishing Co.

MARSHALL, V.F. (1956). Current clinical problems regarding bladder tumors. In *Bladder Tumors, A Symposium*, p. 2. Philadelphia; J.B. Lippincott Company

MITCHELL, R. (1971). Intravesical thiotepa in the treatment of transitional cell bladder carcinoma. *British Journal of Urology*, **43**, 181–184

O'FLYNN, J.D., SMITH, J.M. and HANSON, J.S. (1975). Transurethral resection for the assessment and treatment of vesical neoplasms, A review of 840 consecutive cases, *European Urology*, **1**, 38–40

PAVONE-MACALUSO, M., CARAMIA, G. and RIZZO, F.P. (1974), Chimiothérapie locale dans les néoplasies vésicales. *Journal de radiologie, d'électrologie et des Archives d'électricité médicale*, **55**, 844–848

PAVONE-MACALUSO, M., CARAMIA, G., RIZZO, F.P. and MESSANA, V. (1975). Preliminary evaluation of VM 26: a new epipodophyllotoxin derivative in the treatment of urogenital tumours. *European Urology*, **1**, 53–56

PETO, R., PIKE, M.C., ARMITAGE, P., BRESLOW, N.E., COX, D.R., HOWARD, S.V., MANTEL, N., McPHERSON, K., PETO, J. and SMITH, P.G. (1977). Design and analysis of randomized clinical trials requiring prolonged observation of each patient, II. Analysis and examples. *British Journal of Cancer*, **35**, 1–39

POTTHOFF, R.F. and WHITTINGHILL, M. (1966). Testing for homogeneity II. The Poisson distribution. *Biometrika*, **53**, 183–190

SCHULMAN, C.C., ROZENCWEIG, M., STAQUET, M., KENIS, Y., and SYLVESTER, R. (1976). EORTC randomized trial for the adjuvant therapy of T1 bladder carcinoma. *European Urology*, **2**, 271–273

STAQUET, M. (1976). The randomized clinical trial: a prerequisite for rational therapy. *European Urology*, **2**, 265–270

UICC (INTERNATIONAL UNION AGAINST CANCER). (1974). *TNM Classification of Malignant Tumours, 2nd Edn.*, p. 79. Geneva. Imprimerie G. de Buren S.A.

VEENEMA, R.J., DEAN, A.L. Jr., ROBERTS, M., FINGERHUT, B., CHOWHURY, B.K. and TARASSOLY. H. (1962). Bladder carcinoma treated by direct instillation of thio-TEPA. *Journal of Urology*, **88**, 60–63

VEENEMA, R.J., DEAN, A.L., USON, A.C., ROBERTS, M. and LONGO, F. (1969). Thio-tepa bladder instillation: therapy and prophylaxis for superficial bladder tumors. *Journal of Urology*, **101**, 711–715

WESTCOTT, J.W. (1966). The prophylactic use of thiotepa in transitional cell carcinoma of the bladder. *Journal of Urology*, **96**, 913–918

10

Prophylactic Intravesical Doxorubicin* Instillation after TUR of Superficial Transitional Cell Tumours: 3 Years' Experience

Günther H. Jacobi and J.W. Thüroft

In an attempt to search for topically active, well tolerated and trans-vesically non-reabsorbable cytotoxic agents for intravesical chemo-therapy, doxorubicin has been thoroughly investigated at the University of Mainz Medical School Department of Urology during the last 3 years. At the outset we were able to show, by radioisotope studies, that reabsorption of topically administered doxorubicin through the bladder wall is negligible, and does not lead to any systemic toxicity (Jacobi and Kurth, 1980). Furthermore, intravesical doxorubicin is taken up mainly by normal flat epithelium and exophytic papillary lesions, and to a far lesser extent by muscle. Our clinical trial used prophylactic treatment with doxorubicin at a dose level of 40 mg in 30 ml normal saline monthly, starting 1 month after transurethral resection had cleared the bladder of visible tumour. A total of 38 patients with recurrent superficial tumours (pTis, pTa or pT1 stages, were treated, 15 as part of a randomized trial. In this trial the 15 treated patients received an average total dose of 560 mg doxorubicin, (14 months' treatment) and then stopped treatment and have been followed with 3-monthly cystoscopies for up to 3 years.

Fifteen patients served as untreated controls under randomized conditions and were followed for 27 months. Five of the control patients with repeated recurrences during the trial were changed to

*Adriamycin

doxorubicin treatment after TUR. At present, these patients have been under treatment for 1 year and have received an average total dose of 300 mg (*Tables 10.1 and 10.2*). The 2-year results of this randomized series have been published elsewhere (Jacobi *et al.*, 1979).

Another 15 subjects were treated twice weekly with an increased dose of 50 mg doxorubicin/30 ml saline (average total dose 520 mg) and followed for up to 2 years. In addition, three patients with multifocal carcinoma in situ (pTis) were treated with *curative* rather than *prophylactic* intent.

The overall results are given in *Table 10.2*. It is striking that all 15 patients without chemoprophylaxis (randomized controls) developed

Table 10.1
STAGING OF PATIENTS GIVEN INTRAVESICAL DOXORUBICIN INSTILLATIONS

Number of patients	Stage (UICC)	Study	Follow-up (years)
15	Pa−P1	Randomized DOX	3
15	Pa−P1	Randomized control	
		➜ DOX	1
15	Pa−P1	Non-randomized DOX	1−2
2	P2	Incorrect indication	2.5
3	Pis	Treatment not evaluable	1−3
1	P1	Radiotherapy for	
		prostate carcinoma	2.5

DOX: doxorubicin

Table 10.2

Results	Randomized 40 mg/month doxorubicin	Randomized controls	Controls subsequently given doxorubicin	Non-random doxorubicin 50 mg/2 weeks
Number of patients	15	15	5	15
Total dose doxorubicin (mg)	560	−	300	520
Follow-up (months)	34	27	12	13
Patients with recurrences	7/15	15/15	4/5	3/15
Recurrences per patient	1.6	2.5	2	1
Recurrences of more advanced stage	1/7	7/15	0/4	0/3
Number of patients with recurrences, after doxorubicin	4/7	−	2/4	2/3
Recurrence interval after doxorubicin (months)	6	6	4	7
Interval for 1 recurrence (months)	13/1	9/1	8/1	7/1
Number of recurrences prior to entry on study	4	−	8	5

recurrences, whereas only seven out of 15 did so in the doxorubicin group. The rate of recurrences per patient, the number of recurrences with progress in stage as well as the average recurrence interval (months required per new recurrence) differed markedly in both groups. In the series of five patients given doxorubicin, who originally were allocated to the control group (subsequently given drug treatment), four developed recurrences during a 1-year follow-up. These patients, however, had had twice as many recurrent tumours before doxorubicin had been started, compared with the original group of 15 patients (7/15 recurrences). In the non-randomized group, the rate of recurrence was three out of 15 within 13 months. These data are in agreement with our earlier 2-year results of 5/15 recurrences in the original series (Jacobi *et al.*, 1979).

Two patients with pT2 lesions did not respond to doxorubicin: one patient developed a pT3 carcinoma requiring radical cystectomy; another developed distant metastases and died after 2 years. In the pTis group the lesions were controlled in two patients for 8 months and 3 years respectively (as shown by cytology and random biopsy), but one patient developed a pT4 carcinoma and underwent radical cystectomy.

Untoward reactions with doxorubicin instillations were as follows: 18 patients had chemical cystitis which was treated symptomatically, with diffuse haemorrhage in two instances; one developed epididymitis. In no case did systemic toxicity occur.

In conclusion, doxorubicin is of value in preventing recurrences of superficial (pTa, pTl) urothelial bladder tumours, but does not seem to do so in patients with previous pT2 lesions. Multifocal carcinoma in situ, which is usually treated by radical cystectomy, seems to be controlled by doxorubicin instillation. Further protracted multicentre randomized trials are required to confirm these preliminary data; such trials are being attempted by the EORTC.

REFERENCES

JACOBI, G.H. and KURTH, K.H. (1980). Studies on the intravesical action of topically administered (G-^{3}H)-adriamycin in men: plasma uptake and tumor penetration. *Journal of Urology* (in press)

JACOBI, G.H., KURTH, K.H., KLIPPEL, K.F. and HOHENFELLNER, R. (1979). On the biological behaviour of T1 transitional cell tumours of the urinary bladder and initial results of the prophylactic use of topical adriamycin under controlled randomised conditions. In *Diagnostics and Treatment of Superficial Urinary Bladder Tumours*, pp. 83–94. WHO Collaborating Centre Edition. Stockholm; Montedison Läkemedel

IIB

Treatment of superficial disease: flat carcinoma in situ

11

Histopathology of Carcinoma in situ and the Effects of Cyclophosphamide

E. Molland

HISTOPATHOLOGY OF CARCINOMA IN SITU AND ATYPICAL HYPERPLASIA

There have been numerous descriptions of the histology of flat carcinoma in situ of the bladder (Tis) since Melicow's first report of the lesion (Melicow, 1952). The urothelium is composed throughout of easily recognizable malignant cells which have marked abnormalities of cytoplasm and nucleus (*Figure 11.1*). The latter are often uniformly very large and hyperchromatic; mitotic figures are common and sometimes atypical. Such a lesion has the features of Grade 3 transitional cell carcinoma. The thickness of the epithelium is variable: the atypical cells often show decreased attachment to the basement membrane, and are readily exfoliated, so that urine cytology is a useful diagnostic aid.

Less advanced malignant change in the urothelium is usually classified as atypical hyperplasia. This is characterized by an increase in the number of cell layers, and by nuclear abnormalities such as enlargement and hyperchromatism, but the superficial cell layer is usually preserved and the uniformity of cell size seen in Tis is lacking.

The borderline between these two lesions may be difficult to define. Both may be present, adjacent in the same bladder and both are regarded as potential precursors of infiltrative carcinoma. Recent 'mapping' studies of bladders removed surgically because of invasive carcinoma have shown the presence of multiple foci of atypical hyperplasia, and of Tis at a distance from, or adjacent to, the invasive carcinoma (Koss *et al.*, 1977). Urothelium from such cases, which appears

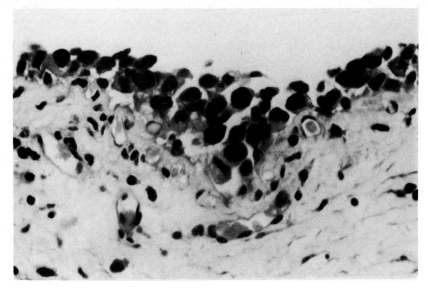

Figure 11.1 Bladder epithelium: flat in situ carcinoma (Tis). 2–3 layers of malignant cells with enlarged, hyperchromatic nuclei. The cells are readily detached from the surface. H and E, × 640

normal by light microscopy, may also show alterations in the luminal surface membrane when examined by scanning or transmission electron microscopy (Newman and Hicks, 1978). Such changes are a feature of invasive and in situ carcinoma in the human bladder and have also been demonstrated in experimental models of bladder cancer; they probably indicate early malignant transformation. Another 'marker' of early malignant transformation is the deletion of tissue-associated blood group antigens. This has been demonstrated in invasive and in situ bladder cancer in man and may also be a feature of histologically normal urothelium adjacent to such lesions (Weinstein *et al.*, 1979).

RELATIONSHIP TO INVASIVE CARCINOMA

An association between atypical hyperplasia, Tis and invasive carcinoma has been established, but there remains uncertainty over a causal relationship. It has been estimated that approximately 70% of cases of Tis develop solid invasive cancer (Koss *et al.*, 1977). However, from clinical experience it is known that a large percentage of invasive tumours are preceded by Grade 1 or 2 papillary lesions, with minimal cytological atypia, the recognition of such neoplastic lesions being based on the exophytic growth pattern and the thickness of the epithelium. No in situ counterpart associated with papillary tumours has yet been identified. In addition, in experimental animals, the majority of papillary and solid transitional cell carcinomas of the bladder arise by malignant transformation from papillomas or papillary hyperplasia (Kunze, 1979).

A further uncertainty lies in the time interval of progression from Tis to invasive carcinoma. An average of 26–33 months has been reported (Melamed *et al.*, 1964), while other figures have varied from 18 to 77 months (Koss *et al.*, 1969).

THE EFFECTS OF CYCLOPHOSPHAMIDE

The following description of the effects of cyclophosphamide is confined to cases of atypical hyperplasia and Tis, diagnosed by multiple field biopsies. Invasive carcinoma, usually Grade 3, was present in some cases in the same bladder, but cyclophosphamide did not have any significant effect on the latter. Cyclophosphamide-induced changes in histologically normal urothelium and in the bladder wall will also be described.

Cyclophosphamide was administered intravenously once every 3 weeks, at a dose of $1g/m^2$ body surface (*see* Chapter 12). Multiple biopsies were taken at 3-monthly intervals, and most cases have now been followed for 2–3 years. Follow-up biopsies were taken in the same way in those cases in which cyclophosphamide had been discontinued. At 3 months there was extensive loss of surface epithelium, although in some biopsies small islands of degenerating tumour cells persisted. In other cases, at 3 months or in subsequent biopsies, the surface epithelium was intact. It was 3–4 cell layers thick, showing marked variability in nuclear size and staining intensity, but lacking the very large size and relatively uniform hyperchromatism of Tis. Nuclei, particularly towards the luminal surface, appeared vesicular with chromatin clumping, and some were vacuolated. There were occasional multinucleate cells with prominent nucleoli (*Figure 11.2*). A prominent feature was ballooning of cytoplasm, especially on the luminal edge, with vacuolation and ill-defined cell margins. In some biopsies the surface epithelium, and particularly the epithelium in Brunn's nests, appeared to be forming a syncytium of necrotic cells, with pyknotic nuclei, often with irregular 'smudged' outlines.

The range of combined nuclear and cytoplasmic abnormalities appeared to be characteristic of cyclophosphamide damage and usually persisted over many months. Many features were similar to the effects of radiation treatment. It is easy to see how the pyknotic nuclei of cyclophosphamide-damaged cells might be mistaken for malignant

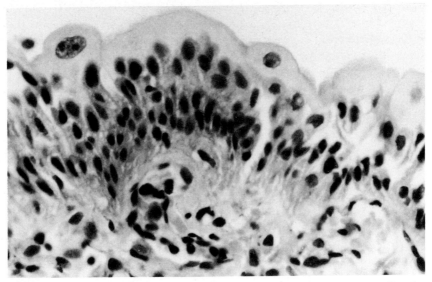

Figure 11.2 Bladder epithelium: effect of cyclophosphamide. 3–4 layers of cells. There is variation in nuclear size and staining. Superficial cells have swollen cytoplasm and large vesicular nuclei. One binucleate cell with prominent nucleoli. H and E, × 640

cells in urine submitted for cytological examination (Forni *et al.,* 1964).

Early biopsies showed telangiectatic vessels in the superficial lamina propria, with much recent haemorrhage. Ulceration of the surface was unusual, and in most cases there was a marked lack of inflammatory cells, although some biopsies showed infiltration of the lamina propria by neutrophils and eosinophils. There was fibrinoid necrosis of the walls of some vessels, but this was not a common finding. In later biopsies there was persistence of haemorrhage in the superficial lamina propria and increasing numbers of thick-walled vessels in the deeper layers (*Figure 11.3*). A characteristic feature was the appearance of large numbers of mononuclear or 'stromal' cells throughout the lamina propria. Some had the characteristics of fibroblasts, and patchy fibrosis in the deep layers of the lamina propria was commonly seen in late biopsies. Pigment-laden macrophages, indicating previous haemorrhage, were also present.

Minor cytological abnormalities of the surface epithelium, increased numbers of stromal cells and abnormal vessels persisted for many months after the end of a course of cyclophosphamide.

Most biopsies included a small amount of bladder wall muscle and, in late specimens, there were usually bands of fibrous tissue extending between muscle bundles, although extensive necrosis of muscle and fibrosis of the wall, such as has been described in children given

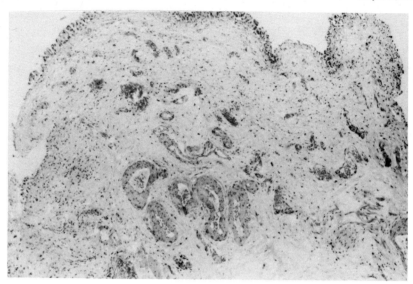

Figure 11.3 Bladder wall: late effects of cyclophosphamide. Persistent abnormalities in surface epithelium,. Oedema and an increase of stromal cells in the lamina propria, with thick-walled vessels more deeply. H and E, × 40

large doses of cyclophosphamide (Johnson and Meadows, 1971) were not observed.

In some cases, where biopsies have been obtained after the end of a course of cyclophosphamide, the reappearance of foci of atypical hyperplasia and eventually of Tis has been observed, usually after an interval of up to 12 months. The recurrent tumour is histologically similar to that seen before therapy and there is no evidence that cyclophosphamide has induced a new malignancy in contrast to the data reviewed by Pearson and Soloway (1978). The histopathology of cyclophosphamide-induced damage is consistent with a direct effect of the drug and its metabolites, excreted in the urine (Philips *et al.,* 1961), on normal and neoplastic transitional epithelium. It also causes vascular injury and damage to superficial interstitial tissue, the effects of which persist after the drug has been withdrawn.

REFERENCES

FORNI, A.M., KOSS, L.G., and GELLER, W. (1964). Cytological study of the effect of cyclophosphamide on the epithelium of the urinary bladder in man. *Cancer,* **17,** 1348–1355

JOHNSON, W.W. and MEADOWS, D.C. (1971). Urinary bladder fibrosis and telangiectasia associated with long-term cyclophosphamide therapy. *New England Journal of Medicine,* **284,** 290–294

KOSS, L.G., MELAMED, M.R. and KELLY, R.E. (1969). Further cytologic and histologic studies of bladder lesions in workers exposed to para-amino-diphenyl. Progress report. *Journal of the National Cancer Institute*, **43**, 233–243

KOSS, L.G., NAKANISHI, I. and FREED, S.Z. (1977). Nonpapillary carcinoma in situ and atypical hyperplasia in cancerous bladders: further studies of surgically removed bladders by mapping. *Urology*, **9**, 442–455

KUNZE, E. (1979). Development of urinary bladder cancer in the rat. In *Carcinogenesis*. Ed. by E. Grundmann, pp. 145–232. (Current Topics in Pathology, Vol. 67). Berlin; Springer-Verlag

MELAMED, M.R., VOUTSA, N.G. and GRABSTALD, H. (1964). Natural history and clinical behaviour of in situ carcinoma of the human urinary bladder. *Cancer*, **17**, 1533–1545

MELICOW, M.M. (1952). Histological study of vesical urothelium intervening between gross neoplasms in total cystectomy. *Journal of Urology*, **68**, 261–279

NEWMAN, J. and HICKS, R.M. (1978). Detection of neoplastic and pre-neoplastic urothelia by combined scanning and transmission electron microscopy of urinary surface of human and rat bladders. *Histopathology*, **1**, 125–135

PEARSON, R.M. and SOLOWAY, M.S. (1978). Does cyclophosphamide induce bladder cancer? *Urology*, **11**, 437–447

PHILIPS, F.S., STERNBERG, S.S., CRONIN, A.P. and VIDAL, P.M. (1961). Cyclophosphamide and urinary bladder toxicity. *Cancer Research*, **21**, 1577–1589

WEINSTEIN, R.S., ALROY, J., FARROW, G.M., MILLER, A.W. and DAVIDSOHN, I. (1979). Blood group isoantigen deletion in carcinoma in situ of the urinary bladder. *Cancer*, **43**, 661–668

12

Systemic Cyclophosphamide in Flat Carcinoma in situ of the Bladder

H.R. England, E.A. Molland, R.T.D. Oliver and J.P. Blandy

Flat carcinoma in situ (Tis) of the bladder has been looked for and found with increasing frequency since it was first described by Melicow and Hollowell in 1952, and its sinister prognostic significance is well recognized. Tumour grade is commonly high, and occasionally Tis may be the only form of malignancy in the bladder, though more frequently it is found in association with invasive tumour. Sometimes there is a history of previous lower-grade tumour, the later development of high-grade Tis being a form of tumour progression.

Treatment has been disappointing. The nature of the lesions make them unsuitable for endoscopic or other local excision and usually they have proved to be radioresistant so that the only really effective treatment has been cystectomy.

When Tis is widespread, symptoms of 'malignant cystitis' are often present. Cystectomy specimens have shown similar changes in the urothelium of the prostatic urethra and ducts in about 20% of patients, while the reported incidence of ureteric involvement ranges from 8% to over 50%. If these patients survive cystectomy for their bladder cancer, an appreciable number develop urothelial tumours of the upper tracts or urethra (Gowing, 1960; Culp et al., 1967; Schade et al., 1970; Sharma et al., 1970; Skinner et al., 1974; Thelmo et al., 1974).

Clearly, the ideal treatment for this disease is an agent which can be given systemically and which can favourably influence the urothelium as a whole. Two years ago we began a small pilot study using cyclophosphamide to treat a series of patients with Tis of the bladder: this communication reports the early results.

PATIENTS AND METHODS

Fifteen patients have been treated (14 men and 1 woman) with ages ranging from 50 to 73 years and a mean age of 62 years. Six patients had severe symptoms of 'malignant cystitis', consisting of frequency

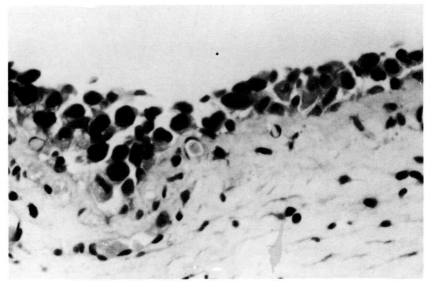

Figure 12.1 Tis-enlarged hyperchromatic nuclei, disorderly pattern of growth and no readily identifiable superficial cell layer

with urgency and often urgency incontinence, as well as bladder and genital pain. Urine cytology was positive in 14 patients and negative in one. Usually six punch biopsies of the bladder mucosa from each patient were examined, and the diagnosis of Tis made only when the epithelium was composed of cells showing definite malignancy (*Figure 12.1*). The extent of mucosal disease was widespread in all 15 patients.

Seven patients had not previously been treated for bladder cancer, the in situ changes being their primary lesion. The other eight had

Table 12.1
PREVIOUS CANCER HISTORY

Histology	pT1	7 patients	G1:- 1
			G2:- 2
			G3:- 4 (associated Tis – 2)
	pT2	1 patient	G2
Treatment	Radiotherapy	5 patients	(Tis persisted:- 2)
	TUR	3 patients	

Tis developed in 6 patients after intervals of 1, 1, 2, 2, 8 and 14 years already received therapy for overt tumour, seven in category pT1 with tumour grades G1 (1 case), G2 (2 cases) and G3 (4 cases), and one in category pT2.G2. In two there was associated Tis at presentation and this persisted after radiotherapy; the six others developed Tis at intervals of 1, 1, 2, 2, 8 and 14 years following treatment of their primary tumour (*Table 12.1*).

Initially, cyclophosphamide was given intravenously every 3 weeks for 6 months and then every 6 weeks for a further 6 months at a dose level of 1g/m² of body surface area. With increasing experience, it seemed that continuing treatment beyond 3 months did not confer any extra benefit, and cyclophosphamide therapy is now stopped at that time.

RESULTS

At 3 months, 12 patients had responded completely, showing negative cytology and biopsies. The remaining three showed a marked reduction in the extent of disease but all still had at least one positive biopsy and in two patients cytology gave positive results. One partial responder had therapy for a further 3 months but a positive biopsy was still obtained.

The most dramatic effect of treatment was the relief of symptoms of 'malignant cystitis'. This began within 48 hours of first receiving cyclophosphamide and was complete in five out of six patients when seen again at 3 weeks. The sixth patient showed substantial improvement but never gained complete relief, probably in keeping with the presence of a positive biopsy at 3 months (*Table 12.2*).

Table 12.2
RESULTS AT 3 MONTHS (15 PATIENTS)

Complete regression of Tis	12 patients (negative cytology and biopsies)
Partial regression of Tis	3 patients (positive cytology: 2; positive biopsy: 3)
Malignant cystitis	5 of 6 patients completely relieved

The change in the plan of therapy has meant that some patients have been treated longer than others; the numbers of injections received and periods of treatment are shown in *Table 12.3*. Also indicated is the type of Tis: whether it occurred *de novo* without preceding malignant bladder tumour (primary), or whether it was concurrent with, or detected after, treatment of a bladder tumour (secondary). Although only one out of three partial responders received treatment beyond 3 months it is probably true that, if a patient does not respond com-

Table 12.3
CYCLOPHOSPHAMIDE DOSAGE AND RESPONSE

Response	Period of treatment (months)	Number of patients	Type of Tis*	
			Primary	Secondary
Complete				
	3	5	3	2
	6	2	–	2
	12	2	1	1
	12	2	–	2
	15	1	1	–
	Total	12	5	7
Partial				
	3	2	2	–
	6	1	–	1
	Total	3	2	1

*Primary Tis = in situ disease with no previous or concurrent bladder tumour
Secondary Tis = in situ disease coincident with, or following cure of a bladder tumour

pletely by that time, he is unlikely to do so, despite further cyclophosphamide treatment.

Of the 12 complete responders, five still have negative cytology and biopsies at 6, 6, 9, 12 and 15 months respectively after stopping therapy; three redeveloped in situ disease 6, 6 and 9 months after cyclophosphamide treatment had stopped, two of whom responded again to further cyclophosphamide and one to intravesical doxorubicin, as recommended by Edsmyr *et al.* (1978); one whose bladder was clear died from a proven second primary carcinoma in the bronchus and three patients have only been treated for three months (*Table 12.4*).

Treatment times of the five patients still free of Tis after stopping therapy varied from 3 to 12 months. Obviously, those who received

Table 12.4
SUBSEQUENT FATE OF COMPLETE RESPONDERS

Result	Number of patients	Time of test (months)
Still clear after stopping therapy	5	6, 6, 9, 12, 15
Becoming positive again	3	6, 6, 9
Not yet followed again	3	
Died	1*	

*Cancer of the bronchus: bladder clear at 6 months on therapy

Table 12.5
DOSAGE AND FATE OF RESPONDERS AFTER TERMINATION OF THERAPY

	Period of treatment (months)	*No. of injections*	*Period clear (months)*	*Type of Tis†*
Patients remaining clear	3	4	15	Secondary
	3	4	12	Primary
	6	8	9	Secondary
	12	10	6	Primary
	12	12	6	Secondary
Patients with recurrent pTis	12	10	6	Secondary
	12	12	6	Secondary
	15	15	9	Primary

†Defined as in Table 12.3

treatment for shorter periods have had the opportunity of remaining disease-free longest. Two patients are still clear at 15 and 12 months after only 3 months cyclophosphamide (*Table 12.5*). This Table also shows that therapy for longer periods is no protection against re-appearance of Tis, three patients becoming positive again after treatment for at least 1 year. Again, the outcome was not affected by the type of Tis concerned.

HISTOLOGY

Histopathological studies revealed two effects of treatment attributable to cyclophosphamide which are described below.

Effect on in situ disease

At an early stage, the bladder surface was extensively denuded or lined by cells showing cyclophosphamide effects (*see below*). There was no evidence of malignancy in the complete responders (*Figure 12.2*), while the partial responders showed tiny foci of residual Tis in one or two biopsies only (*Figure 12.3*). Tissue sections taken at 12 and 15 months in patients with complete response, showed thin but otherwise normal re-epithelialization.

Cyclophosphamide haemorrhagic cystitis

At 3 months, large areas were denuded; persisting cells showed marked enlargement and pleomorphism, and ballooning of cytoplasm, while nuclei were enlarged and irregular (*Figure 12.2*). In the lamina propria,

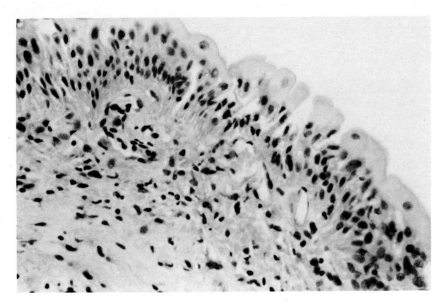

Figure 12.2 Cyclophosphamide effects: well marked ballooning of cytoplasm, no evidence of malignancy

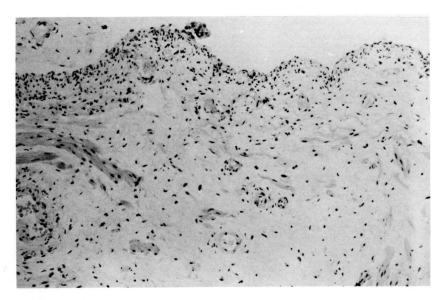

Figure 12.3 Denuded surface with tiny focus of residual Tis after cyclophosphamide − a partial responder (same patient as in Figure 12.1*)*

dilatation and congestion of capillaries was prominent and there were foci of recent haemorrhage. Some sections at 12 and 15 months showed fibrosis of the lamina propria and muscle, which may be a significant side-effect in some patients on long-term treatment (Johnson and Meadows, 1971). Although the number of patients with long-term follow-up is small, non have complained of any change in micturition habit.

Difficulties have been reported in distinguishing malignant epithelium from specific cyclophosphamide-induced effects (Forni *et al.,* 1964; Rubin and Rubin, 1966), but with the knowledge that the patient had received cyclophosphamide it was not difficult to recognize the pleomorphic and rather bizarre changes due to that agent, compared with the relatively uniform hyperchromic cells of Tis.

TOXICITY

The main toxic effect of treatment was nausea and vomiting, coming on some 15 hours after injection and lasting 24–36 hours. In three patients it was severe and they therefore refused treatment after 3 months. Bone marrow depression was minimal and not a problem. Despite the vascular changes seen in bladder mucosal sections, there was no instance of macroscopic haematuria.

DISCUSSION

The majority of bladder tumours which put a patient's life seriously at risk are high-grade, and most of these probably develop from, and are found in association with, areas of flat carcinoma in situ. Unfortunately, further improvement in the treatment of these tumours by conventional radiotherapy and cystectomy is likely to be limited. The use of chemotherapy to treat established distant metastases and/or residual pelvic spread, from which the majority die, has not resulted in any lasting cures, although partial or temporary responses may be achieved (*see* other Chapters).

If Tis can be controlled while it is still pre-invasive and offering no more than a potential threat, some patients may be spared from developing life-endangering invasive tumours and the radical treatment involved thereby. With its very small tumour bulk and high grade, Tis should be the ideal malignancy to treat by chemotherapy, a method well suited also to deal with changes that may be spread throughout the whole urothelium.

If an effective agent were available, suggested areas of use are (1) in primary Tis; (2) in conjunction with radical radiotherapy for infiltrating tumour and associated Tis; (3) for Tis appearing after previously success-ful radical radiotherapy and (4) when in situ changes are found in ureters at cystectomy or in nephro-ureterectomy specimens.

The early experience from our study is encouraging and indicates that, in the short-term, Tis does respond to systemic cyclophosphamide. Primary Tis, or that associated with a current or previous overt tumour, have responded similarly. If a patient is going to respond completely, this becomes apparent at 3 months: prolonging therapy beyond that time did not increase the degree of response, nor, apparently, did it give adequate protection against re-appearance of the disease when therapy was discontinued. The use of cyclophosphamide for the second time in two such cases produced an immediate response, as did doxo-rubicin which was used in one patient.

The advantage of a systemic rather than an intravesical agent is that treatment would also act against changes in the whole urothelium. Perhaps a combination of local and systemic chemotherapy would give the best long-term control.

REFERENCES

CULP, O.S., UTZ, D.C. and HARRISON, E.G. (1967). Experiences with ureteral car-cinoma in situ detected during operations for vesical neoplasm. *Journal of Urology,* **97**, 679–682

EDSMYR, F., BERLIN, O., BOMAN, J., DUCHEK, M., ESPOSTI, P.L., GUSTAFSON, H. and WIKSTROM, H. (1978). Intravesical therapy with Adriamycin in patients with superficial bladder tumours. In *Diagnostics and Treatment of Superficial Urinary Bladder Tumours,* pp 45–51. Stockholm; WHO Collaborating Centre, Karo-linska Hospital

FORNI, A.M., KOSS, L.G. and GELLER, W. (1964). Cytological study of the effect of cyclophosphamide on the epithelium of the urinary bladder in man. *Cancer,* **17**, 1348–1355

GOWING, N.F.C. (1960). Urethral carcinoma associated with cancer of the bladder. *British Journal of Urology,* **32**, 428–438

JOHNSON, W.W. and MEADOWS, D.C. (1971). Urinary-bladder fibrosis and telan-giectasia associated with long-term cyclophosphamide therapy. *New England Journal of Medicine,* **284**, 290–294

MELICOW, M.M. and HOLLOWELL, J.W. (1952). Intra-urothelial cancer: carcinoma in situ, Bowen's disease of the urinary system: discussion of thirty cases. *Journal of Urology,* **68**, 763–772

RUBIN, J.S. and RUBIN, R.T. (1966). Cyclophosphamide hemorrhagic cystitis. *Journal of Urology,* **96**, 313–316

SCHADE, R.O.K., SERCK-HANSSEN, A. and SWINNEY, J. (1971). Morphological changes in the ureter in cases of bladder carcinoma. *Cancer,* **27**, 1267–1272

SHARMA, T.C., MELAMED, M.R. and WHITMORE, W.F. (1970). Carcinoma in situ of the ureter in patients with bladder carcinoma treated by cystectomy. *Cancer,* **26**, 583–587

SKINNER, D.G., RICHIE, J.P., COOPER, P.H., WAISMAN, J. and KAUFMAN, J.J. (1974). The clinical significance of carcinoma in situ of the bladder and its association with overt carcinoma. *Journal of Urology,* **112**, 68–71

THELMO, W.L., SEEMAYER, T.A., MADARNAS, P., MOUNT, B.M.M. and MACKINNON, K.J. (1974). Carcinoma in situ of the bladder with associated prostatic involvement. *Journal of Urology,* **111**, 491–494

13

Intravesical Therapy with Doxorubicin* in Patients with Superficial Bladder Tumours

F. Edsmyr

Doxorubicin (14-hydroxy-daunomycin) is a water-soluble, glycoside antibiotic agent (solubility greater than 10% by weight), prepared either by aerobic fermentation of *Streptomyces peucetius* var. *caesius* or by chemical synthesis from daunomycin (Arcamone *et al.*, 1972). It has been shown to possess an antitumour effect in a variety of situations. The mechanism is mainly by blocking the cell progression from G2 to mitosis (Yagoda *et al.*, 1977).

Doxorubicin is normally administered intravenously, and is rapidly cleared from plasma and deposited in tissues. It is excreted slowly into bile and urine (Yesair *et al.*, 1972). It has been used as induction therapy for many different tumours, such as leukaemia and lymphoma, as well as a number of solid tumours including urological tumours. In metastatic bladder cancer, objective responses have been reported in 0–37% of the cases (Middleman *et al.*, 1971; Bonadonna *et al.*, 1972; O'Bryan *et al.*, 1973; Gottlieb, 1975, Merrin *et al.*, 1975; Slavik, 1975; Weinstein and Schmidt, 1976; De Kernion, 1977; Yagoda *et al.*, 1977). There has been one report suggesting that combined treatment with doxorubicin and cyclophosphamide seems to produce higher response rates (Merrin *et al.*, 1975). This clinical impression is borne out by laboratory screening experiments in the mouse, in which doxorubicin combined with cyclophosphamide proved to be the most successful of several regimes (Soloway, 1975; 1977).

Multiple, low-grade, papillary tumours of the bladder can be controlled by coagulation, transurethral resection or transvesical excision. In the event of frequent recurrences and/or widespread tumours, these

*Adriamycin

methods are often inadequate. Several other methods have been developed. Hydrostatic intravesical pressure treatment has been shown to suppress superficially growing low-grade bladder tumours (Helmstein, 1976). Local cryotherapy has also been tried (Reuter, 1972).

Topical chemotherapy has been applied extensively in this context. Among the agents which have been tested are thiotepa (Jones and Swinney, 1961; Abbassian and Wallace, 1966; Veenema *et al.,* 1969; Edsmyr and Boman, 1970; Mitchell, 1971, Gibson, 1972) bleomycin (Cunningham *et al.,* 1972; Sadaoughi *et al.,* 1973; Smith and McCollum, 1976) and ethoglucid (Riddle and Wallace, 1971; Robinson *et al.,* 1977, Collste *et al.,* 1979), with varying success rates. More recently, doxorubicin has been tried for local treatment of papillomatosis: Pavone-Macaluso and Caramia (1972) reported four cases, with partial regression of tumour growth in three. Banks *et al.* (1977) reported complete remission of recurrent superficial bladder tumour in two of 13 patients.

We report here the preliminary results of an ongoing multicentre study, in which doxorubicin has been given intravesically to patients with transitional cell tumours, some with flat in situ lesions, some with papillary tumours.

MATERIALS AND METHODS

Fifty-eight patients have been admitted to the study at five Swedish institutions − the Radiumhemmet and the Department of Urology at Karolinska Hospital; the Departments of Urology at St Erik's and Huddinge Hospitals (all in Stockholm) and the Department of Urology at the Umea Hospital in Umea.

Before doxorubicin treatment, the patients had been staged according to the TNM classification (UICC, 1974) (*Table 13.1*). In the present report, 'primary' carcinoma in situ (Tis) defines no visible tumour at cystoscopy (pre-invasive carcinoma) or histology and/or malignant cells on cytology. None of the patients in this group had

Table 13.1
T CLASSIFICATION BEFORE DOXORUBICIN TREATMENT

Classification	Number of patients
Tis, primary *	11
Tis, secondary *	19
T1	23
T2	5
Total	58

* See text for explanation.

received previous treatment. 'Secondary' carcinoma in situ denotes patients who had previously been treated with any of the methods outlined below; at the cystoscopy before starting doxorubicin, however, they did not have any visible tumours.

Previous treatment for bladder tumour by transurethral resection, radiotherapy or chemotherapy had been performed in 44 patients, and 14 had not received any previous treatment (*Table 13.2*).

All patients had malignancy established by cytological tests and/or histological examination of biopsy tissue (*Table 13.3*).

Table 13.2
THERAPY BEFORE DOXORUBICIN INSTILLATION

Therapy	Number of patients
Transurethral resection/excision	17
Transurethral resection/excision and chemotherapy	8
Radiotherapy	14
Radiotherapy and chemotherapy	5
Untreated	14
Total	58

Doxorubicin (80 mg) was dissolved in 100 ml of 0.9% NaCl, and instilled in the bladder via a urethral catheter. The catheter was removed and the recumbent patient was instructed to change position every 15 minutes. The solution was retained in the bladder for 1 hour. This procedure was repeated once a month, with the exception of one patient, in whom weekly instillations were initially performed.

Table 13.3
DIAGNOSTIC PROCEDURES BEFORE TREATMENT

Group	Number of patients	Cystoscopy	Tumor verified by: Cytology	Biopsy
Tis, primary	11	11	11	9
Tis, secondary	19	19	19	5
T1	23	23	21	13
T2	5	5	5	3

Urine cytology examinations and peripheral blood cell counts were monitored once a month. Cystoscopy with bladder irrigation was done every 4 months. Positive cytology results and/or cystoscopically visible tumours were defined as treatment failures.

The periods of treatment in this study were variable. In the primary Tis group, 4–26 monthly treatments were given. In the secondary Tis group there have been 1–20 treatments, and in the T1 and T2 groups, 2–9 and 3–10 treatments respectively.

RESULTS

The overall results for the 58 patients are summarized in *Table 13.4.* There were no instances of cystoscopically visible lesions in the primary Tis group. In the secondary Tis group there were three cases in which visible tumour appeared during the treatment period (*Table 13.5*).

Table 13.4

CURRENT RESULTS OF DOXORUBICIN THERAPY REGARDLESS OF DURATION

Group	Number of patients	Cystoscopy		Cytology		Biopsy	
		No tumour	*Partial regression*	*Negative*	*Atypia*	*No tumour*	*Tumour*
Tis, primary	11	11	–	9	1	3	–
Tis, secondary	19	16	–	11	3	1	–
T1	23	10	5	13	3	4	6
T2	5	1	–	3	–	1	1

Table 13.5

CYSTOSCOPY AFTER DOXORUBICIN INSTILLATION THERAPY, REGARDLESS OF DURATION

Tis, primary *No tumour*	*Tis, secondary* *No tumour*	*T1*		*T2* *No tumour*
		No tumour	*Partial regression*	
11/11 (100%)	16/19 (84%)	10/23 (43%)	5/23 (22%)	1/5
			(65%)	

Complete disappearance of carcinoma cells in cytological specimens (cytological remission), occurred in 9/11 patients in the primary Tis group. A partial effect (presence of atypical cells but no carcinoma cells) was seen in one patient in the same group. In the secondary Tis group, 11 out of 19 patients had complete disappearance of carcinoma cells in cytology specimens, while in three, atypical cells persisted (*Table 13.6*).

Table 13.6

CYTOLOGY AFTER DOXORUBICIN INSTILLATION THERAPY, REGARDLESS OF DURATION

Tis, primary		*Tis, secondary*		*T1*		*T2*
Cytological remission	*Atypia*	*Cytological remission*	*Atypia*	*Cytological remission*	*Atypia*	*Cytological remission*
9/11 (82%)	1/11 (9%)	11/19 (58%)	3/19 (16%)	13/23 (57%)	3/23 (13%)	3/5 –
(91%)		(74%)		(70%)		

In the T2 group, complete disappearance of visible lesions was noted in one out of five patients (*Table 13.5*), and complete disappearance of carcinoma cells in cytological specimens was seen in three patients (*Table 13.6*).

Because of the relatively short treatment periods in some of the patients, no definite conclusions can be made about the long-term efficacy of the treatment. When only those patients who received more than five treatments were considered, it appeared that at least four treatments were necessary for primary Tis patients to achieve complete remission, while for the secondary Tis group as many as 11 treatments were necessary. On the other hand there was no difference in the

Table 13.7

CYSTOSCOPY AFTER DOXORUBICIN INSTILLATION THERAPY, $\geqslant 5$ TREATMENTS

Tis, primary No tumour	Tis, secondary No tumour	T1		T2 No tumour
		No tumour	Partial regression	
8/8 (100%)	9/11 (82%)	9/18 (50%)	5/18 (28%)	0/2 —
		(78%)		

Table 13.8

CYTOLOGY AFTER DOXORUBICIN INSTILLATION THERAPY, $\geqslant 5$ TREATMENTS

Tis, primary		Tis, secondary		T1		T2
Cytological remission	Atypia	Cytological remission	Atypia	Cytological remission	Atypia	Cytological remission
7/8 (88%)	1/8 (12%)	7/11 (64%)	2/11 (18%)	10/18 (56%)	3/18 (17%)	1/2 —
(100%)		(82%)		(73%)		

response rate of the patients with T1 and T2 tumours, irrespective of whether they had received more or fewer than five treatments (*Tables 13.7 and 13.8*). From *Table 13.8* it is evident that all of the patients treated for more than five months in the primary Tis group showed evidence of response (including one patient with atypia). Average duration of follow-up in these patients was 12 months.

COMPLICATIONS

While bladder capacity was unchanged in the majority of the patients, a slight reduction of bladder capacity was the most frequent complication in this study, occurring in five patients (*Table 13.9*). Frequency,

Table 13.9

COMPLICATIONS AFTER DOXORUBICIN INSTILLATION THERAPY

Complication	Group	Number of patients
Reduction of bladder capacity		
	Tis, primary	1
	Tis, secondary	1
	T1	2
	T2	1
Discontinuation		
	Tis, secondary	1 (one treatment)
	T1	2 (2 and 6 treatments)

urgency and painful micturition of varying degree occurred in several patients: in three it was significant and treatment had to be discontinued. No bone marrow or systemic side-effects were recorded.

DISCUSSION

The aim of this study was to treat selected patients with monthly doxorubicin instillations for 25 months, followed by treatments every third month. So far, the longest period of treatment is 26 months. The preliminary results demonstrate that Tis lesions respond more readily than macroscopic tumours (T1 and T2), and that the 'primary' (previously untreated) Tis tumours respond better than the 'secondary' (previously treated).

Although the number of patients with T1 and T2 tumours is small and the periods of observation short, doxorubicin seems to compare favourably with previously used topical agents, without evidence of the severe local side-effects reported for ethoglucid (Robinson *et al.*, 1977) or fatal leucopenias associated with thiotepa administration (Abbassian and Wallace, 1966). Further modification of the schedules for doxorubicin instillation, for example, with regard to doxorubicin concentration in the bladder, time dependence, and the influence of urinary pH, are currently under investigation in Stockholm (Eksborg *et al.*, 1980) but no data are yet available from these studies.

REFERENCES

ABBASSIAN, A. and WALLACE, D.M. (1966). Intracavitary chemotherapy of diffuse noninfiltrating papillary carcinoma of the bladder. *Journal of Urology*, **96**, 461–465

ARCAMONE, F., CASSINELLI, G., FRANCESCHI, G., PENCO, S., POL, C., REDAELLI, S. and SELVA, A. (1972). Structure and physicochemical properties of Adriamycin (doxorubicin). In *International Symposium on Adriamycin*. Ed. by S.K. Carter, A. di Marco, M. Ghione, I.H. Krakoff and G. Mathé, p.9. Berlin-Heidelberg-New York, Springer-Verlag

BANKS, M.D., PONTES, J.E., IZBICKI, R.M. and PIERCE, J.M. Jr. (1977). Topical instillation of doxorubicin hydrochloride in the treatment of recurring superficial transitional cell carcinoma of the bladder. *Journal of Urology*, **118**, 757–760

BONADONNA, G., MONFARDINI, S., DE LENA, M., FOSSATI-BELLANI, F. and BARETTA G. (1972). Clinical trials with Adriamycin. Results of three-year study. In *International Symposium on Adriamycin*. Ed. by S.K. Carter, A. di Marco, M. Ghione, I.H. Krakoff and G. Mathé, p. 139. Berlin-Heidelberg-New York; Springer-Verlag

COLLSTE, L., GRANBERG-ÖHMAN, I., BERLIN, T. and VON GARRELTS, B. (1980). Intracavitary Epodyl in diffuse papillomatosis of the urinary bladder. *Scandinavian Journal of Urology*. In press

CUNNINGHAM, T.J., OLSON, K.B., HORTON, J., WRIGHT, A., HUSSAIN, M., DAVIES, J.P. and HARRINGTON, G. (1972). A clinical trial of intravenous and intracavitary bleomycin. *Cancer*, **29**, 1413–1419

DE KERNION, J.B. (1977). The chemotherapy of advanced bladder carcinoma. *Cancer Research*, **37**, 2771–2774

EDSMYR, F. and BOMAN, J. (1970). Instillation of Thio-Tepa (Tifosyl) in vesical papillomatosis. *Acta Radiologica; Therapy, Physics, Biology*, **9**, 395–400

EKSBORG, S., NILSSON, S. -O. and EDSMYR, F. (1980). Intravesical instillation of Adriamycin – a model for standardization of the chemotherapy. *European Urology*, **6**, 218–220

GIBSON, G.R. (1972). Local chemotherapy in bladder cancer. *British Journal of Urology*, **44**, 121

GOTTLIEB, J.A. (1975). Adriamycin: activity in solid tumors. In *Ergebnisse der Adriamycin-Therapie*. Ed. by M. Ghione, J. Fetzer and H. Maier, p. 95. Berlin-Heidelberg-New York; Springer-Verlag

HELMSTEIN, K. (1976). Treatment of bladder carcinoma by a hydrostatic pressure technique. Report on 76 cases. *Panminerva Medica*, **18**, 194–198

JONES, H.C. and SWINNEY, J. (1961). Thiotepa in the treatment of tumours of the bladder. *Lancet*, **2**, 615–618

MERRIN, C., CARTAGENA, R., WAJSMAN, Z., BAUMGARTNER, G. and MURPHY, G.P. (1975). Chemotherapy of bladder carcinoma with cyclophosphamide and Adriamycin. *Journal of Urology*, **114**, 884–887

MIDDLEMAN, E., LUCE, J.K. and FREI, E. (1971). Clinical trials with Adriamycin. *Cancer*, **28**, 844–850

MITCHELL, R.J. (1971). Intravesical Thio-tepa in treatment of transitional cell bladder carcinoma. *British Journal of Urology*, **43**, 185–188

O'BRYAN, R.M., LUCE, J.K., TALLEY, R.W., GOTTLIEB, J.A., BAKER, L.H. and BONADONNA, G. (1973). Phase II evaluation of Adriamycin in human neoplasia. *Cancer*, **32**, 1–8

PAVONE-MACALUSO, M. and CARAMIA, G. (1972). Adriamycin and Daunomycin in the treatment of vesical and prostatic neoplasias. Preliminary results. In

International Symposium on Adriamycin. Ed. by S.K. Carter, A. di Marco, M. Ghione, I.H. Krakoff and G. Mathé, p. 180. Berlin-Heidelberg-New York; Springer-Verlag

REUTER, H.J. (1972). Endoscopic cryosurgery of prostate and bladder tumors. *Journal of Urology,* **107**, 389–393

RIDDLE, P.R. (1973). The management of superficial bladder tumours with intravesical Epodyl. *British Journal of Urology,* **45**, 84–87

RIDDLE, P.R. and WALLACE, D.M. (1971). Intracavitary chemotherapy for multiple non-invasive bladder tumours. *British Journal of Urology,* **43**, 181–184

ROBINSON, M.R.G., SHETTY, M.B., RICHARDS, B., BASTABLE, J., GLASHAN, R.W. and SMITH, P.H. (1977). Intravesical Epodyl in the management of bladder tumors: combined experience of the Yorkshire Urological Cancer Research Group. *Journal of Urology,* **118**, 972–973

SADAOUGHI, N., JOHNSON, R.A., EZDINLI, E.Z., BUSH, I.M. and GUINAN, P. (1973). Intravesical bleomycin in treatment of carcinoma of the bladder. *Journal of the American Medical Association,* **226**, 465

SLAVIK, M. (1975). Adriamycin activity in genito-urinary and gynecologic malignancy. *Cancer Chemotherapy Research,* **6**, 297

SMITH, P.H. and McCOLLUM, C.N. (1976). Intravesical bleomycin in bladder cancer. *Journal of the American Medical Association,* **235**, 906–907

SOLOWAY, M.S. (1975). Single and combination chemotherapy for primary murine bladder cancer. *Cancer,* **36**, 333–340

SOLOWAY, M.S. (1977). Intravesical and systemic chemotherapy of murine bladder cancer. *Cancer Research,* **37**, 2918–2929

UICC (INTERNATIONAL UNION AGAINST CANCER) (1974). *TNM Classification of Malignant Tumors,* 2nd Ed., p. 79. Geneva; WHO

VEENEMA, R.J., DEAN, A.L. Jr., USON, A.C., ROBERTS, M. and LONGO, F. (1969). Thio-tepa bladder instillation: therapy and prophylaxis for superficial bladder tumors. *Journal of Urology,* **101**, 711–715

WEINSTEIN, S. and SCHMIDT, J.D. (1976). Doxorubicin chemotherapy in advanced transitional cell carcinoma. *Urology,* **8**, 336–341

YAGODA, A., WATSON, R.C., WHITMORE, W.F., GRABSTALD, H., MIDDLEMAN, M.P. and KRAKOFF, I.H. (1977). Adriamycin in advanced urinary tract cancer: experience in 42 patients and review of the literature. *Cancer,* **39**, 279–285

YESAIR, D.W., ASBELL, M.A., BRUNI, R., BULLOCK, F.J. and SCHWARTZBACH, E. (1972). Pharmacokinetics and metabolism of Adriamycin and Daunomycin. In *International Symposium on Adriamycin.* Ed. by S.K. Carter, A. di Marco, M. Ghione, I.H. Krakoff and G. Mathé, p. 117. Berlin–Heidelberg–New York; Springer-Verlag

IIIA

Treatment of invasive tumours:
radiotherapy and surgery

14

Carcinoma of the Bladder Treated by Local Interstitial Irradiation

Grant Williams, M.A. Jones, P.A. Trott and H.J.G. Bloom

INTRODUCTION

The long history of interstitial irradiation for carcinoma of the bladder has been reviewed by Dix *et al.* (1970) and by Bloom and Wallace (1971). Various radioactive materials have been used for this purpose, principally radium needles, radon seeds, tantalum-182 wire, gold-198 grains, cobalt-60 needles and iridium-192 wire. All except radon and gold-198 have long half-lives and therefore must be removed from the patient when the calculated dose of radiation to the bladder tumour has been reached. Radon is no longer available in the UK because of radiation hazards in its manufacture. Sources like cobalt-60, tantalum-182 or iridium-192, with relatively long half-lives of 5 years, 111 days and 74 days respectively, can be kept in stock and made available at short notice, while gold-198 with a half-life of only 2.7 days must be ordered specifically for each case. Most implants performed today for bladder cancer are with gold-198 grains. Although tantalum-182 wire is used to a lesser extent, the advantage of this technique is that greater control can be exerted over the positioning of these removable sources in tissues than is possible with small non-removable radioactive grains. This results in a greater degree of flexibility in control of the dose and its distribution within the treated volume (Bloom, 1960).

The observation that bladder tumours may be part of a pan-urothelial disease has provided justification for doubting the value of a purely local treatment such as provided by interstitial irradiation. Before the advent of megavoltage equipment, this technique was used in a number of centres as the most effective means of delivering high doses of irradiation to a tumour of limited size in a deep-seated organ with considerable sparing of surrounding normal tissues.

Cases suitable for interstitial therapy were, of necessity, highly selected. The tumours had to be solitary and limited to the superficial tissues. Because insertion of radioactive sources in the bladder wall must be restricted to one plane (which confines the effective radiation dose to a slab of tissue 1 cm thick) this technique was suitable only for patients with T1 and T2 tumours. The overall diameter of a radioactive implant should not exceed 6 cm, for fear of inducing radiation necrosis. This produces a rim of effectively irradiated normal tissue around a 3–4 cm tumour. Occasional errors in pre-operative staging may lead to some T3 tumours being encountered at operation. When this happens, a decision must be made before the bladder is opened, either to abandon the procedure altogether or to proceed with the implant on the understanding that supplementary external beam therapy will be required.

With care in selection of patients for intersitial therapy, several authors were able to report results which equalled those being achieved by surgical methods for apparently comparable tumours (Jacobs, 1949; Poole-Wilson, 1957; Riches, 1958; Carver, 1959). in 1952, workers at the Royal Marsden Hospital introduced the tantalum-182 wire technique (Wallace *et al.,* 1952), and a repeating gold-grain gun (Hodt *et al.,* 1952) for radioactive implants in the bladder. These innovations increased the safety and the accuracy of the procedure. The first long-term survival data on a series of patients treated with radioactive tantalum were reported by Bloom (1960). Bloom and Wallace (1971) reviewed these results and also those achieved by other techniques of interstitial therapy. The present publication reports our more recent experience with interstitial irradiation using tantalum-182 wires or gold-198 grains in an attempt to assess the place for this treatment, now that megavoltage external beam therapy is generally available.

PATIENTS

Between 1958 and 1976, 180 patients were treated at the Royal Marsden Hospital for transitional cell carcinoma of the bladder by interstitial irradiation, using either gold-198 or tantalum-182 sources, with follow-up for 3–21 years. Thirty-three patients were excluded from this study because of inadequate information in the patients' notes to give a clinical T category (TX, 16 cases) or because tumour tissue was no longer available for pathological review (17 cases).

The available histopathological material (biopsy and/or tissue removed at open operation) in the remaining 147 patients has been independently reviewed by one of us (P.A.T.) and assessed according to the criteria of the UICC classification of 1978. Attention was given to cellular differentiation, invasion beyond the lamina propria and the presence of carcinoma in situ in the adjacent epithelium (*Table 14.1*). It is evident that the clinical category of the group with T1 tumours

Table 14.1
COMPARISON OF CLINICAL T AND BIOPSY STAGE BY HISTOLOGICAL GRADE

Histological grade	T1 pTa	T1 pT1	T1 ≥pT2*	T2 pTa	T2 pT1	T2 ≥pT2*	T3 pTa	T3 pT1	T3 ≥pT2*
G1	22	1	0	0	0	1	0	0	1
G2	10	7	2	2	17	14	0	0	5
G3	0	3	2	0	11	31	0	2	16

*Might be pT2 or greater as it is impossible to determine precise depth of muscle invasion on biopsy

was confirmed by the pathological findings in all except four cases, which showed a more advanced stage with muscle invasion. In only 39% of the patients with T2 tumours was it possible to demonstrate, in the limited material available for review, actual tumour invasion into muscle. However in only two of these patients was there no evidence of any infiltration at all.

RESULTS

Survival according to T stage is recorded in *Table 14.2*. At 5 years the survival rate of patients with T1, T2 and T3 tumours was 69%, 41% and 21%, respectively. For patients with T1 and T2 tumours the depth of tumour invasion and the histological grade were each of comparable prognostic significance (*Tables 14.3, 14.4*).

The occurrence of flat carcinoma in situ (pTis) in the epithelium immediately adjacent to the tumour was, as expected, not found in patients with G1 tumours. When such mucosal changes were associated

Table 14.2
CLINICAL STAGE AND ACTUARIAL SURVIVAL

Clinical stage	Total number of cases	Percentage alive after 5 years	N	Percentage alive after 10 years
T1	47	69	28	40
T2	76	41	39	21
T3	24	21	4	11
Total	147	46	71	25

N= number of patients alive at 5 years and valid for assessment at 10 years by actuarial method

Table 14.3
ACTUARIAL SURVIVAL OF T1 AND T2 PATIENTS ACCORDING TO EXTENT HISTO–
LOGICAL INVASION

Histopathological classification	Total cases	Percentage alive after 5 years	N*	Percentage alive after 10 years
pTa	34	73	21	45
pT1	39	57	16	29
pT2	50	33	13	15

*See footnote *Table 14.2*

Table 14.4
ACTUARIAL SURVIVAL OF T1 AND T2 PATIENTS ACCORDING TO HISTOLOGICAL
GRADE

Histological grade	Total cases	Percentage alive after 5 years	N*	Percentage alive after 10 years
G1	24	78	14	50
G2	52	53	21	25
G3	47	37	15	20

*See footnote *Table 14.2*

Table 14.15
FLAT CARCINOMA IN SITU: INFLUENCE ON 5 YEAR ACTUARIAL SURVIVAL (G2/G3
CASES ONLY)

Classification	pTis negative		pTis positive	
	Total cases	Percentage of patients surviving after 5 years	Total cases	Percentage of patients surviving after 5 years
T1 (G1)	23	82	—	—
T1 (G2/G3)	15	65	9	56
T2 (G1)	1	100	—	—
T2 (G2/G3)	59	39	16	48
Total G1	24	83	—	—
Total G2/G3	74	44	25	50

with G2 or G3 tumours, there was no significant difference in survival for both T1 or T2 cases (*Table 14.5*).

The only other histological factor of prognostic significance was the occurrence of lymph node metastases discovered at the time of implantation in 9/11 patients in whom suspicious pelvic nodes were biopsied. This was associated with an extremely poor prognosis, only one patient surviving beyond 1 year.

After interstitial therapy, 45% of the T1 patients, 38% of the T2 patients and 50% of the T3 patients developed local recurrences in the bladder, which were treated by various procedures as shown in *Table 14.6*. At the time of writing, 21 of the 47 T1 cases, 16 of the 76 T2 and two of the 24 T3 cases are alive, with follow-up varying between 3 – 21 years (*Table 14.7*).

Table 14.6
TREATMENT OF RECURRENT TUMOUR IN THE BLADDER

Number of recurrences and treatment	Original stage T1	Original stage T2	Original stage T3
Recurrences	21/47	29/76	12/34
Closed cystodiathermy	9	12	3
Radiotherapy	0	8	3
Cystectomy	7	3*	1
Symptomatic	5	9	7

*Including 1 partial cystectomy

Table 14.7
STATUS AT LAST OBSERVATION BY INITIAL CLINICAL CATEGORY

Status	Original stage T1 (N = 47)	Original stage T2 (N = 76)	Original stage T3 (N = 24)
Alive (3–21 yr)			
All cases	21 (45%)	16 (21%)	2 (8%)
Disease-free	14 (30%)	15 (20%)	2 (8%)
Dead	26	60	22
Local disease ± metastases	8 (17%)	34 (45%)	16 (67%)
Metastases only	0 (0%)	3 (4%)	3 (13%)
2nd primary	1 (2%)	7 (9%)	0 (0%)
Other causes	17 (36%)	16 (21%)	3 (13%)

The principal causes of death, other than bladder cancer, were respiratory and cardiovascular disease. There was also a high incidence of second malignant tumours unrelated to the bladder.

Complications of treatment were usually minor (*Table 14.8*), and there were only two post-operative deaths (1.4%). The most frequent complication was ureteric reflux, but in only three of the 36 patients in whom this was demonstrated was there any serious, non-lethal alteration in renal function and this was invariably associated with recurrent infection (Williams *et al.,* 1971). Post-operative suprapubic leakage of urine was occasionally a problem but usually ceased within 10 days, although one patient with a T3 tumour died three months post-operatively with fungating tumour. Tumour implant in the scar

Table 14.8
COMPLICATIONS OF TREATMENT

Complication	T1 (N = 47)	T2 (N = 76)	T3 (N = 24)	Total (N = 147)
Operative death	0	2	0	2 (1.4%)
Suprapubic urinary leak	2	6	4	12 (8.2%)
Ureteric reflux	5	23	8	36 (25%)
Scar implant	0	2	1	3 (2%)

was rare and occurred in only three (2%) patients: all three patients had a G3 bladder tumour associated with pTis. The scar recurrences were treated by excision and external beam radiotherapy and one patient survived for 15 years. The 5-year survival rate of the 42 patients who were treated with tantalum-182 (60%) was superior to that of the 105 patients who received gold-198 (42%). This was most evident in patients with T1 tumours. On the other hand, there was a better survival for patients with T3 tumours treated with gold-198 (*Table 14.9*).

Table 14.9
INFLUENCE OF TYPE OF ISOTOPE ON 5-YEAR SURVIVAL

Isotope	Number of cases	T1	Number of cases	T2	Number of cases	T3
Tantalum-182	13	100%	23	55%	6	0%
Gold-198	34	58%	53	35%	18	24%

Table 14.10
INFLUENCE OF AGE ON 5-YEAR SURVIVAL

Stage	Number of cases	<60	Number of cases	60–64	Number of cases	65–75	Number of cases	>75
T1	15	87%	10	60%	13	54%	8	55%
T2	21	52%	16	46%	24	28%	15	33%
T3	10	20%	2	0%	8	38%	4	0%
Total	46	56%	28	47%	45	37%	27	35%
Total*	45	58%	20	65%	34	48%	20	50%

*(Excluding deaths due to causes other than bladder tumour)

Survival was worse with increasing age, mainly because of deaths from disease other than carcinoma of the bladder (*Table 14.10*).

DISCUSSION

The results reported here for tantalum-182 and for gold-198 sources in the treatment of bladder cancer, confirm and enlarge on those published previously from the Royal Marsden Hospital (Bloom 1960; Bloom and Wallace 1971). Precise comparison of these results with those reported from other centres is difficult as most series were treated before the UICC classification was introduced. This problem is exemplified by the report from the London Hospital by Dix *et al.* (1970). Overall survival at 5 years in that series was 57% compared with 46% in the Marsden study. Survival of patients with G1 tumours in the Marsden series (78% at 5 years) was similar to that in patients with papillary differentiated tumours in the London Hospital series (78%). The survival of patients with G3 tumours in the Marsden series or solid anaplastic tumours in the London Hospital series was 37% and 30% respectively.

A more recent study, taking into account the UICC classification, was published from Rotterdam by Werf-Messing (1978). Overall, with the exception of T2 tumours, our results at 5 years were comparable with those of the Rotterdam series (T1 69% vs 75%; T2 42% vs 55%; T3 21% vs 24%). However, the incidence of death from disease other than bladder cancer (29%) and the average age (65 years) in the Marsden series was higher than in the Rotterdam cases (13% and 63 years) and may have contributed to the difference between the two series. Of interest was the lack of prognostic significance of flat in situ change in the mucosa adjacent to the tumour, reported in the present study, a feature also noted by Werf-Messing (1978). This suggests that the wider local effect from interstitial irradiation compared with resection may have exerted some controlling influence on the premalignant changes in the surrounding tissue. We know of no comparable observations in relation to treatment by transurethral resection or cystodiathermy.

There have been no previous reports in which the results of two different interstitial techniques have been compared in the same centre. The somewhat better results using the more precise linear tantalum-182 wire sources compared with the less precise multiple gold-198 grains in T1 and T2 tumours is therefore of considerable interest. On the other hand, in T3 tumours the better survival following the use of gold-198 grains may have been attributable to the more effective, although irregular, irradiation of a larger volume of tissue than was possible with a more precise single plane of tantalum-182 wires.

For the T1 tumours, there is little difference between the 5-year results for interstitial irradiation and those reported for transurethral resection (Miller *et al.,* 1969; Whitmore, 1979). It would seem that, with the ready availability of modern equipment for endoscopic resection, there is no justification for the use of interstitial irradiation for this type of tumour. On the other hand, interstitial therapy may substantially reduce the risk of recurrence in the more aggressive, less well-differentiated superficial tumours. The possible inadequacy of purely endoscopic techniques in patients with high-grade tumours is well brought out by Miller *et al.* (1969) from the Bristol Bladder Tumour Registry. These authors report a mortality rate of 37% from tumour extension among 278 patients treated by transurethral diathermy or resection, compared with only 2% of 466 patients with well-differentiated lesions treated by the same technique. Furthermore, comparison of results of interstitial therapy with those reported for cystectomy alone, radiation alone or combined radiation and cystectomy (*see* general review by Whitmore, 1979) shows that even these more radical procedures appear to be no better for T1 tumours. However, it must be remembered that megavoltage irradiation and cystectomy would not be used for patients with superficial tumours until they had failed simpler treatments such as transurethral cysto-diathermy. At present it would seem that the main role for interstitial radiotherapy is in the management of T2 bladder tumours, following which the results are equal to those reported for more radical procedures including cystectomy (*see* reviews by Hendry and Bloom, 1976; Whitmore, 1979). In addition, with implant techniques there is greater sparing of normal tissues, compared with external beam therapy, and the former, while offering the opportunity to avoid cystectomy, does not preclude the use of more radical procedures if subsequently required.

The limited depth of radiation penetration possible using a single-plane radioactive implant means that this treatment would not be suitable for most patients with T3 tumours, by virtue of the size and thickness of the lesions, and because of the high incidence of lymph node metastases. However, we have treated 24 such cases because they were thought initially to be T2 but were found at operation to be T3, or were deliberately selected for an implant as a palliative procedure. The 5-year survival rate of 21% for these patients was at least comparable to that following radical external beam therapy or cystectomy alone. In the Rotterdam experience with interstitial therapy, for T3 cases Werf-Messing (1968) reported a 5-year survival rate of only 10%. However, as a result of a high incidence of scar recurrence, she added limited pre-operative external beam irradiation (350 rad × 3 immediately before the implant) and reported reduced local recurrences and a surprisingly high 5-year survival rate of 35% for such cases. This encouraged her to explore a policy of more extensive combined therapy, using interstitial therapy and split-course external beam irradiation as follows: 350 rad pre-operative, implant and then, 3 weeks later, 3000 rad in 3 weeks (Werf-Messing 1979, personal communication). Another possible approach for selected T3 tumours would be a combination of interstitial therapy with chemical radiosensitizers or/and cytotoxic agents. In the meantime, we would not recommend interstitial irradiation alone for T3 tumours (Bloom, 1978) because of the high risk of death from pelvic disease in our series, and also that of Werf-Messing (1968), compared with experience following pre-operative external beam therapy and elective cystectomy. An additional argument against interstitial techniques is the obvious ineffectiveness of such treatment in the management of patients with lymph node metastases. In this series, only 1/9 patients found to have histologically confirmed nodal metastases survived for 1 year compared with 34% of patients with persistent positive nodes after whole pelvic irradiation and elective cystectomy in the Institute of Urology Trial (*see* Chapter 17).

CONCLUSIONS

Results in this series of patients with bladder tumours treated by interstitial radiation show that the main indications for this technique is in the management of T2 lesions. However, the local failure rate is 38% and further improvement of results may be achieved by limited supplementary external beam therapy, either before the implant, or after the procedure when more precise information on the extent of the disease is available. There appears to be no advantage for this technique over endoscopic surgery in patients with T1 tumours, unless the observation in this series of possible control of adjacent areas of flat in situ disease can be confirmed. Interstitial therapy alone would appear to be a totally inadequate approach for the majority of T3 tumours. Such lesions warrant a more intensive regional and systemic attack, although future results from using a combination of interstitial irradiation and external beam therapy may provide a challenge to those achieved by pre-operative external beam therapy and elective cystectomy.

REFERENCES

BLOOM. H.J.G. (1960). Treatment by interstitial irradiation using tantalum[182] wire. *British Journal of Radiology,* **33**, 471–479

BLOOM, H.J.G. (1978). Local regional and systemic attack on bladder cancer. *International Journal of Radiation, Oncology, Biology and Physics,* **4**, 533–537

BLOOM, H.J.G. and WALLACE, D.M. (1971). Tumours of the urinary tract. In *Handbuch der Medizinischen Radiologie,* pp. 454–466, Berlin; Springer Verlag

CARVER, J.H. (1959). Interstitial radiation in the treatment of selected cases of cancer of the bladder. *British Journal of Urology,* **31**, 313–316

DIX, V.W., SHANKS, W., TRESIDDER, G.G., BLANDY, J.P., HOPE-STONE, H.F. and SHEPHEARD, B.G.F. (1970). Carcinoma of the bladder: treatment by diathermy snare incision and interstitial irradiation. *British Journal of Urology,* **42**, 213–228.

HENDRY, W.F. and BLOOM, H.J.G. (1976). Urothelial neoplasia: present position and prospects. In *Recent Advances in Urology.* Ed. by W.F. Hendry, Vol. 2, pp. 245–292. Edinburgh; Churchill Livingstone

HODT, H.J., SINCLAIR, W.K. and SMITHERS, D.W. (1952). A gun for interstitial implantation of radioactive gold grains. *British Journal of Radiology,* **25**, 419–421

JACOBS, A. (1949). The treatment of cancer of the bladder by radium. (1949) *British Journal of Radiology,* **22**, 393–398

MILLER, A., MITCHELL, J.P. and BROWN, N.J. (1969). The Bristol Bladder Tumour Registry. *British Journal of Urology,* **41**, supplement February

POOLE-WILSON, D.S. (1957). Surgery and irradiation in the treatment of bladder cancer. *British Journal of Urology,* **29**, 244–250

RICHES, E.W. (1958). Malignant disease of the urinary tract (Lettsomian lectures). *Transactions of the Medical Society of London,* **74**, 77–140

WERF–MESSING, B. VAN DER (1978). Cancer of the urinary bladder treated by interstitial radium implant. *International Journal of Radiation, Oncology, Biology and Physics,* **4**, 373

WALLACE, D.M., STAPLETON, J.E. and TURNER, R.C. (1952). Radioactive tantalum wire implantation as a method of treatment for early carcinoma of the bladder. *British Journal of Radiology,* **25**, 421–424

WHITMORE, W.F. (1979). Management of bladder cancer. In *Current Problems in Cancer,* Vol 4, No. 1. Ed. by R.C. Hickey. Chicago; Year Book Medical Publishers

WILLIAMS, G., WALLACE, D.M., BLOOM, H.J.G. and STEVENSON, J.J. (1971). Vesico-ureteric reflux following interstitial irradiation of the urinary bladder. *Proceedings of the Royal Society of Medicine* (1971). **64**, 64–66

15

Radical Radiotherapy and Salvage Cystectomy in the Treatment of Invasive Carcinoma of the Bladder

H.F. Hope-Stone, J.P. Blandy, R.T.D. Oliver and H. England

INTRODUCTION

Treatment of patients with advanced but operable invasive carcinoma of the bladder is still a subject of considerable controversy. Partial cystectomy, transurethral resection, total cystectomy and radiotherapy have all been used singly in the past (for review, *see* Whitmore, 1979). Whitmore (1975) was the first to demonstrate, by comparison of results from his own sequentially treated patients, that the combination of radiotherapy and radical cystectomy was better than either treatment alone. Subsequently, four other studies including two controlled trials supported this observation (Wallace and Bloom, 1976; Miller, 1977; Slack *et al.*, 1977; Werf-Messing, 1979), and led to greater acceptance of a combination of total cystectomy and radiotherapy as the treatment of choice for T3 bladder cancer. However, in the largest of the randomized trials, the advantage of such combined treatment over radiotherapy alone was demonstrated only in patients who were under the age of 65 years (Wallace and Bloom, 1976). Less attention has been paid to an interesting finding of this study, namely that a small selected group of patients undergoing salvage cystectomy after failed radical radiotherapy, did considerably better than those having pre-operative radiotherapy and elective cystectomy.

Over the past 20 years at the London Hospital, where more than half of the bladder cancer patients were over 65 years old and severe chest disease was frequent, the high morbidity of cystectomy encouraged us to rely almost entirely on radical radiotherapy, reserving cystectomy for those who failed to respond. This paper presents our experience with this approach.

METHODS

Diagnosis and staging

All patients had a chest X-ray, intravenous urogram, blood count and urea and electrolytes, and were staged according to the UICC TNM classification (Wallace *et al.*, 1975), except that only the minority of

Table 15.1
THE LONDON HOSPITAL BLADDER CANCER STUDY

Stage at start of radiotherapy	Number of cases
T1	90
T2	132
T3	220
T4	262

patients proceeding to salvage cystectomy underwent lymphography. *Table 15.1* summarizes the stage of patients at beginning of radiotherapy.

Radiotherapy technique

Megavoltage irradiation with a fixed head Telecobalt unit incorporating a Johns collimator was standard during the period under review. Localization of the tumour was carried out using skin marks and cystogram, with AP, PA and lateral films. A 3-field pin and arc technique was used, and a typical isodose curve is shown in *Figure 15.1*. Field sizes were of the order of 8 × 8 cm, up to 10 × 12 cm, the aim being to treat only the bladder with a 1–2 cm margin around. The bladder was emptied before each treatment. The standard dose of 5000–5500 rad (depending on the field size) was given in 20 daily fractions, 5 days a week, treating all the fields each day. This gave a rectal dose of less than 4500 rad. Patients were treated as outpatients, except when there was co-existing physical disability or inability to tolerate daily travel.

Although 5000–5500 rad was the standard treatment, some patients received higher doses, either as a result of participation in multicentre trials, or preliminary evaluation of new dose schedules. One-third received less than the standard dose, mostly those patients over the age

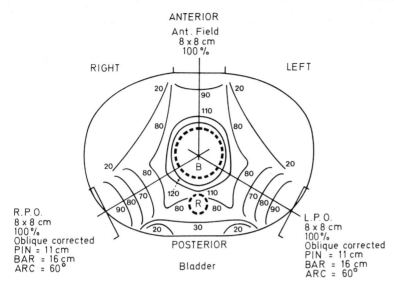

RIGHT   LEFT

ANTERIOR

Ant. Field
8 x 8 cm
100 %

POSTERIOR

Bladder

R.P.O.
8 x 8 cm
100 %
Oblique corrected
PIN = 11 cm
BAR = 16 cm
ARC = 60°

L.P.O.
8 x 8 cm
100 %
Oblique corrected
PIN = 11 cm
BAR = 16 cm
ARC = 60°

Figure 15.1 Calculated isodose curve for treating bladder with cobalt-60

of 70 years with advanced T4 tumours, although a few failed to receive the prescribed dose because of tumour progression during treatment or development of severe local symptoms.

Support of Patients on Radiotherapy

Severe urinary frequency and dysuria were the most distressing symptoms which patients developed during or shortly after therapy. These were controlled by keeping the urine alkaline with mist. sodium citrate, and advising patients to stop taking alcohol while on treatment, although occasionally emepronium bromide or pyridium was necessary. We treated urinary infection before irradiation in order to reduce symptoms and the risk of chronic radiation cystitis. Occasionally, severe symptoms required catheterization during the last few days of treatment, but it was rarely necessary to stop treatment because of urinary symptoms.

Tenesmus and diarrhoea were the other most frequent side-effects, but these were seldom important except in patients who had undergone previous abdominal surgery, or had diverticulitis or ulcerative colitis, in whom the effects of radition were more serious because adhesions restricted bowel mobility. In most patients, the bowel symptoms were controlled by symptomatic treatment with kaolin and morphine mixture, codeine phosphate or small doses of diphenoxylate.

Follow-up

Check cystoscopy was first performed 3 months after completion of radiotherapy, repeated at 3-monthly intervals for the first 2 years, 6-monthly intervals for the next 3 years, and annually thereafter as long as the bladder remained clear of tumour. There were three indications for cystectomy: (1) failure to show any response at 3 months; (2) persistent tumour at 6 months despite previous evidence of response; and (3) local recurrence in the bladder after previous complete response. The surgical technique used in this series has been described elsewhere (Blandy, 1978), and was a standard type of radical cystectomy with ileal conduit diversion, the urethra being removed en bloc only in patients with multifocal tumour.

RESULTS

Computation of Results

Data were extracted from the patients' notes and a computerized actuarial analysis of survival was done using programmes developed from the Vogelback computing centre, Northwestern University Statistical Package for Social Sciences.

Response to Treatment and Survival by Stage and Histology

The complete response rate of patients with T4 tumours was significantly lower than that of all other stages, but there was little difference between T1, T2 and T3 tumours (*Table 15.2*). In terms of survival, although stage T1 patients do significantly better than all other groups,

Table 15.2

INFLUENCE OF T STAGE ON PATIENT'S RESPONSE TO TREATMENT

Stage	N	Complete response (%)	Good partial response (%)	Minor or non-response (%)
T1	82	49	22	29
T2	121	48	26	26
T3	196	42	25	33
T4	224	6	30	64

and stage T4 patients significantly worse, there was no difference between survival of T2 and T3 patients (*Figure 15.2*).

Patients with pure transitional cell carcinoma survived better than

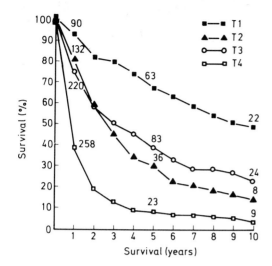

Figure 15.2 Bladder cancer survival and tumour stage

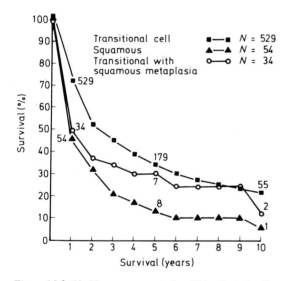

Figure 15.3 Bladder cancer survival and histological cell type

those whose biopsy showed squamous cell carcinoma or squamous metaplasia (*Figure 15.3*).

For all stages, deaths from the local effects of primary tumour were more frequent than death with clinically demonstrable metastases. The incidence of death from local disease was highest in patients with T4 tumours and squamous cell carcinoma (*Tables 15.3, 15.4*).

Table 15.3

DISEASE STATUS AT LAST OBSERVATION*

Status	Percentage of patients			
	T1 N = 90	T2 N = 132	T3 N = 220	T4 N = 262
Alive	48	23	29	4
(% of living patients disease free)	(71)	(87)	(79)	(55)
Dead				
Local disease	21	25	23	40
Local disease + metastases	10	18	15	31
Metastases	2	5	5	8
Other	16	25	23	14

*Follow-up from 5 to 15 years

Table 15.4

DISEASE STATUS AT LAST OBSERVATION: COMPARISON OF SQUAMOUS CARCI–NOMA WITH OTHER BLADDER CANCER

Status	Squamous carcinoma N = 54		All other bladder cancer N = 690	
Alive	6	11%	158	23%
Dead				
Local disease	20	37%	189	27%
Local + metastases	15	28%	138	20%
Metastases	1	2%	41	6%
Other	12	22%	164	24%

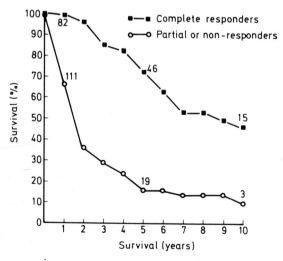

Figure 15.4 Influence of response to radiotherapy on actuarial survival of patients with T3 bladder cancer

Influence of response to treatment on patient survival

The initial response to therapy was the most important prognostic indicator of patient survival, irrespective of stage. When patients responded so well that no residual tumour could be found at cystoscopy 6 months after radiotherapy, 65% were still alive at 5 years, compared with only 14% of those who had shown partial or no response ($P <$ 0.001). This difference between responders and non-responders was demonstrable for all stages, but was most striking for T3 tumours (*Figure 15.4*).

Place of Salvage Cystectomy

Salvage cystectomy was undertaken in 8% of patients in this series, either after failure to respond completely to radiotherapy or on recurrence after an initial complete response. A significant benefit from salvage surgery was demonstrated in the non-responders, i.e. for those who failed to respond completely to radiation. This benefit was demonstrable in all stages (*Table 15.5*). Mortality within the first 3 months

Table 15.5
VALUE OF SALVAGE SURGERY IN RADIOTHERAPY RESPONDER AND NON-RESPONDER PATIENTS

Patient	*T3 cases*		*All stages*	
	Number of cases	*Actuarial survival at 5 years*	*Number of cases*	*Actuarial survival at 5 years*
Complete responder (no surgery)	71	76% (50)*	155	68% (76)
Complete responder (salvage surgery)	7	80% (5)	24	70% (16)
Partial or non-responder (salvage surgery)	16	31% (5)[a]	32	38% (12)
Partial or non-responder (no salvage surgery	71	12% (6)[b]	179	15% (23)

a vs b: $P < 0.001$
*Figures in parentheses denote the number of cases at risk at 5 years

of salvage cystectomy (13/58, 22%) was similar to that found in the small group of patients treated in this period by elective cystectomy after pre-operative radiotherapy (3/18, 17%).

Influence of Radiation Dosage on Response and Survival

Response and survival increased with increasing radiation dose up to 5500 rad. There was no evidence of improvement of results by further increase in the radiation dose (*Table 15.6*). Serious complications of

Table 15.6

INFLUENCE OF RADIATION DOSAGE ON 5-YEAR SURVIVAL

Stage	Radiation dose (rad)			
	< 5000	5000	5500	≥ 6000
T1	16* (75%)†	35 (49%)	30 (90%)	3 (33%)
T2	22 (18%)	61 (25%)	26 (33%)	16 (51%)
T3	57 (28%)	74 (41%)	55 (42%)	32 (40%)
T4	177 (8%)	39 (5%)	19 (8%)	10 (10%)

* No of cases studied
† Survival at 5 years

radiation therapy were infrequent, one patient requiring cystectomy because of severe bleeding and another because of a contracted bladder, both in the absence of tumour. More minor complications were seen in patients who received more than 5500 rad, using a wider field of irradiation to include the iliac nodes for the first 4000 rad.

Patient Age and Survival

This series is unusual in that age was not an absolute contraindication to treatment. The severity of local symptoms and general state of health were the main criteria used to select patients over the age of 75 years for treatment. The oldest patient treated was 91 years old. Although patients under 55 years have survived longest, irrespective of

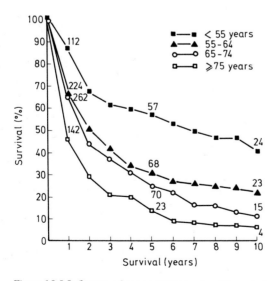

Figure 15.5 Influence of age on patient actuarial survival

Table 15.7

INFLUENCE OF AGE ON 5-YEAR SURVIVAL

Stage		Patient's age (years)		
	< 55	55–64	65–74	> 74
T1	28* (89%)†	29 (55%)	24 (60%)	10 (57%)
T2	18 (70%)	47 (29%)	40 (30%)	28 (0%)
T3	29 (51%)	68 (47%)	85 (33%)	39 (22%)
T4	29 (21%)	75 (6%)	99 (5%)	60 (5%)

* Number of cases studied
† Survival at 5 years

tumour stage, (*Figure 15.5; Table 15.7*) almost half the patients over 75 years old survived 1 year, and 20% were alive at 4 years.

DISCUSSION

The results of treatment of T3 tumours reported here, in an unselected series, following radical radiotherapy with selected salvage cystectomy for all ages (37% uncorrected 5-year survival) are at least comparable to the best that have been achieved using pre-operative radiotherapy and salvage cystectomy reported by others. Among the proponents of primarily planned combined treatment in younger and more selected series, only Miller (1977) (46%, 5-year survival) and Werf-Messing (1979) (45%, 5-year survival) have reported somewhat better results*. The reported operative mortality of cystectomy has fallen to below 10% since the patients reviewed in this study were treated, with the introduction of intravenous feeding, better anaesthesia and more intensive antibiotic therapy (Vinnicombe and Abercrombie, 1978; McCarron and Marshall, 1979). The psychological adjustment of most patients is satisfactory, although the long-term problems of ileal loop diversion, such as chronic pyelonephritis and appliance leakage, are by no means negligible (*see* page 183). In addition, the total loss of sexual potency in the male, although this is something which most patients will accept when faced with the situation, justifies the search for alternative forms of therapy, particularly for the younger patient. As only 8% of the patients in this series underwent cystectomy, it is possible that routine surgery can be avoided. At the same time, these results might have been better if salvage cystectomy had been offered earlier in patients with residual disease, particularly if they had squamous

*Editor's Footnote: the most recent analysis of the Institute of Urology T3 trial reports an uncorrected 5-year survival of 39% (44% corrected) for pre-operative radiation with cystectomy for 77 out of 91 patients who completed pre-operative radiotherapy and cystectomy (*see* Chapter 17).

tumours, in view of the high incidence of death without clinically demonstrable metastases (*Tables 15.3, 15.4*).

The radiation dosage (5500 rad in 28 days) which produced the best survival (42% at 5 years; *see Table 15.6*) used the smallest fields. This might have contributed to the improved results in this series compared with other reports on the use of radical radiotherapy, because most previous studies have used large fields, treating the whole pelvis. The only other direct evidence in favour of using smaller fields comes from the results of pre-operative radiation and cystectomy reported by Werf-Messing (1979), who, while using larger fields than in this series, found an inverse relationship between field size and survival, particularly in patients over 65 years of age (which was the case in more than 50% of patients in this series).

The justification for irradiating the whole pelvis was that there was a lower incidence of lymph node metastases in patients after pre-operative radiotherapy than in those who underwent cystectomy without radiotherapy (Whitmore *et al.,* 1977). Evidence that metastatic nodes do respond to radiotherapy comes from two sources: Wallace and Bloom (1976) observed that the incidence of positive nodes in patients whose primary tumour did not respond to radiotherapy was the same as that in Whitmore's cases of cystectomy without previous radiotherapy, but substantially less when the primary tumour responded to treatment. Turner *et al.* (1976) studied pelvic lymph nodes after cystectomy and correlated the pathological findings with the pre-radiotherapy lymphography: the false-positive rate in patients receiving radiation (5 out of 13 lymphogram-positive patients had no tumour in the lymph nodes) was much higher than that in patients who underwent cystectomy without pre-operative radiotherapy (1 out of 15 lymphogram-positive patients had no tumour). As only one-third of the patients in that series had positive nodes, there might be a case for restricting the use of wide-field therapy to patients with positive lymphograms, in view of the results presented here and the data of Werf-Messing (1979).

The results of T1 tumours in this series (*Figure 15.2*) is as good as that reported by Whitmore *et al.* (1977) (67%, 5-year survival), who showed that radiotherapy added nothing to surgery alone, although he did not have data on the use of radiotherapy alone for this tumour stage. Undoubtedly, the series reported here is highly selected for patients with either undifferentiated tumours or multiple recurrences (less than 10% of all T1 in our own series (Blandy and England, 1979)) and therefore may not be directly comparable with Whitmore's results.

The fact that T2 tumours in this series did no better than T3 tumours is surprising: it may be a reflection of observer error in assessing depth of muscle layer infiltration or of case selection by the referring surgeons of the more unfavourable T2 tumours on the basis of histology or failed previous local treatment. Detailed study of the histology of these patients is currently in progress in an attempt to resolve this problem. If this lack of difference is confirmed, it would suggest that once there is histological evidence of muscle invasion, a patient should be treated radically with radiotherapy and, if there is no early response, salvage cystectomy should be offered even if no mass is palpable bimanually.

Approaches to treating T4 tumours (with less than 10% survival at 5 years) has been little discussed in the literature. Although much of the tumour is extravesical in these patients, the removal by TUR of as much tumour as possible could be of theoretical importance, because removal of bulk might increase the chance of response to either chemotherapy or radiotherapy, both of which are more effective for a smaller volume of disease. Although many of these patients are old and debilitated, for the younger patient there may be a case for treating them all as T3 tumours. If the tumour fails to respond completely after initial radiotherapy, diagnostic laparotomy should be performed to establish the practical possibility of surgery, as 'fixation' on bimanual examination may prove to be only fibrosis or radiation reaction. A comparison of the inoperability rate (15%) in Whitmore's series of patients (*see page 175*), all of whom underwent surgical exploration whatever the T stage, with the incidence of T4 in this series (35%), suggests that several patients might have benefitted.

Chemotherapy has not yet established a place in the standard management of invasive tumours. The results reported elsewhere in this book demonstrate its value as a palliative treatment in patients with metastases, and also recurrent primary tumours (Part IIIB). At present, two adjuvant studies are in progress, one to evaluate methotrexate, and one doxorubicin and 5-fluorouracil (*see* Chapters 25, 26), but it will be another 5 years before definite conclusions can be established.

Chemotherapy is not without risk or unpleasant side-effects. Given the better survival of complete responders to radiotherapy, a more appropriate area in which to explore the value of new drugs (once they have been shown to have action against measurable metastases) might be for the first recurrence after radiotherapy, or in those patients with known residual disease after cystectomy.

This study shows that radical radiotherapy with selective salvage cystectomy in non-responders can achieve results equal to those of routine cystectomy after pre-operative radiotherapy. The use in this study of relatively small fields, restricting radiation to the bladder, draws attention to the problem of evaluating the benefit of extending the irradiation field to include the pelvic lymph nodes because of the lack of true comparative data.

ACKNOWLEDGEMENTS

We are grateful to our colleagues in the North East Metropolitan region for referring patients for treatment; to colleagues in the London Hospital (A. Paris, B. Mantell and G. Mair) for permission to study patients treated by them; and to Steven Evans for performing the computer analysis.

REFERENCES

BLANDY, J.P. (1978). In *Operative Urology,* pp. 124–141. Oxford; Blackwell Scientific Publications

BLANDY, J.P. and ENGLAND, H.E. (1979). Management of superficial bladder cancer. In *Bladder Tumours and Other Topics in Urological Oncology,* pp. 343–346. Ed. by M. Pavone Macaluso, P.H. Smith and F. Edsmyr. New York; Plenum Press

McCARRON, J.P. and MARSHALL, V.F. (1979). The survival of patients with bladder tumors treated by surgery: comparative results of an old and a recent series. *Journal of Urology,* **122**, 322–324

MILLER, L.S. (1977). Bladder cancer: superiority of preoperative irradiation and cystectomy in clinical stage B2 and C. *Cancer,* **39**, 973–980

SLACK, N.H., BROSS, I.D. and PROUT, G.R. (1977). 5-year follow-up results of a collaborative study of therapies for carcinoma of the bladder. *Journal of Surgical Oncology,* **9**, 393–405

TURNER, A.G., HENDRY, W.F., MacDONALD, J.S. and WALLACE, D.M. (1976). The value of lymphography in the management of bladder cancer. *British Journal of Urology,* **48**, 579–586

VINNICOMBE, J. and ABERCROMBIE, G.F. (1978). Total cystectomy – a review. *British Journal of Urology,* **50**, 488–491

WALLACE, D.M. and BLOOM, H.J.G. (1976). The management of deeply infiltrating (T3) bladder carcinoma: controlled trial of radical radiotherapy versus preoperative radiotherapy and radical cystectomy (first report). *British Journal of Urology,* **48**, 587–594

WALLACE, D.M., CHISHOLM, G.D. and HENDRY, W.F. (1975). TNM Classification for urological tumours (UICC) – 1974. *British Journal of Urology,* **47**, 1–12

WERF-MESSING, B. VAN DER (1979). Radiotherapy and cystectomy in treatment of carcinoma of the bladder. In *Bladder Tumours and Other Topics in Urological Oncology,* p. 281. Ed. by M. Pavone Macaluso, P.H. Smith and F. Edsmyr. New York; Plenum Press

WHITMORE, W.F. (1975). Total cystectomy. In *The Biology and Clinical Management of Bladder Cancer.* Ed. by E.H. Cooper and R.E. Williams, p. 193. Oxford; Blackwell Scientific Publications

WHITMORE, W.F. (1979). Management of Bladder Cancer. *Current Problems in Cancer,* **4**, No. 1

WHITMORE, W.F., JR., BATATA, M.A., GHONEIM, M.A., GRABSTALD, H. and UNAL, A. (1977). Radical cystectomy with or without prior irradiation in the treatment of bladder cancer. *Journal of Urology,* **118**, 184–187

16

Radiotherapy in the Management of Bladder Carcinoma

F. Edsmyr

For the evaluation of the results of therapy of cancer patients, it is of immense importance to collect large series which are followed for a long period under the supervision of well-trained teams. The treatments should ideally be given in conjunction with randomized trials.

Few series which deal with radical radiation therapy of patients with bladder carcinomas comply with the above conditions. During the last 10–15 years, six series followed for 5–10 years and which fulfilled most of these criteria, but were not randomized, have been published

Table 16.1
URINARY BLADDER CARCINOMA RADIOTHERAPY: NON-RANDOMIZED TRIALS

Author	Year	Number of patients	Total number of cases followed 5 years	10 years
Werf-Messing	1965	326	292	–
Caldwell et al.	1967	213	65	–
Frank	1970	181	90	–
Miller	1977	348	348	280
Morrison	1975	540	540	–
Edsmyr et al.	1978	598	598	474

(*Table 16.1*). In addition, four randomized studies have been published during the same period. They have compared orthovoltage X-ray therapy versus high voltage irradiation; the tumour response versus radiation dose rate; irradiation given in air versus irradiation with oxygen at a pressure of 303 kPa; conventionally given irradiation, once

139

Table 16.2
URINARY BLADDER CARCINOMA: RANDOMIZED TRIALS

Author	Year	Total number of patients	Follow-up period (years)	Number at 5 years	Type of therapy
Pointon and Evans	1969	234	5	234	Orthovoltage and megavoltage
Morrison	1975	175	2	–	Dose–tumour response
Kirk *et al.*	1976	27	5	27	Air–oxygen (303 kPa)
Edsmyr *et al.*	1978	157	3	157	Superfractionation vs. conventional fractionation

daily, compared with superfractionated irradiation, given three times daily (*Table 16.2*).

Because of the disappointing results from surgical treatment of patients with advanced bladder carcinomas, radiation therapy was introduced in Stockholm in 1957. Before this, the 5-year survival rate for patients treated by surgery alone was 22% for T2 tumours and 3% for T3 tumours.

FIRST SERIES 1957–1970

Material

This report covers 598 patients given radical irradiation between 1957 and 1970 and followed for at least 5 years. The following criteria were used. The patients were clinically free from metastases and had trans-urethral biopsies and/or other surgical procedures, known to have removed only *part* of the tumour. There was no age limit. The mean age was 65 years and the mean interval from onset of symptoms to irradiation was 12 months. All patients had T3 or T4 tumours, or poorly differentiated T2 lesions. In addition, a few more differentiated tumours with extensive involvement of the whole bladder mucosa, although still pathologically staged T1 or T2, were treated.

Tumour characteristics

To ensure similarity between treatment groups, the cases were divided according to prognostic features:

The extent or stage of the disease

The TNM categories recommended by the Union International Contre le Cancer (UICC) in 1974 were followed.

The largest category of patients (47%) were T3. T2 lesions made up 31% and T4, 22%. In practice it was difficult to distinguish between T1 and T2 tumours, and these were grouped together as T1/T2.

Histopathological tumour grade

The tumour grade was assessed by one histopathologist, according to the recommendation of WHO, into grades 1–3. The largest number of patients had tumours of category T3 and grade 3 (*Table 16.3*).

Table 16.3
T CLASSIFICATION COMPARED WITH GRADING

T	*Grade*		*Total*
	2	*3*	
1/2	79	107	186
3	78	205	283
4	24	105	129
Total	181	417	598

Investigations

Routine staging involved intravenous urography, cystoscopy and bimanual palpation under anaesthesia, and biopsy. Bladder-washing cytology before the primary therapy, and at follow-up investigations, was introduced in 1965.

Barium studies were performed in the majority of cases before treatment, and in 130 patients after therapy, at different intervals up to more than 10 years.

A minority of the patients also underwent lymphography, aortography and cavography, introduced as part of special research projects.

Special research project

In a series of 16 patients, the clinical TNM system was compared with a diagnostic surgical staging, including lymphography, aortography, cavography, laparotomy and biopsies from suspicious lymph nodes in the surrounding area (*Table 16.4*).

Investigation of the upper urinary tract in the cases followed over a long period showed that the appearance of the urinary tract obstruction clearly indicated recurrence of the tumour (Edsmyr *et al.*, 1967).

Investigation showed that irradiation itself does not give rise to vesico-ureteric reflux (Edsmyr and Nilsson, 1965).

Table 16.4

FIRST SERIES 1957–70 : COMPARATIVE STAGING

Clinical stage		Surgical stage	
	T2	T3	T4
T1/2	3[a]	2[a]	–
T3	2	6[a]	2
T4	–	–	1

[a]Lymph node metastasis in one patient

A spectrophotometric investigation was made to determine the amount of bone mineral content of the femoral region before, during and after therapy. The results were normal throughout (Dalén and Edsmyr, 1974).

Method of Treatment

Radiotherapy consisted of external irradiation using either cobalt-60 gamma rays (1957–68) or 6 MV X-rays (1969–70). The calculated mean tumour dose was 6000–7000 rad over 7–8 weeks. Weekly tumour doses of 900–1000 rad were given in daily fractions, 5 days a week. An individual irradiation plan was worked out for each case, based on the anatomical outline of the patient in a horizontal section through the centre of the treatment region. The respective positions of the primary tumour, the rectum and hip joints, were determined by means of clinical and roentgenological examinations.

Six different treatment techniques have been used during the first 3 years. With the aim of reducing the integral dose, an increasing number of patients (and all cases after 1961) have been treated by a three-field technique, using two anterior fields with wedge filters and a direct posterior beam field. The length of the fields was 12 cm. One field was treated each day.

The aim in treatment planning was to deliver to the whole bladder and a wide margin a homogeneous dose of irradiation, and to give as low a dose as possible to regions beyond this volume.

In spite of a number of variables, such as dose output from treatment units, the three-dimensional dose distribution, mobility of organs within the patient, possible change of body contour during treatment and inaccuracy in set-up, the dose to the 'tumour volume' was considered to vary within ± 10% of the calculated average dose. The regional lymph node chains were considered to have received 75% of the average bladder tumour dose.

Results of radiotherapy

In order to compare the results from different centres, the same classification and tumour-grading system has to be followed. The two main systems of classification of patients with bladder carcinoma have been the O-D2 system used in the United States and the TNM system recommended by UICC. Six series have been published during the last 10–15 years, non-randomized and followed long-term. Four used the TNM system, where the analysis showed in general the same results with the exception of the series from Rotterdam (Werf-Messing, 1965) (*Table 16.6*). This series is highly selected, as only the more advanced patients in each stage were treated by external beam irradiation (the less advanced cases received interstitial radiotherapy).

Table 16.6
FIVE-YEAR SURVIVAL RATES IN PATIENTS TREATED BY IRRADIATION. NON-RANDOMIZED STUDIES

Author	Year	Number of patients	*Percentage patients and stage*				
			T1	*T2*		*T3*	*T4*
Werf-Messing	1965	292	12	12		5	1
Frank	1970	90	80	57		31	10
Morrison	1975	540	–	41	–	28	7
Edsmyr *et al.*	1978	598	–	32		22	10
			0	A	B1	B2	C	D1 D2
Caldwell *et al.*	1967	65	–	50	–	–	20	– –
Miller	1977	348	–	–	24	21	18	9 0

Among the four randomized series, Pointon and Evans (1969) could not demonstrate any difference in survival using orthovoltage or high voltage units for T1 to T4 tumours. Morrison (1975) showed that the tumour response rate at 2 years varied from 38–80% with tumour doses of 4250–6250 rad. Kirk *et al.* (1976) could not demonstrate any

Table 16.7
RADICAL RADIOTHERAPY: RANDOMIZED TRIALS

Author	Year	Comments
Pointon and Evans	1969	No difference in survival between orthovoltage and megavoltage in T1–T4 tumours (sparse material)
Morrison	1975	Control rates of the local tumour and complication rates. Tumour response at 2 years, 38–80% at doses of 4250–6250 rad.
Kirk *et al.*	1976	Irradiation in air against 303 kPa hyperbaric oxygen. No difference in survivals < 1910 CRE recommended
Edsmyr	1980	See text

difference in survival using irradiation in air compared with treatment in hyperbaric oxygen (*Table 16.7*).

   Although the survival rate is the important consideration for the clinician, it may not always be a good index of the effectiveness of a local method of treatment. It is, therefore, important to consider both survival rate and local tumour control in assessing the effectiveness of therapy (Morrison, 1975; Miller, 1977).

Survival rate

Miller (1977) pointed out that 5-year all-stage survival rates had limited prognostic value in evaluating radiotherapy because of a high failure rate between the fifth and tenth post-radiation years — more than 50%

Table 16.8
URINARY BLADDER CANCER RADIOTHERAPY 1957–1970:
CORRECTED SURVIVAL RATES (KAROLINKSKA HOSPITAL)

Category	Interval	Number of patients	Percentage survival
T1/2	5	188	31 [a]
	10	151	22
T3	5	283	20 [a]
	10	220	14
T4	5	129	10 [a]
	10	103	4

[a] $P < 0.01$

Table 16.9
RADIOTHERAPY 1957–70: CORRECTED SURVIVAL RATES

Grade	Interval	Number of patients	Percentage survival
G2	5	181	26 [a]
	10	161	19
G3	5	417	18 [a]
	10	313	13

[a] $P < 0.01$

Table 16.10
RADIOTHERAPY 1957–70: CORRECTED SURVIVAL RATES,
T1/2 CASES BY GRADE

Interval	Number of patients	Percentage survival of G2	G3
5	187	34	27
10	151	25	20

Table 16.11
RADIOTHERAPY 1957–70: CORRECTED SURVIVAL RATES,
T3 CASES BY GRADE

Interval	Number of patients	Percentage survival of	
		G2	G3
5	283	23	18
10	220	17	16

Table 16.12
RADIOTHERAPY 1957–70: CORRECTED SURVIVAL RATES,
T4 CASES BY GRADE

Interval	Number of patients	Percentage survival	
		G2	G3
5	129	8	10
10	103	5	4

of deaths during this period being due to cancer. Our results, shown in *Tables 16.8–16.12,* indicate that patients with the higher-grade T categories of transitional cell carcinoma have the worse prognosis.

Local tumour control

In the material from Hammersmith Hospital, London (Morrison, 1975) only 15% of patients died of causes other than cancer during the first 5 years. In our material, 8% of patients died of causes other than cancer during the first 5 years, and another 4% during the period 5–10 years after therapy.

Using bladder-washing cytology as a diagnostic method among asymptomatic patients 5 and 10 years after irradiation, there were some who had positive cytology with malignant cells in the bladder-washings. The incidence of this in different diagnostic stage subgroups is shown in *Table 16.13.*

Table 16.13
FIRST SERIES 1957–70: INFLUENCE OF POSITIVE CYTOLOGY
IN PATIENTS WITH NEGATIVE CYSTOSCOPY

Category	Percentage of patients	
	At 5 years	At 10 years
T1/2	21	9
T3	9	11
T4	7	–
T2–T4	14	8

It was often as long as 5 years or more after first discovery of a positive cytological test for cancer cells before exophytic tumour recurrence was detected in the bladder at follow-up cystoscopy; the majority of patients ultimately died from this tumour. A symptom-free patient, without exophytic tumour at follow-up cystoscopy, should have a cytological bladder-washing test at every subsequent follow-up cystoscopy. This may detect an occult tumour or carcinoma in situ from which a new tumour may later arise. The recent reports that carcinoma in situ is highly responsive to systemic or intravesical chemotherapy (Edsmyr 1980; Chapter 13) make routine cytological follow-up even more important.

Quality of life

In the literature, little or no attention has been paid to quality of life after therapy for patients with malignant tumours. We have assessed the general condition of the patients, including the ability to work and

Table 16.14
QUALITY OF LIFE

Years of follow-up	Number of patients	General condition unaffected (%)	Normal bladder capacity (%)	Mean age (years)
5	123	78	88	68
10	45	89	93	71

enjoy a normal social life, and the bladder capacity following radical radiotherapy. The results at 5 and 10 years after treatment were satisfactory (*Table 16.14*).

Cystectomy after radical radiotherapy

In 47 patients, a simple cystectomy with artificial bladder was performed 6 months to 5 years after irradiation (*Table 16.15*). Thirty-six of these patients died of cancer and four of intercurrent disease (*Table 16.16*). The remaining seven lived for more than 5 years after operation; histology of the bladder in these patients showed no evidence of muscle invasion by persisting tumour. The patients who died of recurrent cancer all had deeply infiltrating tumour growth in the muscle layer of the bladder wall.

Table 16.15
CYSTECTOMY AFTER RADICAL IRRADIATION

Interval, irradiation to cystectomy (months)	Number of patients	Percentage
0– 6	2	4.3
6–12	19	40.4
12–18	9	19.1
18–24	4	8.5
24–30	4	8.5
30–	9	19.2
Total	47	100.0

Table 16.16
CYSTECTOMY AFTER RADICAL IRRADIATION

Interval (years)	Number of deaths	
	Cancer	Intercurrent disease
0–1	15	1
1–2	11	1
2–3	5	–
3–4	4	–
4–5	–	–
5–	1	2
Total	36	4

Bowel complications

One hundred and thirty patients were followed with special reference to bowel complications over a 10-year period after radiotherapy. Barium enemas were performed at regular intervals (*Table 16.17*). The seven patients requiring surgery were operated upon within 3 years of irradiation.

Table 16.17
BOWEL COMPLICATIONS AFTER RADICAL IRRADIATION

Reduced distension	10/130
Proctitis	3/130
Diverticulitis	3/130
Strictures not requiring surgery	3/130
Strictures requiring surgical correction	7/598

Autopsy

In this series, the frequency of autopsies was comparable among the group of patients dying of cancer and those dying from intercurrent disease, being approximately 40% in each group.

SECOND SERIES 1971

There is experimental evidence (Littbrand *et al.,* 1975; Littbrand and Edsmyr, 1976) that the radiosensitivity of tissue cells increases with increasing access to oxygen. With the aim of delivering a larger radiation dose to the tumour tissue without undue damage to the surrounding normal tissues, irradiation was given at a higher total dose, but was divided into a larger number of small individual dose fractions. Since 1971, 150 patients have been randomly allocated to receive either three or one fraction daily. There were no significant differences between the two groups in the distribution of clinical stage, tumour grade or mean age.

Method

The treatments were given by 6 MV X-rays using a three-field technique as in the first series. All fields were irradiated at each treatment session.

Scheme 1. 100 rad given 3 times daily at 4-hour intervals, 5 days per week to a total dose of 8400 rad; the patients were given 2 weeks' rest in the middle of the treatment period.

Scheme 2. 200 rad given once daily, 5 days per week to a total dose of 6400 rad; the patients had a rest of 2 weeks in the middle of the treatment period.

Results

In the group treated according to scheme 1 (71 patients), tumour regression after 6 months was observed in 56% of T2 cases, 63% of T3 and 50% of T4; in scheme 2 (79 patients) the corresponding figures were 49%, 37% and 36% respectively.

Complications

Bowel complications necessitating surgery were observed in five patients receiving the superfractionation treatment and in two of the single daily fraction group. These complications appeared 11–36 months after therapy. Colostomy was performed because of stenosis, fistula or bleeding. Diarrhoea and/or frequency of micturition was only transient in the two groups.

Discussion

The results indicate greater tumour sterilization at 6 months following high-dose irradiation using a superfractionation technique. There appears to be no undue damage to the surrounding tissues and no increase in complications. Although there was a difference in survival rates between the two groups at 1 year, in favour of the superfractionation technique, there was no difference demonstrable at 3 and at 5 years.

REFERENCES

CALDWELL, W.L., BAGSHAW, M.A. and KAPLAN, H.S. (1967). Efficacy of linear accelerator X-ray therapy in cancer of the bladder. *Journal of Urology,* **97**, 294–301

DALÉN, N. and EDSMYR, F. (1974). Bone mineral content of the femoral neck after irradiation. *Acta Radiologica (Therapy, Physics, Biology),* **13**, 97–101

EDSMYR, F. and NILSSON, A. -E. (1965). Vesico-ureteric reflux in connection with supervoltage therapy for bladder carcinoma. *Acta Radiologica (Therapy, Physics, Biology),* **3**, 449–456

EDSMYR, F., GIERTZ, G. and NILSSON, A. -E. (1967). Effect of supervoltage therapy for carcinoma of the bladder on the outflow from upper urinary tract to bladder. *Scandinavian Journal of Urology and Nephrology,* **1**, 247–252

EDSMYR, F., ESPOSTI, P. -L., GIERTZ, G. and LITTBRAND, B. (1978). Radiation treatment of urinary bladder carcinoma. *Urological Research,* **6**, 229–232

FRANK, H.G. (1970). Policy and results of treatment by radiotherapy of carcinoma of the bladder in Leeds. *Clinical Radiology,* **21**, 425–430

KIRK, J., WINGATE, G.W. and WATSON, E.R. (1976). High-dose effects in the treatment of carcinoma of the bladder under air and hyperbaric oxygen conditions. *Clinical Radiology,* **27**, 137–144

LITTBRAND, B. and EDSMYR, F. (1976). Preliminary results of bladder carcinoma irradiated with low individual doses and a high total dose. *International Journal of Radiation, Oncology, Biology, Physics,* **1**, 1059–1062

LITTBRAND, B., EDSMYR, F. and REVESZ, L. (1975). A low-dose fractionation scheme for the radiotherapy of carcinoma of the bladder. *Bulletin du Cancer,* **62**, 241–248

MILLER, L.S. (1977). Bladder cancer: superiority of preoperative irradiation and cystectomy in clinical stages B2 and C. *Cancer,* **39**, 973–980

MORRISON, R. (1975). The results of treatment of cancer of the bladder – a clinical contribution to radiobiology. *Clinical Radiology,* **26**, 67–75

POINTON, R.C.S. and EVANS, C.M. (1969). Clinical trials in malignant disease. 8 – Cancer of the bladder. *Clinical Radiology,* **20**, 95–98

WERF-MESSING, B. VAN DER (1965). Telecobalt treatment of carcinoma of the bladder. *Clinical Radiology,* **16**, 165–172

17

Pre-operative Intermediate-Dose Radiotherapy and Cystectomy for Deeply Invasive Carcinoma of the Bladder: Rationale and Results

H.J.G. Bloom

This chapter deals with the treatment of patients with cancer of the bladder which is infiltrating the deep muscle or perivesical tissue (category T3 cases of the UICC or B_2 and C of the Jewett-Marshall classifications). It does not include cases of infiltrating tumour limited to the superficial muscle (T2 of the UICC or B_1 of the Jewett-Marshall categories) which have been discussed elsewhere (Bloom, 1979).

Radical cystectomy alone rarely achieves more than a 20% 5-year survival rate for patients with T3 cancer of the bladder. Similar results have been produced by radical megavoltage irradiation, although recently some centres have reported 5-year survival rates of 28% (*Table 17.1*). These results for external beam therapy can be achieved with less selection, without hospitalization and without the operative mortality and morbidity, including loss of urinary and sexual function, associated with radical cystectomy.

The results of radical radiotherapy depend more upon case-selection based on size of primary tumour, the precise depth of mural infiltration (deep muscle or perivesical) and the general health of the patient than on specific techniques and skills (Bloom, 1978).

Persistent or recurrent local disease in the bladder or pelvis is to be expected in at least 50–65% of patients with infiltrating bladder cancer following radiotherapy, and in 30–40% treated by cystectomy. These

Table 17.1
RESULTS OF RADICAL RADIOTHERAPY FOR T3 BLADDER
CANCER FROM VARIOUS CENTRES DURING PAST 5 YEARS
(1975–79)

Series	Number of patients	Percentage 5-year survival
Edsmyr (1975)	125	20
Goffinet *et al.* (1975)	218	28
Morrison (1975)	45	28
Miller (1977)	137	20
Reddy *et al.* (1978)	53	17
Backhouse (1979)	124	19
Institute of Urology (1979)	85	31[a]

[a] see page 159

figures reflect the current limits of conventional therapeutic endeavour.
For practical purposes the surgeon can cut out no more, and it would
be dangerous to exceed the doses of radiotherapy now generally
employed for radical treatment. It therefore seems logical to explore
the value of combining the two modalities of irradiation and surgery, in
the hope of achieving more than from either one alone. In patients with
bladder cancer, interest in combined treatment has focussed mainly on
irradiation given pre-operatively, which carries certain practical and
theoretical advantages over such treatment given after surgery.

PRE-OPERATIVE RADIOTHERAPY

The possible beneficial effect of irradiating tumours before their
surgical removal is supported by many laboratory experiments (*Table
17.2*). In clinical practice, the aim of pre-operative irradiation is to
reduce tumour bulk and tumour cell viability before surgery. Actively
growing, well-oxygenated cells at the periphery of the tumour, in
efferent lymphatics and as micrometastases in regional nodes, may be
particularly vulnerable to this limited type of treatment.

Table 17.2
EFFECT OF LOW-DOSE PRE-OPERATIVE IRRADIATION ON
SURVIVAL OF C3H MICE WITH TRANSPLANTED GARDNER
LYMPHOSARCOMA (POWERS AND TOLMACH, 1964)

Treatment	Number of mice	Percentage survival
Nil	50	0
500 rad	50	0
500 rad + op.[a]	116	85
Op.	106	53

[a] Immediate excision

Pre-operative radiotherapy is thus directed towards reducing the risk of tumour recurrence arising from just outside the operative field, from incompletely excised tumour within this field, from tumour spilt in the operation wound and in the pelvic cavity, and as a result of cell dissemination in blood vessels and lymphatics during tumour excision and lymph node dissection. Finally, radical operation will remove any residual radioresistant tumour at the primary site and in regional nodes.

In brief, pre-operative irradiation and radical surgery together attempt to overcome the problems of radioresistance associated with radiotherapy alone, and of borderline inoperability, tumour spill and dissemination during operation associated with surgery alone. By this means it is hoped to gain more effective control of disease in the pelvis and a reduction in iatrogenic metastases. However, no matter how successful pre-operative irradiation may be in achieving these aims, it can have no *direct* effect on already existing metastases outside the irradiated volume, and for this type of spread other approaches are required. On the other hand, there is some evidence that irradiation may release antigens from tumour cells, leading to an increase in host immune response (O'Toole *et al.*, 1972a; 1972b). We can only hope that this may have some beneficial controlling influence on limited residual disease in the primary tumour region and at distant metastatic sites.

TREATMENT FACTORS IN PRE-OPERATIVE RADIOTHERAPY

In planning pre-operative radiotherapy, consideration must be given to dose and fractionation of irradiation, the time in which it is given, volume to be treated, interval between completing radiotherapy and surgery, and the extent of operation.

Dose–Time

Doses of between 4500 and 5000 rad in 4.5–5 weeks appear to be greater than 90% efficient in eradicating established subclinical disease in patients with such tumours as squamous cell carcinoma of the head and neck, cervix, adenocarcinoma of the breast and colo-rectum, and teratoma of the testis. There is now evidence that subradical doses of pre-operative irradiation in the range of 4000–4500 rad may grossly reduce, or even appear to eradicate, quite large primary tumours in the bladder, based on pathological examination of the subsequent surgical specimen.

Radiobiological data relating to cell survival in tissue culture suggest that single doses of only a few hundred rads, before surgery, could be sufficient to destroy the reproductive capacity of a high proportion of tumour cells released into the operative field or into vessels during manipulation. This type of treatment may be given on the same day of operation: in fact, it may be given on the way to the operating room. The term 'flash irradiation' would seem to be more appropriate when applied to this type of treatment, rather than to short courses of irradiation extending over several days.

Doses of pre-operative irradiation in the range of 1000–2000 rad given over a few days may be described as 'low-dose', between 4000 and 4500 rad in 4–5 weeks as 'intermediate-dose', and 5000 rad or more as 'high-dose' treatment, the last being generally associated with salvage cystectomy.

After patients with T3 bladder cancer had been given a dose of 350 rad to the whole pelvis on each of three consecutive days before interstitial therapy, Werf-Messing (1978) reported a reduced incidence of wound recurrence (from 23% to nil) and of distant metastases (from 48% to 9%), associated with an increase in 5-year survival rate from 10% to 42%, compared with results achieved by interstitial therapy alone.

Low doses of irradiation may be sufficient to destroy thin columns of advancing, well-oxygenated cancer cells at the tumour periphery and also small foci of such cells in regional nodes. Much greater doses are needed to sterilize established masses of organized tumour tissue where such factors as blood supply, hypoxia and perhaps other, lesser-known, factors relating to radioresistance have to be reckoned with.

Fractionated irradiation over 4 weeks to a total dose of 4000 rad, represents an attempt to attain a progressively increasing anti-tumour effect in a large tumour mass and in substantial lymph node deposits. It is believed that this may be achieved by producing tumour-stromal changes leading to re-vascularization and re-oxygenation, consequent on continuing tumour reduction. It could be argued that, as the main tumour mass will in any case be removed by operation, a limited and more rapid course of pre-operative irradiation should be sufficient to deal with the more vulnerable proliferating and well-oxygenated cell population at the tumour edge and in small nodal deposits. However, it has been estimated that hypoxic areas may exist in quite small tumour volumes even when only a few millimetres in diameter. There is good evidence that the number of tumour cells capable of reproduction decreases exponentially with increasing total dose of fractionated radiotherapy and, therefore, higher dose and more prolonged pre-operative treatment would be expected to have certain advantages over shorter courses of treatment.

Irradiated volume

Pre-operative irradiation must always extend well clear of the operation field and, because doses within normal tissue tolerance are known to be capable of eradicating subclinical disease, it would seem logical, in patients with T3 bladder cancer, to encompass the whole pelvis and regional nodes up to, and including, the common iliac group. However, this type of extended treatment has not yet been established as being superior to smaller volume therapy.

Whitmore *et al.* (1977b) found a reduced incidence of local tumour recurrence in the Memorial Hospital series when larger portals were used for low- or moderate-dose pre-operative radiotherapy (28% with 15 × 15 cm or larger fields, compared with 48% for smaller fields). On the other hand, Werf-Messing (1979) has recently reported that extension of the irradiated volume to include the common iliac nodes in T3 cases did not improve prognosis. Presumably, with nodal deposits at this level, prognosis is determined principally by distant metastases. Furthermore, the survival rate of patients over 60 years of age was reduced when they were treated with large, as opposed to small volume irradiation, but the difference was not statistically significant.

Interval to surgery

It would seem desirable to reduce delay and perform surgery as soon as possible after pre-operative radiotherapy has been completed, in order to avoid cell proliferation in any residual radioresistant tumour. Delay to surgery, however, does not appear to be critical in this clinical situation. For example, in the Rotterdam bladder cancer study, Werf-Messing (1979) reported that a delay of 11–40 days did not affect prognosis adversely, compared with a delay of less than 10 days: the 5-year survival rates were 43% and 48%, respectively. At the Memorial Hospital, Whitmore *et al.* (1977b) found that recurrence rates after 4000 rad were comparable, following delays to surgery of less than, or greater than, 6 weeks. In patients treated at the same centre with 2000 rad, there was no difference for intervals of less than, or more than, 4 days.

Simple or radical cystectomy following pre-operative irradiation

So far, the results of combined pre-operative radiotherapy and cystectomy appear to be at least comparable for both the simple (Werf-Messing, 1975; Miller, 1977) and also the radical operations (Wallace and Bloom, 1976; Whitmore *et al.,* 1977a). This observation may be interpreted in one of two ways. If lymph nodes are positive, it does not matter whether they are removed or not — the patient is doomed. Alternatively, certain patients with strictly limited or subclinical node metastases are cured by the pre-operative irradiation, in which case subsequent lymphadenectomy is unnecessary. Reports of long-term survival following removal of limited nodal metastases (Dretler *et al.*, 1973; Laplante and Brice, 1973) and also of an operative mortality no greater for radical than that for simple cystectomy, argues in favour of the extended operation. At present, we prefer to continue with the radical operation and gather information regarding the state of regional nodes.

RADIOTHERAPY AND IMMUNOLOGICAL ASPECTS

The degree of lymphoreticular reaction in relation to the primary tumour (Pomerance, 1972) and in regional lymph nodes (Herr *et al.*, 1976) in patients with bladder cancer, may reflect a host immune-defence response. Since a well-marked reaction of this type may influence prognosis favourably, there is the spectre of a possibly harmful suppressive effect on lymphoid tissue produced by large-volume irradiation, radical or pre-operative.

In spite of the prolonged decrease in blood lymphocytes (up to 3 or more years) (O'Toole and Unsgaard, 1979) and the temporary reduction of various skin delayed hypersensitivity reactions in patients after radiotherapy, there is no convincing evidence in clinical practice that a reduction in host resistance consequent on regional radiotherapy is likely to have a significantly adverse effect on prognosis. On the contrary, modern megavoltage irradiation, sometimes involving extensive prophylactic node irradiation, has produced improved survival rates for such tumours as head and neck cancer, testicular tumours, gynaecological cancers, rectal carcinoma, Wilms' tumour and lymphomas. Furthermore, there is some evidence that certain therapeutic procedures, including radiotherapy and chemotherapy, ultimately produce an increased immunological responsiveness in cancer patients as their malignant disease is brought under control.

After radiotherapy for bladder cancer, a strong lymphocyte cytotoxicity, previously depressed or absent, may develop and persist for up to 1 year, except in patients with gross residual disease. Patients treated by pre-operative radiotherapy with cystectomy 4—5 weeks later, maintain their lymphocyte cytotoxicity for at least 3—7 months after operation (O'Toole *et al.*, 1972b). This reaction, which may be the result of the liberation of tumour-cell antigenic material by radiation, may produce a beneficial effect against minimal residual disease. This concept implies that pre-operative irradiation over 4 weeks, with an enforced interval of at least 3—4 weeks to surgery, may produce a more effective immunological host reaction than would be possible if operation were carried out immediately after only a few days of radiotherapy. More work is required to evaluate and perhaps to try to enhance this type of host reaction.

Conclusions regarding pre-operative radiotherapy techniques

The optimum factors for pre-operative irradiation combined with surgery for bladder tumours are not known, but from experience gained in recent years, the following major points emerge. To avoid surgical disaster after pre-operative irradiation, such as wound breakdown, disruption of ureteric anastomosis and bowel fistula, it has been recommended that the dose should not exceed 4000—4500 rad in 4—5 weeks, that operation be performed 3—4 weeks after completing radiotherapy, and that division of ureters should be carried out above the irradiated volume with careful selection of a suitable viable-looking ileal loop for the conduit. With these time scales, tissue re-oxygenation can be established during treatment and a substantial decrease in tumour volume can take place during the interval to operation. Surgery is carried out after the acute reaction has subsided, before late irradiation changes set in and before substantial regrowth of cancer cells can occur.

The overall time for this type of combined therapy involving pre-operative irradiation of 4000 rad in 4 weeks, is approximately 12 weeks. From radiobiological considerations, doses of the order of 1000—2000 rad given over a few days immediately before surgery, may also be of value in reducing the risk of local and distant spread. This shorter treatment would be more economical and would have the great merit of enabling patients to return to a normal life more quickly. On the other hand, with such brief treatment there is virtually no time to benefit from an increased vascularity leading to re-oxygenation and therefore to greater responsiveness in the remaining tumour fraction, which would be the case in longer radiotherapy programmes. Nevertheless, from recent reports, limited pre-operative irradiation does appear to be of value. In studies from the Memorial Hospital (Whitmore *et al.,* 1977b) and also from Montreal (Reid *et al.,* 1976) a pre-operative dose of 2000 rad in 4—5 days has given survival rates which, so far, are not inferior to those following 4000 rad in 4 weeks.

INSTITUTE OF UROLOGY T3 BLADDER TRIAL

In 1966, Mr David Wallace and I decided to embark on a randomized prospective trial at the Royal Marsden Hospital to assess the value of pre-operative irradiation and radical cystectomy for deeply infiltrating bladder cancer (Bloom, 1971).

The choice of 4000 rad in 4 weeks for pre-operative irradiation was based on empirical considerations and on the observations of Dr Whitmore and his colleagues at the Memorial Hospital that radical cystectomy after such doses was not associated with a significant increase in life-threatening complications. The interval of 4 weeks between treatment and operation was selected to permit reasonable time for tumour regression and for recovery of normal tissues from irradiation reaction.

In 1968 we were joined by 7 other London hospitals[a] and came under the sponsorship of the Institute of Urology. These hospitals each contributed 7—10% of the cases, while the Royal Marsden, with its earlier start, entered 44%. The study was closed in 1975. Preliminary results on behalf of the cooperating centres were reported by Wallace and Bloom in 1976. This material has recently been updated for a second report (Bloom *et al.,* 1980). Observations regarding the influence of the combined treatment and of radical irradiation on deeply invasive bladder cancer will be largely drawn from this study.

Results

Between 1966 and 1975 a total of 199 patients entered the trial, of which 189 were eligible for analysis. At June 1979, follow-up information was available in all 189 patients for a period of not less than 4

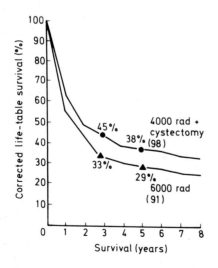

Figure 17.1 Institute of Urology T3 Bladder Carcinoma Trial: corrected life-table survival for all cases randomized to either pre-operative irradiation (4000 rad) and radical cystectomy or radical radiotherapy (6000 rad) (P>0.1)

[a]St. Bartholomews, Charing Cross, Guys, Kings College, The London, Oldchurch and St. Peter's Group.

years. The corrected [a] 5-year actuarial survival rate for all 98 patients, without exclusions, randomized to receive pre-operative irradiation followed by radical cystectomy, was 38%, compared with 29% for 91 patients in the radical radiotherapy group (*Figure 17.1*)(*see* Appendix, p.171).

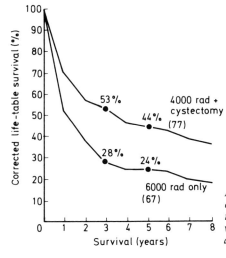

Figure 17.2 Institute of Urology T3 Trial: corrected life-table survival according to actual treatment received – pre-operative irradiation with radical cystectomy or radical radiotherapy alone without salvage cystectomy (P<0.01)

The 5-year survival rate for the 85 patients actually treated by radical radiotherapy was 31%, compared with 44% for 77 patients receiving the planned combined treatment of pre-operative irradiation and radical cystectomy. Of the 85 patients in the radical radiotherapy group, 18 ultimately came to salvage cystectomy with 60% surviving for 5 years. If these patients are removed, only 24% of those treated by radical radiotherapy *alone* remain alive at 5 years, compared with 44% following the planned combined procedure (*Figure 17.2*).

TUMOUR RESPONSE TO RADIOTHERAPY

Pre-operative irradiation

Substantial bladder tumour regression may occur after subradical pre-operative irradiation. From various reports, it appears that 'down-staging' following doses of about 4000 rad in 4 weeks may occur in at least 40% of T3 cystectomy specimens, while in about 30% no residual tumour, or only in situ changes, are found (Prout *et al.*, 1973; Wallace and Bloom, 1976; Whitmore *et al.*, 1977b; Werf-Messing, 1979) (*Table 17.3*). Not surprisingly, following lower doses of irradiation such as 2000 rad with immediate operation, the proportion of cases showing

---

[a]   Age-adjusted rates excluding the theoretically expected deaths from diseases other than cancer of the bladder.

Table 17.3
STAGE REDUCTION ('DOWNSTAGING') OF T3 TUMOURS IN SURGICAL SPECIMEN
FOLLOWING PRE-OPERATIVE IRRADIATION. AFTER 4000–4500 RAD IN 4–4.5
WEEKS IT APPEARS THAT REDUCTION IN STAGE OCCURS IN ABOUT 40% OF CASES,
WHILE COMPLETE REGRESSION OR IN SITU CHANGES ONLY ARE FOUND IN ABOUT
30%

Series	Dose/time (rad/week)	Interval to cystectomy (weeks)	Number of patients	Stage pT0–pT2	pT0–pTis
Prout *et al.* (1973)	4500/4.5	4–15	83	49%	32%
Werf-Messing (1975)	4000/4	1– 6ª	89	68%	32%
Whitmore *et al.*	4000/4	4–12	50	40%	14%
(1977b)	2000/2	1	52	23%	6%
Institute of Urology (1980)	4000/4	4	74	49%	31%

ª Werf-Messing (1979)

tumour regression is reduced (eg. 23% reported by Whitmore *et al.*,
1977b).

In purely surgical cases without previous irradiation one would
expect to find node metastases in some 40–50% of T3 cases. Following
pre-operative radiotherapy in the Institute of Urology trial such metastases were found in only 15 of the 74 cases (20%) in which information regarding lymph nodes was available. In the presence of an
apparently good response of the primary tumour to irradiation, demonstrated by stage reduction, the incidence of positive nodes was only 6%
(2/36), as opposed to 34% (13/38) in radioresistant cases, that is, those
showing no 'downstaging'[b]. This suggests that a good radiation response
in the primary bladder tumour is associated with a good response of
metastases in regional lymph nodes.

This downstaging effect is unlikely to be explained simply by initial
clinical overstaging, because errors of staging are generally in the
direction of *understaging*. Furthermore, the improved response of the
patients showing a reduction in clinical T category following pre-
operative radiotherapy applies, whether the pre-treatment biopsy confirmed muscle invasion by tumour or not (Werf-Messing, 1979).

The failure to find tumour tissue in the surgical specimen following
pre-operative irradiation is, of course, merely an indication of gross
tumour destruction. It does not imply total tumour eradication,
because a limited number of residual malignant cells may be difficult to
find. On the other hand, the discovery of such cells in histological
sections does not necessarily imply that the tumour has not been
effectively sterilized, for the cells may well have lost their reproductive
capacity: irradiation damage may be concealed until they attempt to
undergo division.

[b] These figures, which are based on a new analysis of the pathological data, differ slightly from
those in our previous report (Wallace and Bloom, 1976), when the incidence of positive nodes
in downstaged cases was given as 8% (3/36), and in non-downstaged cases, 37% (15/41).

Radical radiotherapy

Failure to eradicate local disease in patients with infiltrating bladder cancer following radical radiotherapy occurs in at least 50–70% of cases. With doses as high as 7000 rad in 7 weeks, Goffinet *et al.* (1975) reported local failure in 190 of 384 cases (54%). Of the 85 patients treated by radical radiotherapy (6000 rad in 6 weeks) in the Institute of Urology trial the response to irradiation was recorded in 81: 30 (37%) showed no appreciable clinical response to treatment, 19 (23%) had a partial response and, in 32 (40%), complete tumour regression was noted.

PROGNOSIS BY RESPONSE TO RADIOTHERAPY

Pre-operative irradiation

Patients whose tumours respond to pre-operative irradiation have a greater survival than do those showing no such response. Thus, the survival rate in patients with downstaged tumours in the Institute of Urology trial was more than twice as great as that for those patients showing no tumour reduction: at 5 years, 64% of the patients with

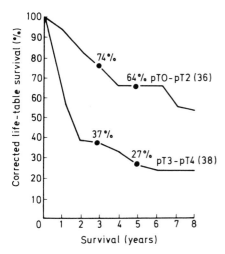

Figure 17.3 Institute of Urology T3 Trial: corrected life-table survival of patients treated by pre-operative irradiation and radical cystectomy according to tumour pathological stage in the surgical specimen. Note the marked difference in survival between downstaged cases ('responders'), compared with those showing no downstaging ('non-responders'). (P<0.01)

pT0-pT2 tumours were alive, compared with only 27% for those with persistent pT3 or pT4 lesions (*Figure 17.3*). A similar trend was reported by Prout *et al.* (1973) and also by Werf-Messing (1979).

Until quite recently, the presence of node involvement in patients with bladder cancer was considered to indicate a hopeless prognosis, and this is supported by the high mortality in patients at the Royal

Marsden Hospital with positive lymphograms (Turner *et al.,* 1976). However, this radiological investigation demonstrates only nodes with gross disease, and our radiological therapeutic endeavours may be of value in patients with nodal micrometastases. There is, in fact, evidence that strictly limited node involvement is compatible with survival for 5 years or more following radical surgery (Dretler *et al.,* 1973; Laplante and Brice, 1973; Clark, 1978).

The 5-year survival rate for node-negative cases treated by pre-operative irradiation and cystectomy in the Institute of Urology trial

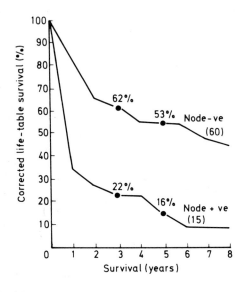

Figure 17.4 Institute of Urology T3 Trial: corrected life-table survival of patients treated by pre-operative irradiation and radical cystectomy according to pelvic node status. Note that 22% of the node-positive cases are still alive at 3 years and 16% at 5 years (P < 0.01)

Table 17.4

INSTITUTE OF UROLOGY T3 TRIAL: CORRECTED LIFE-TABLE SURVIVAL IN PATIENTS TREATED BY PRE-OPERATIVE IRRADIATION (4000 RAD) AND RADICAL CYSTECTOMY, ACCORDING TO RESPONSE OF PRIMARY TUMOUR TO RADIOTHERAPY AND PELVIC NODE STATUS. NOTE THE 3-YEAR SURVIVAL RANGES FROM AS HIGH AS 78% FOR DOWNSTAGED NODE-NEGATIVE CASES TO AS LOW AS 25% FOR THOSE WITH NON-DOWNSTAGED TUMOURS AND POSITIVE NODES.

Downstaged	Nodes	Number of cases [a]	Corrected survival (years) [b] 3	5
Yes	—ve	34	78%	68%
No	—ve	25	43%	32%
No	+ve	13	25%	18%
Yes	+ve	2	(0%)	(0%)

[a] Stage unknown in 3 cases
[b] Life table

was 53%, compared with 16% for those with persistent node involvement (*Figure 17.4*). At the most favourable end of the prognostic scale, we have downstaged primary tumour, node-negative cases with 3- and 5-year corrected survival rates of 78% and 68% respectively, to be compared with only 25% and 18% for unresponsive primary tumour, node-positive cases (*Table 17.4*).

It is important to note that, in 15 patients with persistently positive nodes following pre-operative irradiation, the crude 3- and 5-year survival rates were not negligible, being 22% and 16% respectively (*Figure 17.4*). Reid *et al.* (1976) report a remarkably high 5-year survival rate of 26% among 24 node-positive patients with deeply infiltrating carcinoma, following limited pre-operative irradiation and cystectomy.

Radical irradiation

Prognosis can be related to the degree of tumour response to irradiation, based on cytoscopic appearances and bi-manual examination during the months following radical radiotherapy. Patients in the Institute of Urology trial were classified according to 'complete', 'partial' or 'nil' response. A striking difference was seen at 3 years, the

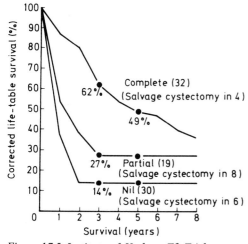

Figure 17.5 Institute of Urology T3 Trial: corrected life-table survival in patients treated by radical radiotherapy according to clinical response as judged at subsequent cystoscopies and bi-manual examinations. The difference between complete and partial or nil response is significant (P < 0.01).

corrected survival rates being 62%, 27% and 14% respectively (*Figure 17.5*). Thus, the survival of patients showing a complete response to irradiation was between four and five times greater than for those showing no such response.

PROGNOSIS BY AGE

The 5-year survival rate* for patients less than 60 years old, receiving the combined treatment, was 49% compared with 25% for radical radiotherapy. The same trend in results was seen in patients aged 60–64 years with 41% and 28% alive, respectively. On the other hand, for patients aged 65–70 years the trend was reversed, with a possible slight advantage for radical irradiation, the 5-year survival rates being 35% and 43% respectively. The difference in treatment results for each of the three age-groups was not statistically significant.

In the Rotterdam study, the 5-year survival rate following pre-operative irradiation and simple cystectomy was 58% for patients under 60 years of age, compared with 40% for older patients (Werf-Messing, 1979).

For patients over 65 years old, we now recommend radical radiotherapy alone, with the possibility of salvage surgery in selected cases if the primary treatment fails.

OPERATIVE MORTALITY FOR COMBINED TREATMENT

In the Institute of Urology study, the operative mortality within 2 months of radical cystectomy following pre-operative radiotherapy was 7.8%, but ranged from 5.5% for patients under 60 years of age to 11% for those aged between 65 and 70 years (Wallace and Bloom, 1976). In the Memorial series, the hospital mortality was 14% for radical cystectomy alone and 11% for the operation performed after 4000 rad (Whitmore *et al.,* 1977a). It is clear that pre-operative irradiation to a dose of 4000 rad, with surgery about 4 weeks later, is not associated with a greater mortality than following surgery alone. The operative mortality for cystectomy alone or after pre-operative irradiation continues to improve and, in recent series in which a two-stage procedure for cystectomy was performed with radiotherapy administered between the stages, the mortality ranged from nil to 2% (Mahoney *et al.,* 1975; Ellingwood *et al.,* 1979).

SALVAGE CYSTECTOMY IN SELECTED CASES

In patients with infiltrating bladder cancer, delayed cystectomy may save lives after radical radiotherapy has failed to control the disease. However, after doses of the order of 6000–7000 rad in 6–7 weeks, the late tissue changes may make delayed radical operation more difficult, and the morbidity and mortality may be appreciably greater than that following early cystectomy after subradical pre-operative radiotherapy.

*Corrected for natural mortality (*see* Appendix, p. 171)

Nevertheless, substantial survival rates have been reported after delayed cystectomy. Thus, Whitmore *et al.* (1977a) report a 5-year survival rate of practically 50% for T2 cases and 30% for T3 cases following late cystectomy after failed radiotherapy.

In the Institute of Urology trial, 18 out of 85 patients treated by radical radiotherapy ultimately came to salvage cystectomy. The operative mortality was 11%. The 5-year survival rate was 60% while at 8 years, 54% were still alive.

It is important to stress that, although patients for salvage cystectomy are indeed radiotherapy failures, they nevertheless represent a highly selected group of people. They must still be operable and medically fit, thereby eliminating the worst failures. On the other hand, some 'good' cases are also excluded because they are the ones that responded well to radiotherapy and therefore are not candidates for surgery.

In considering the role of delayed cystectomy for radical radiotherapy failures, one must consider the following: (1) a palpable mass following radical irradiation, suspected of being residual tumour, may consist of fibrous tissue only; (2) the original tumour may have been eradicated and a new tumour appear, perhaps of lesser stage and malignancy, for which the surgery is carried out; (3) cystectomy may be required for complications of radiotherapy in the absence of tumour recurrence; (4) in any series we must know the fate of all patients *not* treated by the salvage operation — some will be cures but there will be many failures who have become unsuitable for major surgery, either because of their general medical condition or because of advanced disease.

ADVANTAGES OF PRE-OPERATIVE RADIOTHERAPY AND PLANNED CYSTECTOMY COMPARED WITH SALVAGE CYSTECTOMY

Routine cystectomy following pre-operative irradiation has the advantage of removing not only any radioresistant tumour core at an early stage, but also the source of any new tumours. These advantages can be offered to all suitable patients. On the other hand, salvage cystectomy can be performed only in a highly selected group of already failed patients, that is, those with recurrent active local tumours which tend not to disseminate. With planned cystectomy following pre-operative irradiation, patients have the possibility of disease eradication at a relatively early stage although, undoubtedly, some with occult metastases will be included which will render the operation a futile ordeal. At present, the planned combined treatment appears to offer a greater opportunity for cure and less operative risk for a larger number of patients, than does radical radiotherapy with the possibility of delayed cystectomy.

The mortality for salvage cystectomy is falling and is now in the region of 10%. Perhaps further reductions (Vinnicombe and Abercrombie, 1978) may be made and the opportunity for cure increased by recognizing radical radiotherapy failures at an earlier stage and by operating before the disease becomes too advanced and fibrosis well established. Such an approach would result in more patients retaining their bladders, than if post-irradiation cystectomy was performed routinely. If we could assess the likely tumour and host response to irradiation at an early stage, it might become possible to select those patients who will need a cystectomy for cure, without having to wait for obvious recurrence.

Although bladder cancer may appear to respond well to high-dose irradiation, based on cystoscopic appearances and bi-manual examination, viable growth may persist deep in the vesical wall, to recur at some future date (Engel *et al.*, 1969). Nevertheless, good responses gauged simply from clinical examination are associated with an

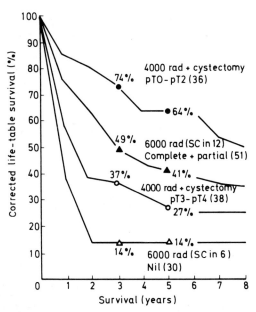

Figure 17.6 Institute of Urology T3 Trial: corrected life-table survival in patients treated by pre-operative irradiation (4000 rad) and cystectomy or by radical radiotherapy, according to tumour response to irradiation. Note that the 5-year results are better following the combined treatment than after radical radiotherapy (even with salvage cystectomy in some cases of the latter group), whether the tumour shows a good response to irradiation or not. The difference in survival between patients showing downstaging in the surgical specimen (pT0–pT2) after 4000 rad and those with a complete or partial response to 6000 rad is significant (P < 0.05). 5C–salvage cystectomy; number of patients in parenthesis

improved prognosis following radical radiotherapy (6000 rad), or as a result of downstaging following pre-operative irradiation (4000 rad). Hence, routine cystoscopy and bi-manual examination after 4000 rad may help to identify potentially 'good' and 'poor' responders to irradiation, following which, cases can be selected, either to continue with radiotherapy to a radical dose, or to proceed to cystectomy.

The programme of radical radiotherapy and selective delayed salvage cystectomy has the merit of avoiding operation in those patients destined to develop early metastases — akin to the situation of some years ago with regard to delayed amputation for osteogenic sarcoma. On the other hand, there must be an appreciable number of cases in which delay to cystectomy is directly associated with further tumour spread, resulting in the opportunity for cure being lost.

In the Institute of Urology trial there was a trend for better results in favour of the planned combined treatment, compared with radical radiotherapy (with salvage cystectomy in some patients), not only for the 'good' responders to irradiation (64% compared with 41% alive at 5 years), but also for the 'poor' responders (27% as opposed to 14% at 5 years) (*Figure 17.6*).

Recurrence of tumour

Pre-operative irradiation and surgery is followed by a reduced incidence of recurrence in the pelvis. After radical radiotherapy alone, the first evidence of tumour recurrence is generally in the bladder and/or pelvis (50–70% of cases). After surgery alone, the proportion of cases that develop pelvic recurrence is also high (28% in the series by Whitmore *et al.*, 1977a). On the other hand, the regional recurrence rate after combined treatment is only between 14% and 17%, the chief cause of failure being distant metastases, often within 12–18 months of operation (Miller, 1977; Prout, 1977; Whitmore *et al.*, 1977a,b; Werf-Messing, 1979). In the Rotterdam study, death with lymph node involvement occurred in only 7% of 96 patients showing downstaging, compared with 40% of 43 presumed radioresistant cases, while distant metastases without node involvement was the cause of death in only 7% of downstaged cases, compared with 19% in resistant pT3 cases (Werf-Messing, 1979).

After cystourethrectomy, the target organ for vesical tumour development has been removed but, of course, urothelial tumours may still develop in the upper urinary tract (Hendry and Bloom, 1976).

Results of other studies concerning pre-operative radiotherapy for T3 bladder cancer

Table 17.5 shows the results of pre-operative irradiation and radical cystectomy in six studies. The 5-year survival rate following 2000 rad and immediate operation is comparable with that following 4000 rad with surgery delayed for several weeks. In these studies, simple cystectomy appears to be no less effective than the radical operation. Miller (1979) has recently compared results following pre-operative doses of 5000 rad in patients at the MD Anderson Hospital with those following 2000 rad in a series at the Memorial Hospital. The greater dose was

Table 17.5
RESULTS OF COMBINED TREATMENT FOR T3 BLADDER CANCER; CRUDE 5-YEAR SURVIVAL RATES FOLLOWING PRE-OPERATIVE IRRADIATION WITH 4000/5000 or 2000 RAD FROM VARIOUS CENTRES WHICH HAVE GIVEN ADEQUATE INFORMATION, PARTICULARLY WITH REGARD TO CLINICAL STAGING. ALL RESULTS ARE BASED ON PATIENTS COMPLETING THE COMBINED TREATMENT

Author	Dose (rad)/ time	Number of patients	Uncorrected percentage 5-year survival
Whitmore *et al.* (1977a, b)	4000/4 wk	50	34
	2000/5 d	52	40
Reid *et al.* (1976)	2000/4 d	92	34
Miller (1977)[a] (simple cystectomy)	5000/5 wk	35	46
Werf-Messing (1975) (simple cystectomy)	4000/4 w	89	50
Institute of Urology[a]	4000/4 w	77	39

[a]Controlled trials

Table 17.6
CRUDE 5-YEAR SURVIVAL FOR RADICAL RADIOTHERAPY AND COMBINED TREATMENT GROUPS IN TWO CONTROLLED STUDIES IN PATIENTS WITH T3 BLADDER CANCER. NO CASES EXCLUDED

Treatment	Author	Number of patients	Uncorrected percentage 5-year survival
Pre-operative radiotherapy (5000 rad/5 wk) + simple cystectomy	Miller (1977)	35	46
Radical radiotherapy (7000 rad/7 wk)		34	22
Pre-operative radiotherapy (4000 rad/4 wk) + radical cystectomy	Institute of Urology Cooperative Trial	98	34
Radical radiotherapy (6000 rad/6 wk)		91	25

associated with a higher incidence of stage reduction and tumour-free cystectomy specimens, together with greater 5-year survival rates of these categories and possibly lower incidence of local failure in the pelvis. Results from two controlled trials in which the data available permit comparison are shown in *Table 17.6.*

FUTURE STUDIES AND PROSPECTS

Because reduction of tumour stage and apparent clearance of pelvic nodes in some T3 cases following pre-operative radiotherapy is associated with improved survival rates following radical cystectomy, it would seem reasonable to pursue the principle of combined treatment with the aim of achieving an even greater incidence and degree of tumour regression before operation. At the same time, one should also be seeking greater tumour control by radiation for those patients unsuitable for major surgery, and also hoping eventually to improve radical radiotherapy results to such an extent that cystectomy becomes necessary only rarely.

Single daily doses of irradiation to deliver 1000 rad per week, generally to a total of 6000 rad, has been a long-standing principle applied to radical radiotherapy for bladder cancer. Alternative irradiation fractionation schedules should be explored with the aim of increasing the tumour lethal effect and improving the therapeutic ratio (i.e. the relative effect on neoplastic and normal tissues). Work in this direction has already been undertaken by Littbrand and Edsmyr (1976) and by Awwad *et al.* (1979).

The treatment of patients with bladder cancer by irradiation under hyperbaric oxygen, in order to overcome radioresistance associated with tumour cell hypoxia, has been disappointing (Cade and McEwen, 1967; Dische, 1973). More recently, the administration of electron-affinic chemical radiosensitizers and the use of fast neutron beams for cancer treatment, give hope of ultimately achieving more effective local-regional control of bladder cancer, but such approaches will still have little or no effect on extra-pelvic disease and distant metastases.

The presence of tumour deposits in the para-aortic nodes from pelvic cancers does not necessarily mean that blood-borne metastases are inevitable (Vongtama *et al.*, 1974; Rotman *et al.*, 1978). Irradiation of the para-aortic nodes may therefore have a role in the treatment of those patients with bladder cancer who have proved or suspected pelvic node involvement, and in whom there may be limited para-aortic disease. However, careful consideration would have to be given to case selection and to dose — time factors, because of the potential risks of 'heavy' irradiation to gastrointestinal tissue.

The period of maximum risk following pre-operative radiotherapy and cystectomy, as with radical radiotherapy alone, is greatest within the first 2 years of treatment: about 50% of patients die during this time. Because pelvic recurrence is uncommon after the combined treatment (14–17%), it may be assumed that half of the patients already have distant spread at the time of, or soon after, the original treatment. Hence there is a limit to what can be achieved by more effective local-regional treatment, and this brings us to consider systemic approaches to bladder cancer, which will be largely dealt with in other sections of this book.

Adjuvant chemotherapy, before or during radiotherapy, and for maintenance, may not only increase the local tumour destructive effect of irradiation, but also control micrometastases outside the radio-surgical volume. Finally, immunotherapeutic measures may destroy minimal residual tumour following irradiation, surgery and chemotherapy.

Our Urological Group has been engaged in a series of single-agent phase 2 chemotherapy studies in patients with advanced bladder cancer (Hall *et al.*, 1974; Turner *et al.*, 1977; Turner *et al.*, 1979). Methotrexate has given an objective response rate of about 50%, but in our hands neither doxorubicin (25 mg/m² intravenously, repeated at three-week intervals), nor bleomycin (5 mg/m² intramuscularly twice weekly) have been of any benefit. At present we are examining the effects of cis-platinum and, although some responses have been observed, we find it poorly tolerated in elderly patients with advanced disease.

Our ultimate aim is to develop a multi-agent chemotherapy programme for the multimodal treatment of patients with deeply infiltrating bladder cancer. In the meantime, and in view of our experience with methotrexate in advanced cases, we have embarked on a controlled trial which includes this drug as a single agent adjuvant. It is given during the 2 weeks before pre-operative irradiation, and then as intermittent maintenance therapy over 12 months following recovery from surgery (*see* Chapter 25).

CONCLUSIONS

Evidence is mounting that, for deeply infiltrating bladder cancer, a combination of pre-operative irradiation and cystectomy produces greater control of the primary tumour and regional nodes and higher survival rates than either modality alone, especially among those patients showing a good response to the preliminary irradiation. The benefit of the combined treatment, however, seems to be restricted to patients under 65 years of age.

The combined treatment appears to be more effective than radical radiotherapy (even with salvage cystectomy in some patients) not only for T3 tumours showing a poor response to irradiation, but also for those with a good response. From experience in the Institute of Urology Trial, it seems that planned combined treatment from the outset is more generally effective than radical radiotherapy with salvage cystectomy for irradiation failures.

The opportunity to increase further the survival of T3 cases following combined treatment may soon become available through the use of chemical radiosensitizers and cytotoxic agents. Finally, let us hope that, in future, the therapeutic effect of radiation can be so enhanced by such means, that local-regional control of bladder cancer will be achieved more effectively and more frequently, with less need for cystectomy.

APPENDIX[a]

Calculation of survival rates and significance testing relating to the Institute of Urology T3 bladder trial

To calculate the survival rates, the standard Actuarial or Life Table method was used, which incorporated a correction for natural mortality based on the method of Berkson and Gage (1950, 1958). The crude rate was divided by an 'expected' rate calculated from the expected mortality given the age, sex and birth cohort of cases constituting each line of the life table, thus yielding a 'corrected' or 'relative' rate.

The standard errors of the results were calculated by the method employed by Greenwood (1926). The standard error so calculated tends to be unreliable where the number of cases is small; comparisons using such groups should be interpreted with caution.

When comparing pairs of patient groups, the difference between the survival rates was divided by the standard error of the difference and the result referred to the normal distribution. Two-tailed tests were used throughout.

REFERENCES

BERKSON, J. and GAGE, R.P. (1950). Calculation of survival rates for cancer. *Proceedings of the Staff Meetings of the Mayo Clinic*, **25**, 270–286

BERKSON, J. and GAGE, R.P. (1958). Specific methods of calculating survival rates of patients with cancer. In *Treatment of Cancer and Allied Diseases*. Ed. by G.T. Pack and I.M. Ariel, Vol. 1, pp. 578–590. London; Pitman Medical Publishing Co. Ltd.

[a]Mr Richard Skeet, Director, South Thames Cancer Registry

AWWAD, H., EL-BAKI, H.A., EL-BOLKAINY, N., BURGERS, M., EL-BADAWAY, S., MANSOUR, M., SOLIMAN, O., OMAR, S. and KHAFAGY, M. (1979). Pre-operative irradiation of T3-bladder carcinoma in bilharzial bladder: a comparison between hyperfractionation and conventional fractionation. *International Journal of Radiation, Oncology, Biology, Physics,* **5**, 787–794

BLOOM, H.J.G. (1971). Recent advances in radiotherapy of carcinoma of the bladder. Proceedings of the 10th International Cancer Congress, Houston, 1970, *Oncology,* **3**, 234–250

BLOOM, H.J.G. (1978). Multi-modal treatment of deep infiltrating (T3) bladder cancer. In *Recent Advances in Clinical Oncology.* Ed by T.A. Hazra and M.C. Beachley, pp. 117–134. New York; Alan R. Liss

BLOOM, H.J.G. (1979). Treatment of infiltrating bladder cancer. *Journal of the Royal Society of Medicine,* **72**, 203–210

BLOOM, H.J.G., HENDRY, W.F., WALLACE, D.M. and SKEET, R. (1980). Treatment of deep infiltrating bladder cancer (T3): Controlled trial of radical radiotherapy versus pre-operative radiotherapy combined with radical cystectomy. Second report on behalf of the Clincial Trials Group, Institute of Urology. *British Journal of Urology,* In preparation

BACKHOUSE, T.W. (1979). A rotation technique for irradiation of the bladder and the results obtained. *Clinical Radiology,* **30**, 259–262

CADE, I., and McEWEN, J.B. (1967). Megavoltage radiotherapy in hyperbaric oxygen. A controlled trial. *Cancer,* **20**, 817–821

CLARK, P.B. (1978). Radical cystectomy for carcinoma of the bladder. *British Journal of Urology,* **50**, 492–495

DISCHE, S. (1973). The hyperbaric oxygen chamber in the radiotherapy of carcinoma of the bladder. *British Journal of Radiology,* **46**, 13–17

DRETLER, S.P., RAGSDALE, B.D. and LEADBETTER, W.F. (1973). The value of pelvic lymphadenectomy in the surgical treatment of bladder cancer. *Journal of Urology,* **109**, 414–416

EDSMYR, F. (1975). Radiotherapy in the management of bladder cancer. In *The Biology and Clinical Management of Bladder Cancer.* Ed. by E.H. Cooper and L.E. Williams, pp. 229–254. Oxford; Blackwell Scientific Publications

ELLINGWOOD, K.E., DRYLIE, D.M., DE TURE, F.A. and MILLION, R.R. (1979). Post diversion precystectomy irradiation for cancer of the bladder. *Cancer,* **43**, 1032–1036

ENGEL, R.M., URTASUN, R.C., JEWETT, H.J. and LOTT, S.J. (1969). Treatment of infiltrating bladder cancer by cobalt-60 radiation: recurrence of tumour in bladder after initial disappearance. *Journal of Urology,* **101**, 859–862

GREENWOOD, M. (1926). A report on the natural duration of cancer. *Ministry of Health. Reports on Public Health and Medical Subjects, No. 33.* London; HMSO

GOFFINET, D.R., SCHNEIDER, M.J., GLATSTEIN, E.J., LUDWIG, H., RAY, G.R., DUNNICK, N.R. and BAGSHAW, M.A. (1975). Bladder cancer: results of radiation therapy in 384 patients. *Radiology,* **117**, 149–153

HALL, R.R., BLOOM, H.J.G., FREEMAN, J.E., NAWROCKI, A. and WALLACE, D.M. (1974). Methotrexate treatment for advanced bladder cancer. *British Journal of Urology,* **46**, 431–438

HENDRY, W.F. and BLOOM, H.J.G. (1976). Urothelial neoplasia: present position and prospects. In *Recent Advances in Urology.* Ed. by W.F. Hendry, Vol. 2, pp. 245–292. Edinburgh; Churchill Livingstone

HERR, H.W., BEAN, M.A. and WHITMORE, W.F. (1976). Prognostic significance of regional lymph node histology in cancer of the bladder. *Journal of Urology*, **115**, 264–267

LAPLANTE, M. and BRICE, M. (1973). The upper limits of hopeful application of radical cystectomy for vesical carcinoma: does nodal metastasis always indicate incurability? *Journal of Urology*, **109**, 261–264

LITTBRAND, B. and EDSMYR, F. (1976). Preliminary results of bladder carcinoma irradiated with low individual doses and a high total dose. *International Journal of Radiation, Oncology, Biology, Physics*, **1**, 1059–1062

MAHONEY, E.M., WEBER, E.T. and HARRISON, J.H. (1975). Post-diversion pre-cystectomy irradiation for carcinoma of the bladder. *Journal of Urology*, **114**, 46–49

MILLER, L.S. (1977). Bladder cancer: superiority of preoperative irradiation and cystectomy in clinical stages B2 and C. *Cancer*, **39**, 973–980

MILLER, L.S. (1979). Pre-operative irradiation for bladder cancer: the 2000 versus 5000 rad controversy. In *Cancer of the Genitourinary Tract*. Ed. by E.D. Johnson and M.L. Samuels, pp. 81–88. New York; Raven Press

MORRISON, R. (1975). The results of treatment of cancer of the bladder: A clinical contribution to radiobiology. *Clinical Radiology*, **26**, 67–75

O'TOOLE, C. and UNSGAARD, B. (1979). Clinical status and rate of recovery of blood lymphocyte levels after radiotherapy for bladder cancer. *Cancer Research*, **39**, 840–843

O'TOOLE, C., PERLMANN, P., UNSGAARD, B., MOBERGER, G. and EDSMYR, F. (1972a). Cellular immunity to human urinary bladder carcinoma: I. Correlation to clinical stage and radiotherapy. *International Journal of Cancer*, **10**, 77–91

O'TOOLE, C., PERLMANN, P., UNSGAARD, B., ALMGARD, L.E., JOHANSSON, B., MOBERGER, G. and EDSMYR, F. (1972b). Cellular immunity to human urinary bladder carcinoma: II. Effect of surgery and pre-operative irradiation. *International Journal of Cancer*, **10**, 92–98

POWERS, W.E. and TOLMACH, L.J. (1964). Pre-operative radiation therapy: biological basis and experimental investigation. *Nature*, **201**, 272–273

POMERANCE, A. (1972). Pathology and prognosis following total cystectomy for carcinoma of the bladder. *British Journal of Urology*, **44**, 451–458

PROUT, G.R. (1977). The role of surgery in the potentially curative treatment of bladder carcinoma. *Cancer Research*, **37**, 2764–2770

PROUT, G.R., SLACK, N.H. and BROSS, I.D.J. (1973). Preoperative irradiation and cystectomy for bladder carcinoma. In *7th National Cancer Conference Proceedings*, pp. 783–791. Philadelphia; J.B. Lippincott

PROUT, G.R. (1976). The surgical management of bladder carcinoma. *Urologic Clinics of North America*, **3**, 149–175

REDDY, E.K., HARTMAN, G.V. and MANSFIELD, C.M. (1978). Carcinoma of the urinary bladder: role of radiation therapy. *International Journal of Radiation, Oncology, Biology and Physics*, **4**, 963–966

REID, E.C., OLIVER, J.A. and FISHMAN, I.J. (1976). Pre-operative irradiation and cystectomy in 135 cases of bladder cancer. *Cancer*, **8**, 247–250

ROTMAN, M., MOON, S., JOHN, M., CHOI, K. and SALL, S. (1978). Extended field para-aortic radiation in cervical carcinoma: the case for prophylactic treatment. *International Journal of Radiation, Oncology, Biology, Physics*, **4**, 795–799

TURNER, A.G., DURRANT, K.R. and MALPAS, J.S. (1979). A trial of bleomycin versus adriamycin in advanced carcinoma of the bladder. *British Journal of Urology,* **51**, 121–124

TURNER, A.G., HENDRY, W.F., MACDONALD, J.S. and WALLACE, D.M. (1976). The value of lymphography in the management of bladder cancer. *British Journal of Urology,* **48**, 579–586

TURNER, A.G., HENDRY, W.F., WILLIAMS, G.B. and BLOOM, H.J.G. (1977). The treatment of advanced bladder cancer with methotrexate. *British Journal of Urology,* **49**, 673–678

VINNICOMBE, J. and ABERCROMBIE, G.F. (1978). Total cystectomy – a review. *British Journal of Urology,* **50**, 488–491

VONGTAMA, V., PIVER, S.M., TSUKADA, Y., BARLOW, J.J. and WEBSTER, J.H. (1974). Para-aortic node irradiation in carcinomas. *Cancer,* **34**, 169–174

WALLACE, D.M. and BLOOM, H.J.G. (1976). The management of deeply infil-trating (T3) bladder carcinoma: controlled trial of radical radiotherapy versus preoperative radiotherapy and radical cystectomy. *British Journal of Urology,* **48**, 587–594

WERF-MESSING, B. VAN DER (1975). Carcinoma of the bladder T3 NXMO treated by preoperative irradiation followed by cystectomy. Third report of Rotterdam Radiotherapy Institute. *Cancer,* **36**, 718–722

WERF-MESSING, B. VAN DER (1975). Cancer of the urinary bladder treated by interstitial radium implant. *International Journal of Radiation, Oncology, Biology and Physics,* **4**, 373–378

WERF-MESSING, B. VAN DER (1979). Preoperative irradiation followed by cystec-tomy to treat carcinoma of the urinary bladder category T3NX, 0–4 MO. *International Journal of Radiation, Oncology, Biology, Physics,* **5**, 394–401

WHITMORE, W.F., BATATA, M.A., GHONEIM, M.A., GRABSTALD, H. and UNAL, A. (1977a). Radical cystectomy with or without prior irradiation in the treat-ment of bladder cancer. *Journal of Urology,* **118**, 184–187

WHITMORE, W.F., BATATA, M.A., HILARIS, B.S., REDDY, G.N., UNAL, A., GHONEIM, M.A., GRABSTALD, H. and CHU, F. (1977b). A comparative study of 2 pre-operative radiation regimens with cystectomy for bladder cancer. *Cancer,* **40**, 1077–1086

18

Pre-Operative Low-Dose Radiotherapy and Cystectomy

Willet F. Whitmore, Jr.

Pre-operative irradiation with cystectomy in the management of selected patients with bladder cancer was started approximately 20 years ago, with the realization that neither radiation therapy nor cystectomy produced satisfactory levels of local control in selected patients with bladder cancer, and with the largely empirical hope that an appropriate combination of these two procedures might yield better results than either alone. In the intervening years, accumulating experimental and clinical evidence has more or less confirmed the usefulness of such integrated therapy. The experimental support for integrated treatment regimens has been reviewed (Powers and Palmer, 1968; Perez, 1970). A number of clinical experiences (Miller and Johnson, 1973; Prout et al., 1973; Werf-Messing, 1973, 1975; Reid et al., 1973; Wallace and Bloom, 1976; Whitmore et al., 1977a, b) specifically support the usefulness of pre-operative radiotherapy and cystectomy in patients with bladder cancer, but questions regarding total dose, dose fractionation, field size, overall treatment time for irradiation, and interval between irradiation and operation, remain. At the Memorial Sloan-Kettering Cancer Center (MSKCC) two different pre-operative radiation regimens were explored in the interval 1959–71, and this report is an analysis of certain aspects of this experience.

MATERIALS AND METHODS

Between 1949 and 1971, 342 patients with bladder cancer at MSKCC underwent radical cystectomy, usually with bilateral pelvic lymph node dissection.

Group 1   One hundred and thirty-seven patients had radical cystectomy alone in the interval 1949–59.

Group 2   One hundred and nineteen patients received 4000 rad, in 20 fractions of 200 rad each over 4 weeks, to fields generally encompassing the true pelvis, with radical cystectomy 4–12 weeks later (average 46 days) (1959–66).

Group 3   Eighty-six patients received 2000 rad in five fractions of 400 rad over a one-week period to portals encompassing the true pelvis ('flash' radiotherapy) with radical cystectomy within 2 weeks (average 2 days) (1966–71).

For radiation therapy, megavoltage photon beam equipment (2 MV X-ray, cobalt-60 teletherapy, or 6 MV linear accelerator) was used. Treatment was usually administered through anterior and posterior parallel opposed portals, but occasionally by rotation or by multiple fields. Pelvic portal sizes varied, the average being 13 X 13 cm in both groups (Whitmore *et al.*, 1977a, b). The mean total normal tissue dose (Ellis, 1969) in group 2 was 1173 rets compared with 850 rets in group 3.

The indications for cystectomy were: (1) *Superficially infiltrating tumours (Tis, T1, T2) unsuitable for conservative management.* The therapeutic policy at MSKCC has been, and remains, that conservative treatment (usually by transurethral resection) provides essentially as good a prospect of control of *existing* low-stage (Tis, T1, T2) tumours as does more radical therapy (Whitmore, 1979b). Tumour multicentricity in space and/or time, and/or tumour location (prostatic urethra), however, may make conservative treatment impractical or impossible. Successive tumour occurrences ('recurrences') of increasing grade tend also to increase the inclination towards aggressive treatment (radical cystectomy). (2) *Deeply infiltrating tumours (T3, T4) unsuitable for segmental resection.* High-stage (T3, T4) tumours are considered to be unsuitable for segmental resection when there is existing or previous multicentricity, or close proximity to the bladder neck. Although less than 5% of patients with T3 or T4 lesions will prove to be suitable for segmental resection, 5-year survival rates in appropriately selected patients are similar to those attained in patients with similar stage tumours treated by radical cystectomy (Whitmore, 1979a, b).

It has been general policy to explore surgically all medically fit patients with local or regional lesions potentially suitable for cystectomy, regardless of the apparent degree of local fixation (T4). The surgical finding of non-resectable local extensions, or of metastasis outside the pelvis, or of extensive lymph node metastasis within the pelvis, has generally led to a decision against cystectomy and this has occurred in approximately 15% of all patients surgically explored in anticipation of cystectomy.

All patients were subjected to a general evaluation which included complete history and physical examination, complete blood count, urinalysis, posteroanterior and lateral X-ray films of the chest, serum electrolyte and liver profiles, blood urea nitrogen and/or creatinine determinations and such other blood and radiographic studies as seemed indicated. Liver and bone scans and radiographic skeletal surveys were not routine staging techniques and were performed only for specific indications. Lymphangiography was not employed at all.

The clinical and pathological staging classification used was the Marshall modification of Jewett's classification (Marshall, 1952) which relates to the TNM system in the fashion set forth by Skinner (1977). Clinical staging was based upon the findings of cystoscopy, bi-manual examination and appropriate biopsies performed under anaesthesia and upon adjunctive information derived from intravenous urograms. Pathological staging was based upon the histological study of surgical specimens following radical cystectomy and bilateral pelvic lymph node dissection. The discrepancies between the clinical and pathological staging for each of the groups have been discussed elsewhere (Whitmore *et al.*, 1977a, b). Pelvic recurrences were defined as soft tissue recurrences within the pelvis, with or without involvement of contiguous bone, and extrapelvic recurrences (or distant metastases) included all other sites of vesical neoplasm. Low-stage neoplasms include Tis, T1 and T2 lesions, and high-stage neoplasms include T3 and T4 lesions. The majority of low-stage lesions were T2 tumours (42/66 group 1; 36/58 group 2; 22/29 group 3) and the majority of high-stage lesions were T3 tumours (26/32 group 1; 15/26 group 2; 9/14 group 3).

Histological grading of tumours recognized benign papilloma (none in this series) and four grades of carcinoma. Carcinomas were grouped as low-grade (grade 1 or 2) or high-grade (grade 3 or 4). Most low-grade lesions were grade 2 and most high-grade lesions were grade 3.

A valid criticism of the data derived from this experience is that a historical control group of patients having cystectomy alone is compared with chronologically consecutive groups of patients having pre-operative irradiation and cystectomy. Although this criticism can hardly be dismissed, the following considerations strengthen the validity of the comparisons to be made: (1) the indications for, and technique of, radical cystectomy were constant; (2) all cases were managed in the same institution under the supervision of the same individuals; (3) the methods and system of clinical and pathological staging remained constant; (4) analyses of the three groups relative to patient age, sex, tumour grade and stage, tumour configuration (papillary or solid), tumour multicentricity, and previous therapy has not revealed any conspicuous differences which might suggest selection bias; (5) as a generalization, it is apparent that tumour grade and tumour stage are the principal determinants of end results in patients with bladder cancer, regardless of therapy (Whitmore, 1979a, b). Using the same system of grading and staging, there is no apparent evidence that other selection biases may influence end results. The validity of this argument is enhanced by the fact that reported end results of different methods of treatment over the past 20–30 years have remained remarkably constant when stage is the common denominator in the survival analysis (Whitmore, 1979a, b).

RESULTS AND DISCUSSION

In *Table 18.1* are shown the overall 5-year survival results in the three groups. Control of neoplasm was without doubt higher in the irradiated than in the non-irradiated patients. The proportion of deaths from causes other than bladder cancer was similar in the three groups.

Table 18.1
RADICAL CYSTECTOMY WITH OR WITHOUT PRE-OPERATIVE IRRADIATION: 5-YEAR RESULTS

Status at 5 years	Group 1 patients		Group 2 patients		Group 3 patients	
	Number	%	Number	%	Number	%
Alive without tumour[a]	45	33	50	42	36	42
Dead with recurrence	66	48	47	40	35	41
without recurrence[b]	25	18	22	18	15	17
Lost to follow-up	1	1	–		–	
Total	137		119		86	

[a] Later recurrence in 1 in group 1, 5 in group 2, and 1 in group 3.
[b] Treatment complications in 19 in group 1, 13 in group 2, and 8 in group 3.

Table 18.2
FIVE-YEAR SURVIVAL FOLLOWING RADICAL CYSTECTOMY WITH OR WITHOUT PRE-OPERATIVE IRRADIATION ACCORDING TO CLINICAL STAGE AND HISTOLOGICAL GRADE

Group	Low clinical stage				High clinical stage			
	Low-grade		High-grade		Low-grade		High-grade	
1	26/43	60%	9/23	39%	5/24	21%	4/46	9%
2	23/35	66%	11/23	48%	7/19	37%	10/42	24%
3	12/20	60%	3/9	33%	12/29	41%	9/28	32%

In *Table 18.2* are shown the 5-year survival rates in the three groups relative to tumour stage and tumour grade. There was a progressive decrease in survival as tumour grade and stage increased. Survival rates are clearly better with low-grade than with high-grade tumours, with either low-stage or high-stage lesions. Among patients with low-grade, low-stage tumours, the survival rates are similar and reasonably good in all three groups. In patients with high-grade, low-stage tumours, no significant difference in survival was demonstrated between the irradiated and non-irradiated patients. In patients with high-stage tumours there is a clear improvement in survival in the irradiated compared with the non-irradiated patients. Survival rates are better with the low-grade than with the high-grade lesions, but the relative improvements with pre-operative irradiation may have been slightly greater with high-grade than with low-grade lesions. Pre-operative irradiation thus appeared to reduce the impact of T stage upon survival.

Table 18.3
RADICAL CYSTECTOMY WITH OR WITHOUT PRE-OPERATIVE IRRADIATION. PELVIC RECURRENCE ALONE IN FIVE OR MORE YEARS, ACCORDING TO CLINICAL STAGE AND HISTOLOGICAL GRADE

Group	Low clinical stage				High clinical stage			
	Low-grade		High-grade		Low-grade		High-grade	
1	7/43	16%	5/23	22%	6/24	25%	20/46	43%
2	4/35	11%	3/23	13%	3/19	16%	9/42	21%
3	2/20	10%	0/9	0%	4/29	14%	6/28	21%

Table 18.3 shows the incidence of pelvic recurrence alone in 5 or more years relative to stage and grade in each of the groups. A progressive increase in pelvic recurrence is noted as grade and stage increase. The incidence of pelvic recurrence is generally reduced in groups 2 and 3, compared with group 1, in the corresponding grade and stage categories. This reduction in pelvic recurrences is relatively greatest with the high-grade, high-stage tumours and least with the low-grade, low-stage tumours. Irradiation tends to reduce the impact of T stage on pelvic recurrence rate.

In *Table 18.4* is shown the incidence of extrapelvic recurrence alone in 5 or more years for each of the groups, relative to tumour grade and

Table 18.4
RADICAL CYSTECTOMY WITH OR WITHOUT PRE-OPERATIVE IRRADIATION. EXTRA-PELVIC RECURRENCE ALONE IN FIVE YEARS OR MORE, ACCORDING TO CLINICAL STAGE AND HISTOLOGICAL GRADE

Group	Low clinical stage				High clinical stage			
	Low-grade		High-grade		Low-grade		High-grade	
1	0/43	0%	3/23	13%	2/24	8%	8/46	17%
2	3/35	9%	6/23	26%	4/19	21%	10/42	24%
3	5/20	25%	3/9	33%	6/29	21%	5/28	18%

stage. In group 1, the incidence of extrapelvic recurrence alone as a cause of treatment failure is less than in any of the respective groups receiving pre-operative irradiation. In reducing pelvic recurrence alone as a cause of treatment failure, patients receiving pre-operative irradiation are at risk of death attributable to distant spread.

Werf-Messing (1973) was the first to point out the beneficial effect of tumour downstaging on the end results of integrated treatment. In *Table 18.5,* survival rates at 5 years for the different groups are indicated for those tumours in which the pathological stage following

Table 18.5
FIVE-YEAR SURVIVAL FOLLOWING RADICAL CYSTECTOMY
WITH OR WITHOUT PRE-OPERATIVE IRRADIATION, ACCOR-
DING TO P–T RELATIONSHIP

Group	$P < T$		$P \geqslant T$	
Group 1	2/6	33%	43/130	33%
Group 2	27/48	56%	24/71	34%
Group 3	10/23	43%	26/63	41%

radiotherapy was less than the initial pre-radiotherapy clinical stage ($P < T$) and for those in whom the pathological stage was the same as, or greater than, the clinical stage ($P \geqslant T$). Such down staging is unlikely to be due to errors in clinical assessment, because in patients not receiving pre-operative irradiation, clincial overstaging was uncommon and occurred in only 6 of the 136 patients in whom satisfactory data were available. It must be concluded that the greater incidence of stage reduction in the irradiated groups was largely attributable to an effect of irradiation. The discrepancy is larger in group 2 than in group 3. This is only to be expected, because the radiation dose was larger and the interval between radiation and cystectomy longer in group 3 than in group 2, thereby providing a larger dose of radiation and a longer interval for tumour downstaging to become evident.

Comparison of the survival rates in downstaged ($P < T$) patients with non-downstaged patients ($P \geqslant T$) reveals the best survival in group 2 patients with downstaged tumours. However, although overall survival rates were improved in group 3 patients as well, the apparent equivalence of survival rates between the downstaged and nondownstaged patients in group 3 must be due to the 'flash' nature of the pre-operative irradiation, because the dose and the interval between radiation and cystectomy were relatively small and provided little opportunity for *demonstrable* downstaging to occur. Nevertheless, the survival rates both in the downstaged and non-downstaged categories of group 3 patients are better than in the corresponding categories of the group 1 patients. This interpretation is supported by analyses of the pelvic recurrence rates alone in the different groups at 5 or more years, relative to whether or not demonstrable tumour downstaging occurred. The results are consistent in demonstrating the lowest pelvic recurrence rates in patients whose tumours were downstaged as a consequence of irradiation.

Hospital mortality in group 1 was 14%, in group 2, 11% and in group 3, 9%, and was roughly equally divided between cardiopulmonary deaths and deaths attributable to sepsis. Complications possibly due to pre-operative irradiation consisted principally of delayed healing of infected wounds, and were not appreciably different for group 2 or group 3 patients.

The data do not demonstrate any material difference in survival rates or local recurrence rates between apparently comparable patients who received 4000 rad in 4 weeks and those who received 2000 rad in 1 week, before operation. The principal advantage of so-called 'flash' pre-operative irradiation is the shortened treatment time, which has physical, psychological and economic advantages for the patient. A disadvantage of 'flash' radiation therapy is that it reduces the capability for recognition of that fortunate proportion of patients in whom tumour downstaging as a consequence of such irradiation results in an improvement in prognosis. The latter distinction will become increasingly important as useful adjuvants are developed, and should encourage efforts to distinguish the radioresponsive from the non-radioresponsive cases, which are independent of the gross morphological characteristics necessary to make such distinctions at present.

SUMMARY AND CONCLUSIONS

MSKCC experience in a selected group of patients treated by radical cystectomy, with or without two different regimens of pre-operative irradiation, in the period 1949–71, suggests that: (1) pre-operative irradiation improves the survival rates in patients with clinically high-stage tumours, probably by improving the local control rates compared with cystectomy alone; (2) the favourable effects of pre-operative irradiation are at least largely limited to those patients in whom tumour downstaging (P < T) can be demonstrated; (3) either 4000 rad in 4 weeks or 2000 rad in 1 week, before operation, yields equivalent results with such integrated treatment in terms of tumour control, operative mortality and morbidity. The practical advantages of the 'flash' regimen make it currently the method of choice at MSKCC; (3) the optimal method of irradiation in integrated programmes of treatment has yet to be established definitively.

REFERENCES

ELLIS, F. (1969). Dose, time and fractionation. A clinical hypothesis. *Clinical Radiology,* **20**. 1–7

MARSHALL, V.F. (1952). The relation of the preoperative estimate to the pathologic demonstration of the extent of vesical neoplasms. *Journal of Urology,* **68**, 714–723

MILLER, L.S. and JOHNSON, E.D. (1973). Megavoltage irradiation for bladder cancer: alone, post-operative or preoperative? In *Proceedings of the 7th National Cancer Conference,* pp. 771–782, Philadelphia; J.B. Lippincott

PEREZ, C.A. (1970). Preoperative irradiation in the treatment of cancer. *Frontier Radiation Therapy and Oncology,* **5**, 1–29

POWERS, W.E. and PALMER, L.A. (1968). Biologic basis of preoperative radiation treatment. *American Journal of Roentgenology and Radium Therapy,* **102**, 176–192

PROUT, G.R., JR., SLACK, N.H. and BROSS, I.D. (1973). Preoperative irradiation and cystectomy for bladder carcinoma, IV: results in a selected population. In *Proceedings of the 7th National Cancer Conference,* pp. 783–791. Philadelphia; J.B. Lippincott

REID, E.C., OLIVER, J.A. and FISHMAN, I.J. (1973). Preoperative irradiation and cystectomy in 135 cases of bladder cancer. *Urology,* **8**, 247–250

SKINNER, D.G. (1977). Current state of classification and staging of bladder cancer *Cancer Research,* **37**, 2838–2842

WALLACE, D.M. and BLOOM, H.J.G. (1976). The management of deeply infiltrating (T3) bladder carcinoma: controlled trial of radical radiotherapy versus preoperative radiotherapy and radical cystectomy (first report). *British Journal of Urology,* **48**, 587–594

WERF-MESSING, B. VAN DER (1973). Carcinoma of the bladder treated by preoperative irradiation followed by cystectomy. *Cancer,* **32**, 1084–1088

WERF-MESSING, B. VAN DER (1975). Carcinoma of the bladder T3 N_X M_0 treated by preoperative irradiation followed by cystectomy. *Cancer,* **36**, 718–722

WHITMORE, W.F., JR., BATATA, M.A., GHONEIM, M.A., GRABSTALD, H. and UNAL, A. (1977a). Radical cystectomy with or without prior irradiation in the treatment of bladder cancer. *Journal of Urology,* **118**, 184–187

WHITMORE, W.F., JR, BATATA, M.A., HILARIS, B.S., REDDY, G.N., UNAL, A., GHONEIM, M.A., GRABSTALD, H. and CHU, F. (1977b). A comparative study of two preoperative radiation regimens with bladder cancer. *Cancer,* **40**, 1077–1086

WHITMORE, W.F., JR. (1979a). Surgical management of low stage bladder cancer. *Seminars in Oncology,* **6**, 207–216

WHITMORE, W.F., JR. (1979b). Management of bladder cancer. *Current Problems in Cancer,* Vol. 4, No. 1

19

Life with an Ileal Conduit: Results of Questionnaire Surveys of Patients and Urological Surgeons

M.A. Jones, Brigid Breckman and W.F. Hendry

INTRODUCTION

Since its popularization by Bricker in 1950, the ileal conduit has become the most common method of urinary diversion. Much has been written about the technical problems of the operation, but less attention has been paid to the practical difficulties which patients face in trying to cope with a new way of life. Adjustment to life with an ileal conduit requires close cooperation between patient, surgeon and nursing staff if the patient is to return to a normal life. To assess the problems experienced by patients and staff, two questionnaire surveys were undertaken.

METHODS OF SURVEY

Survey of patients

Thirty-four unselected patients attending the follow-up clinic at the Royal Marsden Hospital were asked to complete a questionnaire. There were 21 men and 13 women, and their ages ranged from 46 to 83 years with a mean age of 65 years. The indications for surgery are shown in *Table 19.1*. The patients completed the questionnaire at home and returned it at their next clinic attendance, where it was checked. No patient refused to participate in the survey.

Table 19.1
INDICATIONS FOR SURGERY

Indication	Number of patients
Bladder cancer	19
Gynaecological malignancy and fistula	4
Rectal cancer	1
Irradiation cystitis	5
Neurogenic bladder	2
Gynaecological incontinence	2
Prostatic cancer and Crohn's disease	1

Survey of urologists

Fifty-seven completed questionnaires were received from British Association of Urological Surgeons members out of a total of 151 sent out, a response rate of 38%. Their geographical distribution covered a wide area of the British Isles.

RESULTS

Survey of patients

We were interested in the patients' knowledge about their condition, and who had explained it to them before surgery (*Table 19.2*). The majority of those suffering from malignant disease had accurate knowledge about their condition, but it was disturbing to note that none of the patients suffering from non-malignant disease had a clear idea of the reason for surgery. In 27 of 34 cases the pre-operative counselling had been performed by the consultant.

Twenty-one of 34 patients felt that the quality of their lives had been improved by surgery (*Table 19.3*). Not surprisingly, patients

Table 19.2
PRE-OPERATIVE COUNSELLING

Question	Type of disease/ Counsellor	Accurate	Answer Inaccurate	Don't know
Do you know why you had a stoma made?	Malignant	22	4	5
	Non-malignant	0	1	2
	Consultant	19	0	8
Who explained your operation to you?	Senior Registrar	1	3	0
	Sister	1	0	0
	Nurse	1	0	0
	Stomatherapist	1	0	0

Table 19.3
HOW DO YOU FIND LIFE SINCE YOUR OPERATION?

Indications for surgery	Patient's answer		
	Better	Worse	No change
Planned trial	5	1	3
Salvage/other disease	6	2	4
Irradiation cystitis	5	0	0
Urinary fistula	3	0	1
Neurogenic bladder	1	0	1
Gynaecological incontinence	1	0	1

suffering from irradiation cystitis or incontinence gained the greatest benefit. However, one patient who had suffered from gross stress incontinence, and a second with a urinary fistula, felt that there had been no change in the quality of their lives.

A survey of the pattern of appliance usage showed that 27 of 34 patients had tried more than one appliance. Dislike of the appliance or leakage attributable to material failure were the reasons for change in 25 of 34 patients. Poor supplies, allergy and fitting difficulties were the reasons given in the remaining nine cases. Thirty of 34 patients expressed satisfaction with their present appliance.

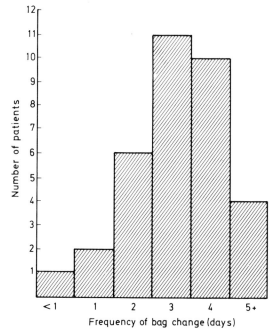

Figure 19.1 Frequency of bag change in days

Table 19.4
PROBLEMS WITH APPLIANCE LEAKAGE

Cause of problem	Severity of problem	
	Minor *(> 1 per month)*	*Major* *(> 1 per week)*
Parastomal hernia	1	1
Gulley/recessed stoma	1	2
Night drainage	2	0
Incisional hernia	1	1
Appliance failure	2	0
Unknown	2	0

Only four patients felt that their stoma care tuition had been poor, and these had been taught before the services of a full-time stoma-therapist had been available. All 28 of 34 patients taught by the stoma-therapist expressed satisfaction.

The frequency of bag change is shown in *Figure 19.1*. The majority of the patients were able to wear their appliance for 2–4 days without changing the bag. Only one patient had to change more than once a day, and he had a very large parastomal hernia. Thirteen of the patients experienced significant problems with urinary leakage, and four of these had severe problems (*Table 19.4*). In seven out of 13, leakage was

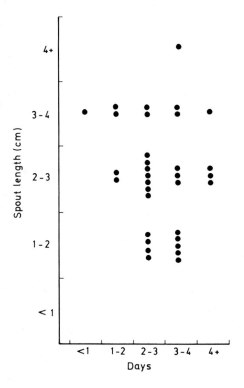

Figure 19.2 Frequency of bag change related to stoma length

associated with 'contour' problems due to abdominal hernias or recession of the stoma. However, there was no relationship between the length of the stoma and the frequency of bag change (*Figure 19.2*).

Thirteen of 29 patients who had been at work before surgery had returned within 4 months, and all those able to do so had returned at 6 months (*Figure 19.3*). Nine patients were forced to retire or to take

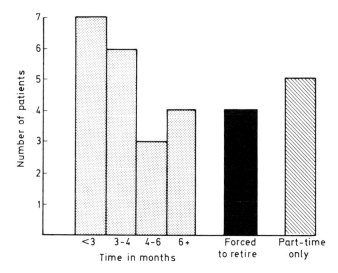

Figure 19.3 Time in months before return to work and incidence of partial or complete retirement after operation

part-time work. However, 21 of 34 patients had restricted their social activities since having a stoma. The causes of this were fear of damaging their stoma (9), appliance consciousness (3) and fear of leakage (9). Of the patients sexually active before surgery, six of 19 men retained some activity, but all were impotent. None of the three women previously active resumed sexual activity after surgery, although none had undergone cystectomy.

Survey of 57 urologists

The number of ileal conduits made in the years 1976–7 and 1977–8 is shown in *Table 19.5*. The average number of stomas made per surgeon per year was seven, of which four were combined with cystectomy. The 1- and 5-year survival figures of 82% and 56% indicate an increasing volume of stoma care work in the future. One hundred and twenty-eight admissions were necessary to treat complications arising in these patients: 43 required revision of the stoma, and there were 85 other urinary complications.

The appliance training of these patients was performed by stoma-therapist (24), nursing sister (39), surgeon (18), appliance fitter (18) and registrar (7). The most popular appliance was the Hollister (*Table 19.6*) and 31 of 57 surgeons made it their first choice. Twenty of 51 surgeons had no stomatherapist and 14 of 20 felt that they would like

Table 19.5
NUMBER OF ILEAL CONDUITS (SURVEY OF 57 BAUS* MEMBERS)

	Number constructed Period		Cystectomy	Children	Estimated survival (%)	
	1976–77	*1977–78*	*(per annum)*	*(per annum)*	*1 year*	*5 years*
Total	402	387	250	36.5		
Average	7.0	6.8	4.5	–	82	56
Range	0–19	0–15	0–13	0–27		

Table 19.6
TYPES OF APPLIANCES (SURVEY OF 57 BAUS* MEMBERS)

Appliances	Types used†	Surgeon's first preference
Down's		
Rubber	17	3
Plastic	27	5
Salts		
Rubber	10	3
Plastic	8	3
Coloplast	10	5
Carshalton	2	
Cutifix		
Simpla	6	
Hollister	49	31
Others	2	

† 4 used 4)
23 used 3)   or more types

Table 19.7
PROBLEMS MOST COMMONLY ENCOUNTERED (SURVEY OF 57 BAUS* MEMBERS)

Problem	Number of patients	Problem	Number of patients	Problem	Number of patients
Skin	19	Retraction	6	Fitting	1
Leakage	17	Stenosis	2	Hair	1
Encrustation	4	Hernia	1	Allergy	1
Bleeding	3	Stones	1	Smell	1
Supply	2	Infection	1	Psychological	1

one. *Table 19.7* shows that skin problems and leakage together accounted for over half of all stoma problems. In this survey, stones and infection were encountered infrequently. It can be seen that most of the problems could have been handled by a competent stoma-therapist, and relatively few (11 of 61) required surgical attention.

* British Association of Urological Surgeons

Table 19.18
FURTHER STUDIES (SURVEY OF 57 BAUS MEMBERS)*

Areas for study	Number interested
Appliances, skin	10
Social, family	8
Psychosexual	8
Children, old people	2
Stoma care	2
Cost	1
Surgery, infection	2

* Wish to participate in further study: Yes, 39; No, 13

Ten of 39 surgeons who felt that they would like to participate in a further study identified appliance and skin problems as the areas they would most like to see covered (*Table 19.8*). Sixteen of 39 felt that social, family and psychosexual problems had received insufficient attention and merited further investigation.

DISCUSSION

From the figures provided by urologists on the numbers of new ileal conduits they are creating annually, and the numbers of patients expected to live for 5 years, it appears that stoma problems will require increasing time and resources in the future. The most important stoma problems that concerned patients and staff were those of urinary leakage and its consequent effects on the skin. When severe, the majority of these problems were found to be related to 'contour problems' in our patients, such as recessed stomas and parastomal hernias.

Witherington *et al.* (1977) stressed the importance of correct siting of the stoma and the avoidance of parastomal hernias by careful closure of the abdominal wall. They considered the ideal length of the stoma to be 1 cm, but from our data we would recommend a *minimum* length of 1 cm. The flush or recessed stoma tends to contract still further, and most patients are unable to see it well enough to apply a bag properly (Jeter, 1976). Although some of the wetting problems in our series were caused by appliance failures, the majority of severe 'contour problems' could probably have been avoided by closer attention to technical detail in making the stoma.

In addition to the difficulties of coping with their appliances, patients who have a stoma may experience profound psychological changes in the perception of their 'body image' (McCawley *et al.,* 1975). Common fears are those of odour, leakage, and loss of sexual attractiveness and performance. Fear was the single feature most important in inhibiting our patients' social lives, and may reflect a failure of explanation on our part.

All our patients felt that pre-operative discussion of sexual problems had been inadequate and that no guidance had been offered after surgery. Compared with a recent study by Bergman *et al.* (1979), who found that 74% of their patients remained sexually active after cystectomy, our results are disappointing. Although age and general fitness play a large part in the resumption of sexual activity after surgery, the principal inhibiting factors in our patients, particularly in the women, were associated with feelings of embarrassment about the stoma or doubts about personal cleanliness.

We conclude that many of the leakage problems associated with the ileal conduit can be eradicated by careful surgical technique. An acceptable quality of life can be enjoyed by patients with an ileal conduit, but aftercare and rehabilitation can be greatly facilitated by close cooperation with a skilled stomatherapist. Further study is needed into the social and psychosexual problems of our patients.

ACKNOWLEDGEMENT

We would like to express our appreciation to the patients and members of BAUS who replied to the questionnaires.

REFERENCES

BERGMAN, B., NILSSON, S. and PETERSÉN, I. (1979). The effect on erection and orgasm of cystectomy, prostatectomy and vesiculectomy for cancer of the bladder. A clinical and electromyographic study. *British Journal of Urology,* **51**, 114–120

BRICKER, E.M. (1950). Bladder substitution after pelvic evisceration. *Surgical Clinics of North America,* **30**, 1511–1521

JETER, K.F. (1976). The flush versus the protruding urinary stoma. *Journal of Urology,* **116**, 424–427

McCAWLEY, A., MANNIX, JR., H. and McCARTHY, D.D. (1975). The psychological problems of ostomates. *Connecticut Medicine,* **39**, 151–155

WITHERINGTON, R., AMIE, J. and MULKEY, A.P. (1977). Making of a stoma. *Urology,* **9**, 69–71

IIIB

Treatment of invasive tumours: chemotherapy as salvage treatment

20

Phase II Trials of Single Agents and Combination Regimens in the Treatment of Urothelial Tract Tumours: Memorial Hospital Experience

Alan Yagoda

Evaluation of the efficacy of chemotherapeutic agents in the treatment of urothelial tract tumours — transitional cell carcinoma of the renal pelvis, ureter, bladder, urethra and prostate — has been hindered by the lack of objectively measurable lesions (Yagoda, 1977). The pattern of tumour recurrence, i.e. osseous, pelvic, rectal and intra-abdominal metastases, impedes accurate objective evaluation and only recently have Phase II studies, particularly disease-orientated trials, specifically entered patients with indicator lesions — lung, liver, lymph node, skin and subcutaneous metastases. While metastases from bladder cancer to these latter sites are uncommon, recent data in patients with stages B_1, B_2 or C tumour (Jewett — Strong — Marshall) who relapse after pre- or post-operative irradiation and radical cystectomy, indicate a decrease in incidence of local recurrence and an increase in distant metastases (Whitmore *et al.*, 1977). Thus, a higher incidence of measurable indicator lesions can be expected with improvement in local disease control and with increased patient survival.

Since 1975, at the Memorial Hospital, chemotherapeutic agents have been systematically evaluated employing six primary and three secondary disease-orientated Phase II protocols in patients with bladder cancer who had objective measurable metastases. Initially, patients selected for protocols had only indicator lesions; subsequently, patients with lymph nodes and intra-abdominal or pelvic masses which had been verified by biopsy and which were measurable in two dimensions by computerized transaxial tomography, also were accepted. This Chapter summarizes the Memorial Hospital experience of 311 cases with objectively measurable urothelial tract tumours.

MATERIALS AND METHODS

Initially, the history of each patient was taken, and a complete physical examination was performed, with all accessible lesions measured by two or more diameters. Pathological material was reviewed by the Department of Pathology. Routine biochemical and roentgenographic studies included automated blood and platelet counts, blood urea nitrogen, serum creatinine, chemical screening profile, 5′-nucleotidase, carcino-embryonic antigen (CEA) and posterior/anterior and lateral chest X-rays. In addition, selected cases had roentgenographic bone surveys, intravenous pyelograms or loopograms and lymphangiograms, radionuclide liver and bone scans, 24-hour urine creatinine clearance tests, audiograms and computerized transaxial tomograms (CTT). All roentgenographic studies were evaluated independently by Dr R.C. Watson, Chief of the Department of Diagnostic Radiology. Appropriate measurements and diagnostic tests were performed before each protocol and at 3–6 week intervals.

Table 20.1
RESPONSE CRITERIA

Code	Criteria
CR	Complete disappearance of all measurable, radiological and biochemical abnormalities.
PR	Soft tissue lesions: >50% decrease in the sum of the products of two or more perpendicular diameters of all lesions for >1 month. Abdominal or pelvic masses: >75% decrease by physical examination and/or >50% by CT in the sum of the products of two or more perpendicular diameters for >1 month. Hepatomegaly: >50% decrease in the sum of all available measurements by physical examination and >50% decrease in all biochemical abnormalities and filling defects on scan for >1 month. (In addition, if the pre-treatment carcino-embryonic antigen (CEA) level is abnormal, a >50% decrease is required.)
MR	Minor remission: 25–49% decrease in tumour size, or biochemical abnormalities for >1 month or >50% for <1 month.
STAB	Stable: 25% decrease or increase in tumour size or biochemical abnormalities for >3 months.
PROG	Progression: >25% increase in tumour size or biochemical abnormalities or a mixed response.

Response criteria employed in all clinical trials are outlined in *Table 20.1*. It should be noted that complete remission (CR) required disappearance of all objective lesions confirmed by systematic restaging with all available diagnostic procedures. When indicator lesions were intra-abdominal or in the pelvis, laparotomy was required to document CR, and total clinical and radiological disappearance of such lesions was not sufficient to classify patients as having achieved CR status. For example, AA, a 62-year-old female who received cis-diamminedichloride platinum II (DDP) and cyclophosphamide (CYCLO) in December 1976 for transitional cell carcinoma of the bladder metastatic to the lung and pelvis (documented by computerized transaxial tomogram), achieved CR (clinically) for 2 years. However, at laparotomy, multiple small liver metastases and sheets of tumour were found in the pelvic area. Patients who had a mixed response, minor remission (MR) and stabilization of disease (STAB) are never included in the overall objective response rate; rather, they are listed as non-responders (Progression). Duration of response was measured from the beginning of the protocol until progression of disease occurred. Although response was evaluated during, and at the completion of, each protocol, final evaluation was made only after perusal of all available information, 4–8 months later.

Adequacy of trial was defined as two doses with or without haematologic depression, or one dose with active progression of disease and 1 month's survival. Leucopoenia indicated a white blood cell count $\leqslant$ 4500 cells/mm³ and thrombocytopoenia, a platelet count $\leqslant$ 175 000 cells/mm³. Toxicity was evaluated as 1+, (mild), 2+ (moderate), 3+ (severe, life-threatening) and 4+ (drug-related death). The Karnofsky Performance Scale (PS) was employed to evaluate subjective changes.

PROTOCOLS

Drugs, dosages and routes of administration are outlined in *Table 20.2*. In Protocol I, doxorubicin (DOX) was administered intravenously in a single bolus every 3 weeks to 33 patients and in an intermittent schedule to 18 patients (Yagoda *et al.*, 1977). In Protocol II the initial dose of DOX and CYCLO was modified depending on the degree of myelosuppression: subsequent doses were re-adjusted upwards to DOX/CYCLO 60/450, 60/600, 75/700, or downwards to 35/350 mg/m² (Yagoda *et al.*, 1978).

Initially, DDP (Protocol III) was administered every 3–4 weeks in doses of 1.25 or 1.6 mg/kg; subsequently, the standard dose was 70 mg/m² (Yagoda *et al.*, 1976). Criteria for patient selection in Protocols III–IV included a creatinine clearance of $\geqslant$ 55 ml/min or a blood urea nitrogen $\leqslant$ 25 mg % (normal 20 mg %), and a serum creatinine $\leqslant$ 1.5 mg %

(normal 1 mg %) and no known platinum allergy or significant hearing deficit. After a one-hour infusion of 250–750 ml of 5% dextrose saline i.v., DDP was administered within a 10-minute period and adequate i.v. fluids were continued for 6–12 hours thereafter. Over 85% of patients were hospitalized and most received sufficient intravenous fluids to maintain a urine output of 100–125 ml per hour. Patients with border-line renal function received 12.5 g of mannitol i.v. at the time of drug administration. In Protocol V, patients who had extensive irradiation were given DOX, 30 mg/m², as the initial dose, but dose modification permitted increases to 45 and 60 mg/m². Patients who had no previous

Table 20.2
BLADDER CANCER: PRIMARY PROTOCOLS

| Protocol | Drugs (mg/m²) | | |
	DDP	CYCLO	DOX
I	–	–	8–12
			45–75
II	–	350–700	37–75
III	65–70	–	–
IV	70	250–1000	–
V	70	–	30–60
VI	70	250	30–45

chemotherapy or limited irradiation (2000 rad in 5 days, before operation) were started at 45 mg/m² (Yagoda, 1979a,b). Data obtained in the murine bladder cancer model indicated synergism when DOX was given 48–72 hours after DDP (Soloway and Murphy, 1979): thus, in Protocol VI, DDP, CYCLO and DOX were administered sequentially on days 1, 2 and 3 every 3–4 weeks and, so far, 27 patients have been treated, 26 of whom are evaluable.

Secondary disease-orientated Phase II protocols, in patients who eventually had progression of disease with Protocols I–VI, included treatment with methotrexate (MTX), neocarzinostatin (NCS) and PALA (N-phosphonoacetyl-L-aspartic acid). Two MTX schedules were used: 250 mg/m² infused i.v. over 4 hours, followed 24 hours later by citrovorum factor rescue, 15 mg p.o. every 6 hours for 12 doses, and 0.5–1.0 mg/kg i.v. weekly. Patients who received the high-dose schedule were given adequate hydration to induce an hourly urine out-put >100 ml before, during and 12–24 hours after, drug administration. In addition, sufficient p.o. and i.v. sodium bicarbonate was administered to keep the urine alkaline. Any rise in serum creatinine (above 1.8 mg %) was treated vigorously with higher doses of citrovorum factor. Two weeks later, maintenance therapy was begun with MTX 0.5–1.5 mg/kg i.v. weekly. NCS, a new antitumour antibiotic, was administered in doses of 1500–2750 u/m² in a half-hour infusion daily for five consecutive days every 6–7 weeks. Antihistamine drugs were used to decrease drug-related chills, pyrexia and allergic reactions. PALA, an intermediate enzyme inhibitor of aspartate transcarbamylase, was administered in doses of 2.5–4.5 gm/m² i.v. weekly.

Tertiary drug protocols included bleomycin (BLEO) 0.25–0.5 mg/kg, daily by continuous infusion for 7–9 days or until mucositis occurred, and CYCLO 25–40 mg/kg i.v. every 3 weeks or 3 mg/kg per day, p.o.

PATIENT CHARACTERISTICS

Patient characteristics in Protocols I–VI are outlined in *Table 20.3*. Some variations are evident, such as an increasing performance status (PS) from Protocol I to Protocols III–VI, and a decreasing incidence of previous irradiation and chemotherapy from Protocols I–III compared with IV–VI. Although patient selection was relatively strict, perusal of all information at conclusion of the study including autopsy

Table 20.3
PATIENT CHARACTERISTICS

Characteristics	Protocol					
	I (N = 51)	II (N = 20)	III (N = 38)	IV (N = 40)	V (N = 30)	VI (N = 23)
Age (years)	63	57	62	62	63	58
	(39–79)	(39–75)	(39–77)	(30–79)	(35–77)	(47–75)
Males (%)	74	70	87	62	76	82
Performance status	60	70	75	80	80	80
	(20–90)	(40–90)	(20–100)	(20–90)	(50–100)	(40–100)
Tumour grade III (%)			70	70	73	81
Prior therapy						
Radiotherapy (%)	96	90	79	87	76	62
Chemotherapy (%)	55	30	34	8	21	8
Ileal conduit (%)	50	55	37	48	27	39
Natural history						
Time from symptoms to			2.0	3.0	2.0	1.5
diagnosis (months)			(0–120)	(0–82)	(0–80)	(0–75)
Time from diagnosis to	32	13	19.5	16	26	23
protocol (months)	(1–120)	(1–63)	(0.5–144)	(0–168)	(1–137)	(2–165)
Time from protocol to	4	6	4.5	6	6	7
follow-up (months)	(1–70)	(1–34)	(1–24)	(1–35+)	(1–22)	(1–15+)

information occasionally led to the reclassification of a few patients from the 'measurable' to the 'evaluable' categories; however, *Table 20.4* indicates that, in most instances, the criteria for admission to these protocols — indicator lesions — were met. The accuracy of computerized transaxial tomograms in defining intra-abdominal and pelvic lesions in two dimensions was evaluated in Protocols III and IV and, subsequently,

Table 20.4
PATIENT CHARACTERISTICS (continued)

Characteristics	Protocol					
	I (N = 51)	II (N = 20)	III (N = 38)	IV (N = 40)	V (N = 30)	VI (N = 23)
Indicator lesions						
Lung	25	14	15	17	14	10
Nodes						
supraclavicular mass	22	6	15	10	12	4
Liver	4	0	2	5	1	2
CTT	0	0	2	4	3	7
Evaluable	0	0	4	3	0	0
Measurable parameters						
Lung	25	14	15	17	14	10
Nodes	32	10	19	16	15	5
Liver	28	0	6	10	6	3
CTT	4	2	2	10	10	13
CEA	0	0	4/9	21/28	8/20	8/15

the number of patients with such indicator lesions entered into Phase II studies has increased. All measurable lesions are outlined in *Table 20.4*. The CEA has been found to be a useful marker in documenting response; 57% of patients had an increase $\geq$ 5 ng % and, in almost all cases, a decreasing CEA level correlated with response.

RESULTS

Two hundred and six patients were entered in Protocols I–VI, 61 in secondary and 44 in tertiary protocols. Adequate trials were obtained in 89% of cases. DOX, used alone, yielded clinically useful remissions (CR + PR) in only 16% of cases, but in patients who had no previous chemotherapy the response rate increased to 27%. Objective regression of disease was rapid, occurring within 3–4 weeks and persisting for 1–5 months. Most responses were observed within two doses or 6 weeks. Four patients achieved MR status for 6 weeks and four additional patients given the intermittent schedule responded, compared with four out of 28 given bolus administration. While there was one patient whose disease progressed after two doses of 45 mg/m^2 and which subsequently responded to 75 mg/m^2, the only CR occurred in a patient who received 45 mg/m^2. In the latter case, death resulted from acute congestive heart failure after a total doxorubicin dose of 430 mg/m^2, and at post-mortem examination no evidence of residual disease was found, although cardiomyopathy, possibly drug-related, was observed on histological examination. The combination of CYCLO and DOX was disappointing; only three of 18 patients achieved PR status (*see Table 20.5*).

Table 20.5
PRIMARY PROTOCOLS: RESPONSE

Protocol	All patients			Previously untreated with chemotherapy			Previously treated		
	Number entered	Number evaluated	CR/PR (%)	Number entered	Number adequate	CR/PR (%)	Number entered	Number adequate	CR/PR (%)
I	18	15	7	10	7	0	8	8	13
II	33	28	18	13	11	27	20	17	12
III	20	18	17	14	12	17	6	6	17
IV	38	35	37	25	23	52	13	12	8
V	40	35	46	38	34	44	2	1	100
VI	30	26	54	24	21	43	6	5	60
	27	26	50	24	23	48	3	2	67

DDP used on its own, produced clinically significant remissions in 37% of patients, and in previously untreated cases the response rate approached one in every two patients (*Table 20.5*). Responses were rapid, generally occurring within 7–21 days, and were noted in irradiated and non-irradiated tumour-bearing sites. However, some patients continued to have recurrent carcinoma in situ or new lesions intravesically despite sustained response to systemically administered DDP. Dose-limiting but not dose-dependent toxicities were anorexia and vomiting. In fact, occasionally a patient given three or more doses of DDP became nauseous and vomited before the next drug administration. Standard anti-emetic therapy was ineffective. Many patients who did respond to DDP refused additional doses, or requested that intervals between doses be delayed for 6–8 weeks; most responses, therefore, were unmaintained. The average duration of response was 5 months and unmaintained remissions persisted for an average of 10 weeks. A few patients did obtain prolonged remissions of up to 9 months' duration without additional therapy.

The combinations of DDP + CYCLO, DDP + DOX and DDP + CYCLO + DOX have produced response rates of 46, 54 and 50% respectively (*Table 20.5*). However, in previously untreated patients, remission rates with combination DDP protocols are identical to those which could be obtained with DDP used singly. Patient entry continues into Protocol VI. At this time there appears to be no advantage associated with DDP-combination regimens because the incidence of complete remission has not increased, whereas toxicity has increased and patient acceptance has fallen.

MTX induced a 36% response rate in 28 cases (*Table 20.6*). Remissions were rapid, usually within 7–14 days, and persisted for 4–6+

Table 20.6
SECONDARY AND TERTIARY PROTOCOLS: RESPONSE

Protocol	Number adequate	CR/PR (%)
Methotrexate (MTX)	28	36
Neocarzinostatin (NCS)	19	5
N-phosphono-acetyl L-aspartic acid (PALA)	18	0
Cyclophosphamide (CYCLO)	11	9
Vinblastine (VLB)	10	20
5-fluorouracil (5-FU)	6	17
Vincristine (VCR)	5	0
Bleomycin (BLEO)	4	0
Melphalan (MEL)	2	0
Hydroxyurea (HU)	2	0
6-mercaptourine (6MP)	1	0
Cyclophosphamide, doxorubicin (CAV)	1	0
Cis-diamminedichloride platinum II + methotrexate (DDP+MTX)	1	0
4'-(9-acridinylamino)-methanesulphone- m-anisidine (AMSA)	17	20

months. Most responses were obtained with doses as low as 0.25–1.0 mg/kg i.v. weekly and have been noted in previously treated patients. So far, only one of 19 patients has responded to NCS (Natale *et al.,* 1980). Although no patient has shown a clinically significant response to PALA, three have had minor remissions.

The low response rate with tertiary protocols is not surprising because the majority of patients have had extensive prior chemotherapy (*Table 20.6*). Previous data from clinical trials in patients with other solid tumours indicate few remissions in previously treated cases.

DOSES AND TOXICITY

The median number of doses and mg/m² in Protocols I, II, V and VI is outlined in *Table 20.7*. Data of Protocols III and IV have already been published (Yagoda *et al.,* 1976; 1978). The incidence of non-haematological and haematological toxicities is presented in *Tables 20.8* and *20.9,* respectively. The intermittent schedule of DOX did produce more mucositis and diarrhoea, but less nausea and vomiting than with bolus administration. DOX induced alopecia, anorexia and nausea, which were dose-dependent and almost universal with higher

Table 20.7
TOTAL NUMBER OF COURSES AND DOSES

Protocol	Drug(s)	Schedule(s)	Number of doses*	Total dose (mg/m²)*
I	DOX	8 mg/m² × 1,2,8,9 → 4 weekly	6.5 (3–10)	70 (35–111)
		15 mg/m² × 1,2,3,8,9,10 → 4 weekly	8 (5–40)	145 (92–940)
		45–60 mg/m² 3 weekly	3 (1–14)	165 (45–590)
II	DOX	45–60 mg/m² 3 weekly	4 (1–10)	184 (45–430)
	CYCLO	450–600 mg/m² 3 weekly		1824 (450–4050)
IV	DOX	30–60 mg/m² 3 weekly	3.5 (1–10)	165 (30–495)
	DDP	70 mg/m² 3 weekly		200 (60–590)
VI	DOX	30–45 mg/m² 3 weekly	3 (1–7)	135 (45–270)
	CYCLO	250 mg/m² 3 weekly		750 (250–1750)
	DDP	70 mg/m² 3 weekly		210 (70–490)

* Median. Range in parentheses

Table 20.8
NON-MYELOSUPPRESSIVE TOXICITY (%)

| Side-effects | Protocol and number of patients | | | | |
| | I | | II | V | VI |
	(N = 18)	(N = 33)	(N = 20)	(N = 30)	(N = 23)
Nausea/vomiting	25	75	100	100	100
Mucositis	75	9		4	
Alopecia	83	90	100	100	100
Cardiac effects	8	9			8
Neuropathy				7	4
Renal effects				36	57
Chills, fever				18	13
Tumour pain				4	8
$\downarrow Ca^{++}$, $\downarrow Mg^{++}$				7	
Tinnitis				13	
Metallic taste				4	

doses. Severe toxicity, rated as 3+ and 4+, occurred in one-third of cases, perhaps because most patients were over 65 years of age, had advanced disease, extensive previous therapy with poor haematopoietic reserve and, frequently, a history of recurrent urinary tract infections with compromised renal function. These factors, coupled with increasing doses of DOX which produced moderate leucopoenia, rapidly led to sepsis. Electrocardiographic changes were noted in only 12% of cases, but most patients received $< 300 \, mg/m^2$. One patient who achieved prolonged STAB had no cardiac toxicity in spite of a total dose of 950 mg/m^2. DOX was stopped in some patients because of minor ST-T wave changes which eventually reverted to normal. Protocol II produced an increased incidence of 3+ toxicity which required hospitalization in 39% of patients because of severe myelosuppression. In addition, haemorrhagic cystitis was noted, which was attributed to the effect of CYCLO on the irradiated bladder.

The major side-effects associated with DDP protocols were nausea and vomiting. Occasionally, hypomagnesaemia, hypocalcaemia, peripheral neuropathy and tinnitus were observed. Any abnormal increase in the blood urea nitrogen or serum creatinine was noted and, although some evidence of renal dysfunction occurred in 25–57% of patients, in the majority of cases impairment was minimal and could be attributed to renal obstruction, pyelonephritis, or the concomitant use of aminoglycoside antibiotics. However, in some cases deterioration of renal function had to be attributed to DDP. In a few patients who were responding to DDP, poor renal function prevented further therapy when progression of disease occurred. As expected, the incidence of thrombocytopoenia and leucopoenia was more common in DDP combination regimens.

With increased doses, all patients who received MTX developed mild to moderate mucositis which was taken to indicate an adequate

Table 20.9
MYELOTOXICITY

Myelotoxic effects

			Protocol and number of patients				
	(N = 18)	*I* *(N = 33)*	*II* *(N = 20)*	*III* *(N = 38)*	*IV* *(N = 40)*	*V* *(N = 30)*	*VI* *(N = 23)*
Leucopoenia ($4.5 \times 10^3/m^3$)							
%	67	60	70	17	65	67	89
Median	2.6	2.5	2.2	3.2	2.8	2.2	2.6
	(0.9–4.5)	(0.8–4.3)	(0.5–3.9)	(1.9–4.2)	(0.8–4.4)	(0.2–4.2)	(0.2–4.4)
Thrombocytopoenia ($175 \times 10^3/m^3$)							
%	50	42	37	23	61	42	67
Median	161	145	144	145	145	118	130
	(12–175)	(51–169)	(100–172)	(100–173)	(24–174)	(12–174)	(31–170)

Range in parentheses

dosage of drug. Because many patients already had some evidence of renal dysfunction secondary to tumour, pyelonephritis, the use of aminoglycoside antibiotics or previous treatment with DDP, surprisingly low doses of MTX resulted in mucositis and leucopoenia. However, only three episodes of severe MTX-induced toxicity required hospitalization.

NCS was generally tolerated well, but one patient had moderate pancytopoenia which persisted for 10 months, two patients had acute allergic reactions and one, reversible hepatic toxicity. Although pulmonary fibrosis and toxicity had been reported with NCS, none occurred in the 19 patients with urothelial tract tumours. PALA induced mild nausea, anorexia, vomiting, mucositis, gastrointestinal disturbances (i.e. diarrhoea) and leucopoenia. Skin rashes were frequent, with severe desquamation in one-third of cases. In fact, five patients required hospitalization and one death could be attributed to sequelae of PALA administration. In addition, seizures were observed in patients with metastatic cerebral lesions.

DISCUSSION

Phase II clinical trials at Memorial Hospital indicate that transitional cell carcinoma of the urothelial tract is a chemotherapeutically responsive tumour. The most active agent is DDP, with response rates approaching almost 50% in previously untreated patients. A review of the literature, coupled with the present series, finds an overall response rate of 42% in 81 adequately treated cases. Data available at present do not indicate any additive or synergistic benefit with the use of DOX, CYCLO, 5-fluorouracil and combinations of these agents in DDP-containing regimens. Response rates of all DDP combination regimes are almost identical to the results (or within the 95% confidence limits) which can be obtained with DDP used singly (Yagoda, 1980). An increase in survival is found in patients who respond to DDP regimens, compared with non-responders (*Figure 20.1*), but survival curves for responders in all four protocols are almost identical.

Other chemotherapeutic agents which have demonstrated antineoplastic activity against this tumour include MTX and DOX. It is noteworthy that MTX responses have occurred in patients who previously have had chemotherapy. A potentially useful combination could be DDP + MTX, but both drugs require normal renal function. The MTX trial at Memorial Hospital confirms the results found by the Royal Marsden Hospital group (Hall *et al.*, 1974; Turner *et al.*, 1977). DOX has been one of the most thoroughly studied drugs in cases of this tumour and although earlier trials indicated remission rates as high as 55%, the overall response rate is 24% in 175 cases (Yagoda, 1980). The duration of remission has been short, averaging 3 months, although some patients have shown responses for 28–52+ weeks.

NCS in previously treated patients has no role in the treatment of disseminated bladder cancer, although Sakamoto *et al.* (1978) have described some beneficial effects in patients with local disease. So far, the results with PALA have been disappointing, although this drug had exhibited excellent antineoplastic activity in a carcinogen-induced bladder cancer model in mice (Soloway and Murphy, 1979). Response rates with tertiary single-drug protocols which have used such drugs as cyclophosphamide, vinblastine and bleomycin, have been few, but additional trials are needed in previously untreated patients to evaluate their efficacy fully.

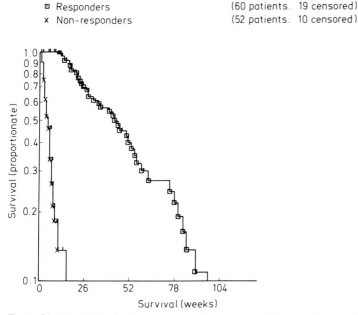

Figure 20.1 Survival of patients with bladder cancer receiving DDP: responders compared with non-responders

Further studies using single agents are needed: such trials should be performed in patients with bladder cancer who have measurably objective two-dimensional lesions, so that a clear end-point of response can be documented. While there are few such patients, the use of computerized transaxial tomography, and possibly of transrectal sonography, may significantly enlarge the patient population available for clinical studies. While a true comparison between activity of two agents used singly or in combination can be made only in prospective randomized extended Phase II or Phase III trials, so far, all studies have failed to induce a sufficiently high complete remission rate. However, the poor prognosis in patients with high-grade Stages B_1, B_2, C and D_1 tumours after pre-operative irradiation and radical cystectomy, suggests the need for some type of adjuvant treatment. With the response rates currently achieved, using DDP, DOX and MTX, it is not unreasonable to start controlled, prospective, randomized trials involving pre- or post-operative adjuvant chemotherapy in high-risk patients with bladder cancer.

REFERENCES

HALL, R.R., BLOOM, H.J.G., FREEMAN, J.R., NAWROCKI, A. and WALLACE, D.M. (1974). Methotrexate treatment for advanced bladder cancer. *British Journal of Urology*, **46**, 431–438

NATALE, R.B., YAGODA, A. and WATSON, R.C. (1980). Phase II trial of neocarzinostatin in patients with bladder and prostatic cancer: toxicity of a 5-day i.v. bolus schedule. *Cancer*, **45**, 2836–2842

SAKAMOTO, S., OGATA, J., IKEGAMI, K. and MAEDA, H. (1978). Effects of systemic administration of neocarzinostatin, a new protein antibiotic, on human bladder cancer. *Cancer Treatment Reports*, **62**, 453–454

SOLOWAY, M.S. and MURPHY, W.M. (1979). Experimental chemotherapy of bladder cancer — systemic and intravesical. *Seminars in Oncology*, **6**, 166–183

TURNER, A.G., HENDRY, W.F., WILLIAMS, G.B. and BLOOM, H.J.G. (1977). The treatment of advanced bladder cancer with methotrexate. *British Journal of Urology*, **49**, 673–678

WHITMORE, W.F., Jr., BATATA, M.A., HILARIS, B.S., REDDY, G.N., UNAL, A., GHONHEIM, M.A., GRABSTALD, H. and CHU, F. (1977). A comparative study of two preoperative radiation regimens with bladder cancer. *Cancer*, **40**, 1077–1086

YAGODA, A. (1977). Future implications of phase 2 chemotherapy trials in ninety-five patients with measurable advanced bladder cancer. *Cancer Research*, **37**, 2775–2780

YAGODA, A. (1979a). Phase II trials in bladder cancer at Memorial Sloan-Kettering Cancer Center, 1975–1978. In *Cancer of the Genitourinary Tract*. Ed. by D.E. Johnson and M.L. Samuels, Raven Press; New York

YAGODA, A. (1979b). Phase II trials with cis-diamminedichloride platinum II in the treatment of urothelial cancers. *Cancer Treatment Reports*, **63**, 1565–1572

YAGODA, A. (1980). Chemotherapy of matastatic bladder cancer. *Cancer*, **45**, 1879–1888

YAGODA, A., WATSON, R.C., GONZALEZ-VITALE, J.C., GRABSTALD, H. and WHITMORE, W.F., Jr. (1976). Cis-dichlorodiammineplatinum (II) in advanced bladder cancer. *Cancer Treatment Reports*, **60**, 917–923

YAGODA, A., WATSON, R.C., GRABSTALD, H., BARZELL, W.E. and WHITMORE, W.F. Jr. (1977). Adriamycin and cyclophosphamide in advanced bladder cancer. *Cancer Treatment Reports*, **61**, 97–99

YAGODA, A., WATSON, R.C., KEMENY, N., BARZELL, W.E., GRABSTALD, H. and WHITMORE, W.F., Jr. (1978). Diamminedichloride platinum II and cyclophosphamide in the treatment of advanced urothelial cancer. *Cancer*, **41**, 2121–2130

21

Cis-platinum Combination Treatment for Bladder Cancer

Stephen D. Williams, Lawrence H. Einhorn and John P. Donohue

INTRODUCTION

Chemotherapy of urothelial malignancy has been discouraging. Doxo-rubicin (DOX), 5-FU, cyclophosphamide (Carter and Wasserman, 1975), and methotrexate (Turner *et al.*, 1977) appear to have moderate activity. More recently, cis-platinum (DDP) has been recognized as having definite single-agent activity (Yagoda *et al.*, 1976) and several combination regimens employing this agent have been evaluated (Sternberg *et al.*, 1977; Troner, 1979; Yagoda, 1980). These have confirmed the feasibility and beneficial effects of DDP-based treatment but, remarkably, none have yielded response rates or remission durations higher than that expected from DDP alone (Yagoda *et al.*, 1976; 1980).

In 1976, we started to evaluate the combination of DDP + DOX + 5-FU. This combination was chosen because of the potential synergism of DDP and DOX (Vogel *et al.*, 1976). In addition, the combination of DOX + 5-FU has been reported to be useful in such patients (Cross *et al.*, 1976; Samal *et al.*, 1977). Our initial results have already been reported (Williams *et al.*, 1978). This Chapter updates our results to include the first 44 patients so treated.

PATIENTS AND METHODS

Forty-four patients with unresectable or metastatic urothelial cancer were treated with the combination of DDP + DOX + 5-FU. Charac-teristics of the patient population are outlined in *Table 21.1*. No patient had been given chemotherapy previously. A few patients had no readily measurable disease. All patients were unsuitable for other types of therapy and gave their informed consent.

Pre-treatment evaluation included routine laboratory studies and radiographs, radioisotope bone scan, abdominal ultrasonography and, frequently, cystoscopy and bi-manual examination under anaesthesia.

Two different treatment schedules were employed. At first, DDP was given at a dose level of 20 mg/m² for 5 days and DOX and 5-FU at dose levels of 50 mg/m² and 500 mg/m² respectively on day 1 of each course. Dose levels of DOX or 5-FU were 40 mg/m² and 400 mg/m² for patients over 65 years of age, or those who had received prior

Table 21.1
PATIENT POPULATION

Number	44
Male	38
Female	6
Median age (years)	62 (range 42–76)
Histology	
Transitional	40
Squamous	2
Adenocarcinoma	2
Prior radiotherapy	25

radiotherapy. Three such courses were given at 4-week intervals and then the second treatment schedule was used. In this, DDP was given at a single dosage of 50–100 mg/m² and DOX and 5-FU were given as above. Twenty-nine patients received the first schedule and 14 received 1-day DDP only. The choice of treatment schedules was made in a non-random fashion and, in general, patients receiving 5-day DDP initially had a more favourable prognosis.

Intravenous hydration with normal saline or one-half normal saline in dextrose was given to all patients. For the 5-day schedule, this was begun on the evening before treatment and continued at 100 ml/hour. For the 1-day schedule 500–1000 ml were given on the treatment day, usually in the out-patient department. Mannitol and diuretics were not used.

During the study, blood count, blood urea and creatinine measurements were obtained before each treatment. In general, creatinine clearances were not obtained. Tumours were usually measured every 4 weeks and never less frequently than every 8 weeks. Treatment was continued until disease progression was noted or toxicity (usually nausea and vomiting) precluded further therapy.

Partial remission was defined as a 50% decrease in measurable tumour.

RESULTS

Toxicity

Toxic manifestations of this treatment are outlined in *Table 21.2*. Nausea, vomiting and alopecia were universal and quite troublesome. Four patients refused further treatment because of prolonged vomiting. Ten patients required transfusion during treatment, presumably related to haematuria and chronic myelosuppression from DDP in this elderly

Table 21.2
TOXICITY

Side-effects	Number of patients (%)
Nausea, vomiting	43 (100)
Alopecia	43 (100)
Transfused	10 (23.6)
Symptomatic hearing loss	3 (7.0)
Fever, leucopoenia	1 (2.3)
Creatinine > 2.5 mg%	5 (11.6)
Cardiotoxicity	0
Refused subsequent treatment	4 (9.3)
Drug-related deaths	0

patient population. Nephrotoxicity was quite acceptable, particularly as the majority of these patients had abnormal baseline renal function. One patient, however, developed clinically significant renal failure (not requiring dialysis) from which he recovered. There were no drug-related deaths.

Therapeutic response

Response, remission duration, and survival are shown in *Table 21.3*. It should be remembered that the patients receiving 1-day DDP in general were those with a less favourable prognosis and thus differences in response rate and duration probably are not due to differences in efficacy of the treatment regimens.

Overall response rate was 46.2% and all remissions were only partial. Remission duration tended to be brief but was usually associated with gratifying subjective benefit. Responding patients appeared to gain little or no increase in survival after treatment.

Of particular interest is a small subgroup of eight patients who, during their initial evaluation, were thought to be possible candidates for radical surgery if they attained a good response to chemotherapy. Of these, six were explored after chemotherapy and four were resected

Table 21.3
THERAPEUTIC RESPONSE

Characteristics	Duration of treatment		
	One day*	Five days*	Total
Number	15	29	44
No measurable disease	3	1	4
Early death	0	1	1
Evaluable	12	27	39
CR†	0	0	0
PR⌀	4 (33.3%)	14 (51.9)	18 (46.2%)
Remission duration (months)	4.3	6.6	6.1
Survival responders (months)	9	11.5	10.9
Survival group (months)	8	9.0	8.7

* Treatment schedule of DDP; † CR = complete remission; ⌀ PR = partial remission

for 'cure', with radical cystectomy and urinary diversion by ileal conduit. Of these four patients, one remained disease-free for 18 months and then developed a pelvic recurrence. One patient is disease-free but follow-up is minimal (5 months) and two other patients developed rapidly progressive metastases in the early post-operative period. At first presentation, both of these latter patients had bulky pelvic disease and small extra-pelvic metastases. The extra-pelvic disease regressed totally with chemotherapy, and residual pelvic disease was surgically removed. The other six patients initially had tumour confined to the pelvis.

DISCUSSION

The response rate of our study is remarkably similar to that reported by Yagoda *et al.* (1978) with DDP + cyclophosphamide (47%) and by Troner (1979) with DDP + cyclophosphamide + DOX (33%). The latter regimen is similar to that reported by Sternberg *et al.* (1977) to have a 90% response, although the patient population in this study is small. Likewise, the duration of remission in our study is brief, a point which has also been noted by others (Yagoda *et al.*, 1978).

It is a matter of concern that these results are similar to those seen when DDP is given as a single agent to patients who have not received previous chemotherapy (Yagoda *et al.*, 1976). Thus, we believe there is serious doubt as to whether combination chemotherapy is any better than DDP alone, although a random prospective trial is needed to answer this question. Such a study is in progress.

We also believe that there is little, if any, survival benefit associated with this chemotherapy. Accordingly, we now reserve such treatment for patients with significant symptoms referrable to this disease.

Of the spectrum of bladder cancer, there is a group of patients with resectable disease who are at high risk of recurrence, presumably due to the presence of micrometastases. It is reasonable to consider the use of post-operative adjuvant chemotherapy in such patients. We have done a pilot study of such an approach in a small group of patients and have found it difficult, but feasible. However, the marginal response rate and the lack of complete remission casts doubt on the potential benefit of currently available chemotherapy. Once again, random prospective trials are needed.

A few patients who present with locally unresectable disease will be made resectable with chemotherapy. Our results imply that this approach should not be used in patients with known metastases even if these respond completely to chemotherapy. The number of patients with pelvic disease only who become resectable is low. Nevertheless, we would still consider such patients for surgery if they appear to have responded well to chemotherapy. We hope that a few of these patients, whose prognosis is otherwise dismal, may enjoy long-term disease-free survival.

Chemotherapy with DDP represents a definite improvement in the management of patients with advanced urothelial cancer. There remains much to be learned, however, and additional active agents are urgently needed.

ACKNOWLEDGEMENT

This study was supported in part by Public Health Service Grant RR 00750 and American Cancer Society CF 3678

REFERENCES

CARTER, S.K. and WASSERMAN, T.H. (1975). The chemotherapy of urologic cancer. *Cancer,* **36**, 729–747

CROSS, R.J., GLASHAN, R.W., HUMPHREY, C.S. (1976). Treatment of advanced bladder cancer with Adriamycin and 5-fluorouracil. *British Journal of Urology,* **48**, 609–615

SAMAL, B., BAKER, L., IZBICKI, R., McDONALD, B. and SAMSON, M. (1977). Phase I-II trial of Adriamycin and 5-fluorouracil. *Proceedings of the American Society of Clinical Oncology,* **18**, 312, (abstract)

STERNBERG, J.J., BRACKEN, R.B., HANDEL, P.B, and JOHNSON, D.E. (1977). Combination chemotherapy (CISCA) for advanced urinary tract carcinoma. *Journal of the American Medical Association,* **238**, 2282–2287

TRONER, M.D. (1979). Cyclophosphamide, adriamycin and platinum (CAP) in the treatment of urothelial malignancy. *Proceedings of the American Association for Cancer Research,* **20**, 117, (abstract)

TURNER, A.G., HENDRY, W.F., WILLIAMS, G.B. and BLOOM, H.J.G. (1977). The treatment of advanced bladder cancer with methotrexate. *British Journal of Urology,* **49**, 673–678

VOGEL, S., OHNUMA, T., PERLOFF, M., and HOLLAND, J.F. (1976). Combination chemotherapy with Adriamycin and cis-diamminedichloroplatinum in patients with neoplastic diseases. *Cancer,* **38**, 21–26

WILLIAMS, S.D., ROHN, R.J., DONOHUE, J.P. and EINHORN, L.H. (1978). Chemotherapy of bladder cancer with cis-diamminedichloroplatinum, Adriamycin, and 5-fluorouracil. *Proceedings of the American Society of Clinical Oncology,* **19**, 316, (abstract)

YAGODA, A. (1980). Chemotherapy of metastatic bladder cancer. *Cancer,* **45**, 1879–1888

YAGODA, A., WATSON, R.C., GONZALEZ-VITALE, J.C., GRABSTALD, H. and WHITMORE, W.F. (1976). Cis-dichlorodiammine-platinum (II) in advanced bladder cancer. *Cancer Treatment Reports,* **60**, 917–923

YAGODA, A., WATSON, R.C., KEMENY, N., BARZELL, W.G., GRABSTALD, H. and WHITMORE, W.F. (1978). Diamminedichloride platinum II and cyclophosphamide in the treatment of advanced urothelial cancer. *Cancer,* **41**, 2121–2130

22

The Contribution of the EORTC (European Organisation for Research and Treatment of Cancer) Urological Group and the Yorkshire Urological Cancer Research Group (YUCRG) to the Management of Invasive Bladder Cancer

P.H. Smith and A. Akdas

INTRODUCTION

The present EORTC Urological Group was formed in 1976 from two pre-existing groups within the same organization — one largely French and Italian in membership, the other English and Belgian. Both groups had recognized the problems presented by the treatment of invasive bladder cancer and were actively investigating the potential role of cytotoxic chemotherapy in urological cancer. Within the last three years, certain British members of the group, largely resident in Yorkshire and known as the Yorkshire Urological Cancer Research Group (YUCRG) have carried out studies additional to those of the EORTC. The results of both form the basis of this Chapter.

The management of invasive bladder cancer remains controversial but the emphasis is moving away from the use of cystectomy or radio-therapy alone and towards the combination of pre-operative radio-therapy and cystectomy (Wallace and Bloom, 1976; Prout, 1977;

Whitmore, 1977). Although the 5-year survival rate following this combined local therapy is approximately 10% higher than after radical radiotherapy used alone, it is increasingly recognized that invasive bladder cancer is a systemic disease which logically deserves some form of systemic therapy – possibly by cytotoxic chemotherapy (De Kernion, 1977; Smith and YUCRG, 1979).

The aim of the EORTC Urological Group and of the YUCRG has been to develop a chemotherapeutic regime suitable for adjuvant therapy.

CLINICAL STUDIES

The choice of drugs was based on the paper by Carter and Wasserman (1975) demonstrating that doxorubicin (DOX) and 5-fluorouracil (5-FU) were the most effective drugs then evaluated. In the last 4 years we have carried out a Phase II study and a toxicity study and implemented two adjuvant studies.

EORTC phase II study*

Sixty-three patients with advanced bladder cancer were treated with four cycles of DOX and 5-FU using a protocol in which after an initial evaluation DOX 50 mg/m² and 5-FU 500 mg/m² were given 3-weekly for four cycles until the final evaluation. Of the 52 evaluable patients there were 21 objective remissions (four complete and 17 partial). In addition symptomatic improvement occurred in many patients, even when objective response was not seen and toxicity was minimal (EORTC Urological Group B, 1977).

YUCRG toxicity study*

In this study, 18 consecutive patients with Category T3 NX MX (UICC, 1974) bladder cancer were treated with the same regime – radical radiotherapy followed by a gap of 1–3 months, then DOX 50 mg/m² and 5-FU 500 mg/m² 3-weekly for a maximum of 11 cycles.

Chemotherapy was started 1 month after completion of radiotherapy when possible, and not later than three months. It was decided to give up to a maximum of 11 cycles at 3-weekly intervals (maximum 550 mg/m² DOX). All patients received at least four cycles with

*Coordinator M.R.G. Robinson, Pontefract

minimal toxicity, but thereafter toxicity became a limiting factor in one-third of the patients – in four patients because of gastrointestinal side-effects not relieved by anti-emetics and in two because of cardiac problems (Glashan *et al.,* 1977).

YUCRG adjuvant study (Protocol 771)*

Encouraged by the results of the first two studies the YUCRG has implemented a randomized adjuvant study to compare the effect of DOX and 5-FU in the same doses as above, compared with no additional treatment, in patients with category T3 NX MO bladder cancer, not over 75 years of age and with no clinical evidence of cardiac disease which would preclude the administration of DOX. Radical radiotherapy was followed by DOX or 5-FU (a minimum of 4 cycles every 3 weeks) or by no additional treatment. By June 1979, 88 patients had been entered into this study and it is hoped to produce a preliminary evaluation in 12–18 months.

EORTC adjuvant study (Protocol 30782)†

The YUCRG adjuvant study was not attractive to surgeons of the EORTC Urological Group in other countries, in part because of differences in the ready availability of high-standard radiotherapy, and in part because of attitudes towards cystectomy as the primary treatment of invasive bladder cancer. As a result a further adjuvant study has been prepared within the EORTC Urological Group. The EORTC study is designed to evaluate the role of adjuvant DOX + 5-FU after radical cystectomy for category P3, N–, N+ (N1, N2) MO bladder cancer.

In fact, there will be two separate studies as surgeons in Italy wish to use radical cystectomy as the primary treatment, while those in France and Spain prefer to give pre-operative radiotherapy using 1500 rad (750 rad daily × 2) 2–7 days before radical cystectomy. Patients are subsequently randomly allocated to a regime of DOX + 5-FU, or no additional treatment.

It has also been suggested that the previous regime used an inadequate amount of 5-FU and, in this study, the doses of the drugs have been modified. It is proposed to give in a 28-day cycle 40 mg/m² DOX on Day 1, followed by 5-FU 500 mg/m² i.v. (or i.m.) on days 2, 3, and 4, and then 300 mg/m² i.m. on days 8, 15, and 22, either monthly for 1 year or until a total dose of 500 mg/m² DOX has been given.

*Coordinator B. Richards, York
†Coordinator J.A. Martinez-Pineiro, Madrid

SIGNIFICANCE OF T AND P CATEGORY REDUCTION

Since our work started, several authors have emphasized the importance of P category reduction in patients treated by radical cystectomy following pre-operative radiotherapy as a factor in predicting survival Werf-Messing, 1975; Wallace and Bloom, 1976). In Leeds we have recently looked at the influence of T category reduction upon the survival of patients following radical radiotherapy. The overall results following T category reduction by radiotherapy are so similar to those

Table 22.1
SURVIVAL FOLLOWING COMPLETION OF RADICAL RADIOTHERAPY IN CATEGORY
T2 AND T3 BLADDER CANCER IN LEEDS (1972–74)

Total number of patients			With T reduction (to TO or T1) Survival		Without T reduction Survival	
Category	Number	Number	3 years	5 years	Number	3 years
T2	16	11	8 (72%)	6 (54%)	5	0
T3	33	16	10 (62%)	5 (30%)	17	0
Total	49 (100%)	27 (55%)	18 (66%)	11 (39%)	22	0

following pre-operative radiotherapy and cystectomy as to question the advisability of continuing to use cystectomy as a routine adjuvant to radiotherapy in patients with invasive bladder cancer (*Table 22.1*). It is especially pertinent to observe that of the seven patients who died between 3 and 5 years after the completion of radiotherapy, only two had evidence of tumour in the bladder at the time of their last cystoscopy (Smith *et al.*, 1980).

SURVIVAL AFTER RADIOTHERAPY AND CYTOTOXIC CHEMO-THERAPY

Several cytotoxic agents have now been shown to have activity in patients with invasive bladder cancer (Smith and YUCRG, 1980) and *Figure 22.1* shows that there is now some evidence from the 3-year survival data of the YUCRG Toxicity Study that the combination of radical radiotherapy and adjuvant chemotherapy may be at least as effective as the combination of radiotherapy and cystectomy. The figure contains the YUCRG survival data superimposed upon those of the Institute of Urology trial (Wallace and Bloom, 1976). If this preliminary evidence can be confirmed in the current EORTC and YUCRG adjuvant studies, the future will hold great promise.

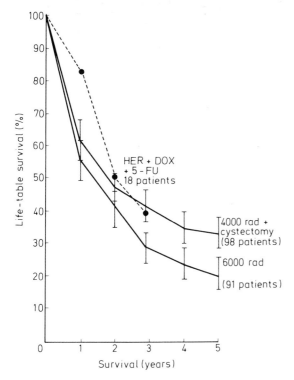

Figure 22.1 Comparison of survival of 18 patients treated on YUCRG adjuvant chemotherapy toxicity study (Glashan et al., *1977) with survival in Institute of Urology and Royal Marsden Hospital trial of pre-operative radiotherapy plus cystectomy versus radical radiotherapy plus salvage cystectomy (Wallace and Bloom, 1976, published by permission of the authors)*

CONCLUSIONS

Although the place of cytotoxic chemotherapy is not yet clearly defined, there is no doubt that the combination of DOX and 5-FU has activity and is not too toxic for use immediately after radical radio-therapy in the primary management of invasive bladder cancer. There is some preliminary evidence to suggest that this combination of therapy may be as effective as the combination of radiotherapy and cystectomy and the results of the trials of adjuvant chemotherapy recently implemented by the YUCRG and the EORTC Urological Group are urgently required.

REFERENCES

CARTER, S. and WASSERMAN, T.H. (1975). The chemotherapy of urologic cancer. *Cancer,* **36**, 729–747
DE KERNION, J.B. (1977). The chemotherapy of advanced bladder carcinoma. *Cancer Research,* **37**, 2771–2774

EORTC UROLOGICAL GROUP B   (1977). The treatment of advanced carcinoma of
the bladder with a combination of Adriamycin and 5-fluorouracil. *European
Urology,* **3**, 276–278

GLASHAN, R.W., HOUGHTON, A.L. and ROBINSON, M.R.G. (1977). A toxicity study
of the treatment of T3 bladder tumours with a combination of radiotherapy
and chemotherapy. *British Journal of Urology,* **49**, 669–672

PROUT, G.R. JR. (1977). The role of surgery in the potentially curative treatment
of bladder carcinoma. *Cancer Research,* **37**, 2764–2770

SMITH, P.H., AKDAS, A., CAMPBELL-ROBSON, L., FRANK, H.G. and WILLIAMS, R.E.
(1980). Radiotherapy and chemotherapy in the management of invasive bladder
cancer. In preparation.

SMITH, P.H. and YORKSHIRE UROLOGICAL CANCER RESEARCH GROUP (1980).
An approach to cytotoxic chemotherapy in carcinoma of the bladder. *Journal
of the Royal Society of Medicine,* in press

UICC (INTERNATIONAL UNION AGAINST CANCER) (1974). *TNM Classification of
Malignant Tumours.* Second Edition. Genève; Imprimerie G. de Buren S.A.

WALLACE, D.M. and BLOOM, H.J.G. (1976). The management of deeply infiltrating (T3) bladder carcinoma: controlled trial of radical radiotherapy versus
pre-operative radiotherapy and radical cystectomy (First report). *British Journal
of Urology,* **48**, 587–594

VAN DER WERF-MESSING, B.H.P. (1975). Carcinoma of the bladder T3 NX MO
treated by pre-operative irradiation followed by cystectomy (third report of
the Rotterdam Radiotherapy Institute). *Cancer,* **36**, 718–722

WERF-MESSING, B. VAN DER (1975). Carcinoma of the bladder T3 NX MO
metastatic lesions. *Cancer Research,* **37**, 2756–2758

23

Methotrexate

Alan G. Turner

INTRODUCTION

Methotrexate has long been considered as an active chemotherapeutic agent in bladder cancer, since Sullivan (1962), using the drug as a continuous intra-arterial infusion, noted in each of three cases of advanced primary bladder cancer 'a sustained clinical benefit and decrease in tumour size'. This observation was confirmed by Burn (1966) who also gave the drug by continuous intra-arterial infusion, and by Altman *et al.* (1972) who, using an intermittent intravenous dose, noted that four out of 11 patients (36%) responded, one showing a 'complete regression of visible tumour' and three showing 'obvious regression of tumour mass, it becoming both smaller and softer'.

A study was therefore instituted at the Royal Marsden Hospital in 1970, using methotrexate given as an intermittent intravenous dose. Hall *et al.* (1974) reported results from the first 42 patients treated, with a response rate of 26%. This study was extended, using higher dosage and folinic acid rescue, and the results which were originally published elsewhere (Turner *et al.*, 1977) are reviewed in this Chapter in the light of more recent experience in the use of chemotherapy in bladder cancer.

PHARMACOLOGY

Methotrexate is a folic acid antagonist. It acts by binding dihydrofolate reductase, thus inhibiting the conversion of folic acid to tetrahydrofolate. The consequent depletion of reduced folate prevents the metabolic transfer of 1-carbon units in a variety of biochemical reactions, including those involved in the synthesis of RNA and DNA. The drug, therefore, is highly cell-cycle dependent, acting specifically

219

during DNA synthesis (S phase). Cells undergoing rapid division with many cells in the S phase are, therefore, most susceptible.

Recent studies with high-dose methotrexate have suggested that high dosage may prevent protein synthesis and that some cells are arrested in the G phase. They are, therefore, prevented from reaching the S phase (Mauer, 1975) and thereby protected from methotrexate. This may produce methotrexate-resistant tumours.

Some dose schedules incorporate a folinic acid rescue at a certain time after methotrexate administration. Folinic acid is converted to tetrahydrofolate which enters the reduced folate cycle and bypasses the methotrexate-induced block.

Excretion of the drug is predominantly renal, 41% of an intravenous dose being excreted within 6 hours, 90% within 24 hours and 95% within 30 hours (Henderson *et al.,* 1965; Pratt *et al.,* 1974). With low plasma concentrations, methotrexate may be reabsorbed by the kidney, but at higher levels it is both filtered and actively secreted by the renal tubular cells (Huffman *et al.,* 1973). Impairment of renal function will cause retention of the drug, and it has been shown that toxicity is related to length of time of exposure rather than to the actual dose (Miller *et al.,* 1961; Goldie *et al.,* 1972).

CLINICAL EXPERIENCE

During the period 1970–77, 61 patients with advanced local or metastatic bladder cancer were treated with methotrexate at the Royal Marsden Hospital London.

Three different two-weekly regimes were used:

(A) methotrexate 50 mg intravenously, with *NO* folinic acid rescue;
(B) methotrexate 100 mg intravenously, with *NO* folinic acid rescue;
(C) methotrexate 200 mg intramuscularly with folinic acid rescue (21 mg i.m.) at 6, 12 and 24 hours.

The regimes A and B without folinic acid were given on an outpatient basis, but regime C was given to inpatients because of the need to give folinic acid rescue intramuscularly, as the oral form was not available when the study was started.

PATIENTS

Patients with advanced local disease that had not responded to, or had recurred after, radiotherapy, and patients with metastatic disease, were considered for therapy. The indications and the numbers of patients for each treatment schedule are recorded in *Table 23.1.*

Pre-treatment investigations of haemoglobin, white blood cell (WBC) count, platelet count, urea and creatinine concentrations, glomerular filtration rate (GFR), either creatinine clearance or EDTA clearance, chest X-ray, bone scan or skeletal survey were performed. If the GFR was found to be below 80 ml/min, then the dose of methotrexate was reduced and folinic acid rescue given.

Table 23.1
DISTRIBUTION OF PATIENTS ACCORDING TO EXTENT OF DISEASE AND TREAT–MENT SCHEDULE

Indications	Treatment schedule*		
	A (N = 23)	B (N = 22)	C (N = 16)
Local disease	14	8	6
Metastatic disease	5	11	6
Local and metastatic disease	4	3	4
Number of courses received	10.9	18.0	13
(range)	(3–47)	(3–64)	(3–49)

* See text for dose levels

Before each treatment, WBC and platelet estimations were performed. If the WBC count was below $3 \times 10^9/\ell$ and/or the platelet count was below $100 \times 10^9/\ell$, then the treatment was not given. Counts were checked 2 weeks later and, if satisfactory, treatment was recommenced.

If side-effects occurred, treatment was delayed unless they were severe, when treatment was abandoned.

In presentation of the results, patients who received only one or two courses were excluded. All these patients died of terminal disease, not of methotrexate toxicity.

RESULTS

Although both objective and subjective responses were noted, only objective responses are considered in the analysis of the results.

Objective responses are defined as *complete:* a complete regression of tumour lasting at least 6 months, or *partial:* objective reduction in size of metastatic deposits as seen radiologically and/or downstaging of local bladder tumours, the latter being assessed under general anaesthesia and confirmed by more than one observer on more than one occasion.

An example of complete regression of lung deposits following treatment with methotrexate can be seen in *Figures 23.1 and 23.2.* Total regression of lung metastases was confirmed on lung tomography.

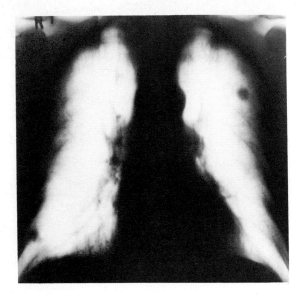

Figure 23.1 Pre-treatment chest X-ray of patient with metastatic carcinoma of the bladder

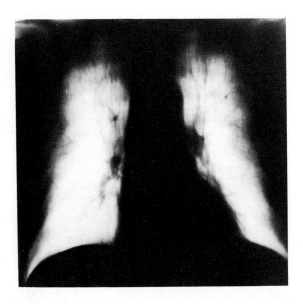

Figure 23.2 Post-treatment chest X-ray of same patient as shown in Figure 23.1

Complete responses

Four complete responses were noted and the site and duration of responses are shown in *Table 23.2*. There were no complete responses in the 50 mg dose group, three in the 100 mg group and one in the 200 mg with rescue group. The patient who had a complete response in bone was initially admitted paralysed because of a spinal deposit; he

Table 23.2
INFLUENCE OF TREATMENT SCHEDULE ON DURATION OF REMISSION IN MONTHS, AT SITES SHOWN

Site	Response	Treatment schedule*		
		A	B	C
Local	CR	—	—	—
	PR	89	4, 7, 26	4, 6, 34
Lung	CR	—	19	22
	PR	6	8, 8, 12	4, 3, 4
Bone	CR	—	18	—
	PR	—	2, 4, 12	3, 3
Skin	CR	—	7	—
	PR	2	3	—
Nodes	CR	—	—	—
	PR	—	4	4

* See text for details of treatment.
CR = complete response; PR = partial response

is now able to walk and has returned to work. Another patient receiving 200 mg with rescue, who achieved complete response in the lung, stopped treatment with methotrexate after 12 months. Subsequently, a solitary spinal deposit developed and the patient died 22 months after initial treatment. At post-mortem examination the lungs were found to be clear.

Partial responses

There were a larger number of partial responses, the site and duration of which are shown in *Table 23.2*. The patient with a local response for 89 months on the 50 mg regime is still alive, the methotrexate being stopped after 47 courses. He was originally staged as T3 but, after radiotherapy, was found to be totally inoperable at laparotomy. He was then started on methotrexate; the local tumour mass, although reduced substantially, persisted even after the treatment was stopped. The median duration of response was 6 months (*Table 23.2*) and overall complete plus partial response rate was 13% in the 50 mg group, 56%

Table 23.3
INFLUENCE OF TREATMENT SCHEDULE ON COMPLETE PLUS PARTIAL RESPONSE, BY SITE OF DISEASE

Site and response	Treatment schedule		
	A	B	C
Local primary tumour	1/18	3/11	3/10
Lymph nodes	0/5	1/5	1/5
Lung	1/1	4/6	4/6
Bone	0/2	4/6	2/7
Skin	1/1	2/2	0/0
Complete response	0/23	3/22	1/16
	13%	56%	50%
Partial response	3/23	9/22	7/16

in the 100 mg group and 50% in the 200 mg with rescue group (*Table 23.3*). Lung metastases responded more frequently than those in any other site (*Table 23.3*).

Subjective responses

Five of the 15 patients with bone metastases experienced dramatic pain relief after administration of methotrexate. In each case, the pain was from bony secondaries but, despite marked pain relief, there was no obvious healing of the deposits. These responses are in addition to the six patients who showed objective healing.

Toxicity

Toxic effects of the drug in the doses used were uncommon (*Table 23.4*). The effects were divided into mild and severe. In the mild cases,

Table 23.4
TOXIC SIDE-EFFECTS

Side-effects	Methotrexate every 2 weeks		
	50 mg	100 mg	200 mg with rescue
Mild (missed a dose)			
Mouth ulcers	9/23	8/22	–
Skin rash	1/23	–	–
Severe (treatment abandoned)			
Marrow toxicity	–	–	1/16
Lung perfusion defect	–	–	1/16
Severe mucositis	1/23	1/22	–
Skin necrosis	–	1/22	–

therapy was temporarily stopped but, in severe cases, treatment was abandoned. The skin necrosis that occurred was when methotrexate was given concurrently with radiotherapy.

DISCUSSION

Until recently there have been only sporadic reports on the effectiveness of chemotherapeutic agents in bladder cancer. In their review, Carter and Wasserman (1975) considered that only three agents were of proved value and that many more had been inadequately studied because the number of patients in each report were small. The agents considered to be of value were doxorubicin, mitomycin C and 5-fluorouracil. Since their paper, there have been many further reports of the effectiveness of single agents and various combinations (*see* Chapters 20–24).

The data reported here demonstrate that methotrexate as a single agent is as effective as any other cytotoxic drug tested in patients with metastatic bladder cancer. Recent confirmation of these results has come from Yagoda (*see* Chapter 20) who reported a 36% response rate in 28 patients who have relapsed after previous treatment with cis-platinum.

From the experience gained in the study reported further consideration should be given to various points:

Local disease

The response of the local bladder tumour to methotrexate is disappointing. In this study, of 39 patients in whom there was local tumour stage T4, only 7 (18%) showed response (*Table 23.3*). In each case it was only a partial response or downstaging of the tumour.

These observations agree with those from previous studies by Sullivan (1962), Burn (1966), Altman *et al.* (1972) and Hall *et al.* (1974), although there were two instances of complete responses in these papers.

As methotrexate is excreted in the urine, the drug has also been given intravesically, but with no effect (Abbassian and Wallace, 1966).

In conclusion, therefore, the effect of methotrexate on the local tumours is poor. This may be because previous radiotherapy has reduced the effectiveness of the drug (Johnston, 1966) or the fact that the tumour has reached an advanced stage and is resistant to all forms of treatment (Irvine, 1966). Combination of methotrexate and radiotherapy in the primary treatment may therefore increase the response of the local tumour.

Disseminated disease:

Methotrexate is more effective against metastases compared with local disease. In this study, 33 patients received methotrexate for metastases and 16 (48%) showed responses, four of which were complete and 12 partial (*Table 23.3*). In our original report (Hall *et al.*, 1974) this different response rate for metastatic disease compared with local disease was also demonstrated.

Dosage

As methotrexate is excreted through the kidneys, the pre-treatment assessment of renal function is essential for control of toxicity. A single injection in patients with reduced renal function may give plasma levels comparable to a 24-hour continuous infusion (Price, 1977). This is important, as it has been shown that toxic effects depend on the length of exposure to the drug (Goldie *et al.*, 1972). Methotrexate can also cause tubular damage (Condit *et al.*, 1969) and hence renal function must be checked during therapy. The regimes used in this study had no effect on renal function.

There was a suggestion of a dose-related increase of response rate shown in this study, although there was no increase when the dose was changed from 100 mg to 200 mg, the latter with folinic acid rescue.

No experience has been reported in bladder cancer with the extremely large doses used in osteogenic sarcoma. Tumour resistance to methotrexate may be attributable to one of the following mechanisms: reduction of cell-membrane permeability to the drug (Fischer, 1959); increased synthesis of the target enzyme (Bertino *et al.*, 1961; Fischer, 1961) or detoxication of the drug (Jacobson and Cathie, 1960). It is possible that use of extremely high doses may overcome these problems and will be considered for future studies as Goldie *et al.* (1972) have given doses up to 20 000 mg by infusion over 24 hours with folinic acid rescue to patients with advanced malignant disease, and observed no serious toxic effects.

Toxicity

Methotrexate in this study was well tolerated and had few of the unpleasant side-effects of other agents. The higher incidence of toxicity seen in the 50 mg group (*Table 23.4*) was due to inexperience of use, as the drug was initially used on a weekly basis. With the weekly regime, the incidence of neutropoenia and mucositis was so high that a two-weekly regime was adopted. Harding *et al.* (1977) have since shown that the incidence of neutropoenia was reduced if each course of methotrexate was separated by at least 8 days, but there was *no* alteration in the antitumour effect. The only side-effect other than those noted in *Table 23.4* was nausea, which responded well to anti-emetics.

Severe side-effects were uncommon. Nesbit *et al.* (1976) found serious side-effects in hepatic, pulmonary and skeletal systems after long-term methotrexate. These were not observed in our study.

Patients with bladder cancer are of the older age group and thus drug tolerance may be poor. Methotrexate was well tolerated, which contrasts with other agents where toxic effects caused abandonment of treatment in a high percentage of cases (Turner *et al.*, 1979) or patient refusal to have further courses of treatment (Yagoda *et al.*, 1976; Glashan *et al.*, 1977). When contemplating chemotherapy, this point must be given careful consideration.

CONCLUSION

From this study it is concluded that methotrexate is a valuable chemo-therapeutic agent in the management of advanced bladder cancer. It is a safe, well-tolerated drug with few side-effects and can be used on an outpatient basis. For these reasons it may be a useful agent in combination with already established treatment regimes and has now been incorporated into a trial by the London and Oxford Cooperative Cancer Group as an adjuvant to radiotherapy and surgery in the management of stage T3 tumours (*see* Chapter 25).

REFERENCES

ABBASSIAN, A. and WALLACE, D.M. (1966). Intracavitary chemotherapy of diffuse, non-infiltrating papillary carcinoma of the bladder. *Journal of Urology,* **96**, 461–465

ALTMAN, C.C., McCAGUE, N.J., RIPEPI, A.C. and CARDOZO, M. (1972). The use of methotrexate in advanced carcinoma of the bladder. *Journal of Urology,* **108**, 271–273

BERTINO, J.R., HUENNEKENS, F.M. and GABRIO, M. (1961). Increased activity of leukocyte dihydrofolic reductose in amethopterin treated patients. *Clinical Research,* **9**, 103

BURN, J.I. (1966). Intra-arterial infusion in malignant diseases of the pelvis. In *Second Symposium on Methotrexate in the Treatment of Cancer.* Ed. by P.M. Worrall and H.J. Espiner, pp. 58–63. Bristol; Wright

CARTER, S.K. and WASSERMAN, T.H. (1975). The chemotherapy of urologic cancer. *Cancer,* **36**, 729–747

CONDIT, P.T., CHANES' R.E. and JOEL, W. (1969). Renal toxicity of methotrexate. *Cancer,* **23**, 126–131

FISCHER, G.A. (1959). Amethopterin-nutritional resistance characteristics of leukaemic clones. *Cancer Research,* **19**, 372–376

FISCHER, G.A. (1961). Increased levels of folic acid reductose as a mechanism of resistance of amethopterin in leukaemic cells. *Biochemical Pharmacology,* **7**, 75–77

GLASHAN, R.W., HOUGHTON, A.L. and ROBINSON, M.R.G. (1977). A toxicity study of the treatment of T3 bladder tumours with a combination of radiotherapy and chemotherapy. *British Journal of Urology,* **49**, 669–672

GOLDIE, J.H., PRICE, L.A. and HARRAP, K.R. (1972). Methotrexate toxicity: correlation with duration of administration, plasma levels, dose and excretion pattern. *European Journal of Cancer,* **8**, 409–414

HALL, R.R., BLOOM, H.J.G., FREEMAN, J.E., NAWROCKI, A. and WALLACE, D.M. (1974). Methotrexate treatment for advanced bladder cancer. *British Journal of Urology,* **46**, 431–438

HARDING, B., CULVENOR, J. and MacLENNAN, I.C. (1977). Effects of varying the interval between courses of methotrexate on its myelotoxic and anti-leukaemic activities. *British Journal of Cancer,* **35**, 40–51

HENDERSON, E.S., ADAMSON, R.H. and OLIVERIO, V.T. (1965). The metabolic fate of tritiated methotrexate, II. Absorption and excretion in man. *Cancer Research,* **25**, 1018–1024

HUFFMAN, D.H., WAN, S.H., AZARNOFF, D.L. and HOOGSTRATEN, B. (1973). Pharmacokinetics of methotrexate. *Clinical Pharmacology and Therapeutics,* **14**, 572–579

IRVINE, W.T. (1966). In *Second Symposium on Methotrexate in the Treatment of Cancer,* Ed. by P.M. Worrall and H.J. Espiner, pp. 68. Bristol; Wright

JACOBSON, W. and CATHIE, I.A.B. (1960). The inactivation of folic acid antagonists by normal and leukaemic cells. *Biochemical Pharmacology,* **5**, 130–142

JOHNSTON, I.D.A. (1966). An assessment of intra-arterial infusion with methotrexate in the treatment of malignant disease of the head and neck. In *Second Symposium of Methotrexate in the Treatment of Cancer.* Ed. by P.M. Worrall and H.J. Espiner, pp. 52–57. Bristol; Wright

MAUER, A.M. (1975). Cell kinetics and practical consequences for therapy of acute leukaemia. *New England Journal of Medicine,* **293**, 389–390

MILLER, E., SULLIVAN, R.D., YOUNG, C.W. and BURCHENAL, J.H. (1961). Clinical effects of continuous infusion of antimetabolites; prevention of toxicity of 5-fluoro-2-deoxyuridine by thymidine. *Proceedings of the American Association for Cancer Research,* **3**, 251

NESBIT, M., KRIVITT, W., HEYN, R. and SHARP, H. (1976). Acute and chronic effects of methotrexate on hepatic, pulmonary and skeletal symptoms. *Cancer,* **37**, 1048–1054

PRATT, C.B., ROBERTS, D., SHANKS, E. and WARMATH, F.L. (1974). Clinical trials and pharmacokinetics of intermittent high dose methotrexate 'leucovorin rescue' of children with malignant tumours. *Cancer Research,* **34**, 3326–3331

PRICE, L.A. (1977). Personal communication

PROUT, G.R., SLACK, N.H. and BRASS, I.D.J. (1972). Preoperative irradiation and cystectomy for bladder carcinoma: Results in a selected population. In *7th National Cancer Conference Proceedings,* pp. 783–793. Lippincott

SULLIVAN, R.D. (1962). Intra-arterial methotrexate therapy: the dose duration and route of administration studies of methotrexate in clinical cancer chemotherapy. In *First Symposium on Methotrexate in the Treatment of Cancer.* Ed. by R. Porter and E. Wiltshaw, pp. 50–55. Bristol; Wright

TURNER, A.G., DURRANT, K. and MALPAS, J.S. (1979). A trial of bleomycin versus Adriamycin in advanced carcinoma of the bladder. *British Journal of Urology,* **51**, 121–124

TURNER, A.G., HENDRY, W.F., WILLIAMS, G.B. and BLOOM, H.J.G. (1977). The treatment of advanced bladder cancer with methotrexate. *British Journal of Urology,* **49**, 673–678

YAGODA, A., WATSON, R.C., GONZALEZ-VITALE, J.C., GRABSTALD, H. and WHITMORE, W.F. (1976). Cis-dichlorodiammineplatinum (II) in advanced bladder cancer. *Cancer Treatment Reports,* **60**, 917–923

24

Effect of Chemotherapy on Locally Recurrent Invasive Bladder Tumours

R.T.D. Oliver

The benefits of elective cystectomy after radiotherapy are most clearly established in patients under the age of 65 years (Wallace and Bloom, 1976). The fact that more than 50% of patients with bladder cancer present at an older age, and that the patients most disturbed by the enforced loss of sexual function after cystectomy are under 65 years old, means that there would be considerable advantage in the development of treatments which did not involve cystectomy.

Most of the data on chemotherapy in the accompanying Chapters in this book are from studies of treatment of measurable metastases. This undoubtedly produces important screening information for detecting active drugs, but as yet has produced little improvement in patient survival. Persistent or recurrent primary tumour after initial treatment is the major problem after radical radiotherapy, and exceeds the incidence of clinically detectable metastatic disease, as demonstrated in *Table 24.1*, which shows the tumour status at last observation in the patients whose survival analysis is reported in Chapter 15. At least two-thirds of patients dying of bladder cancer have persistent problems relating to the primary tumour. To the urologist, this may be a strong argument in favour of cystectomy. To the oncologist, the more important observation relates to the one patient in four treated by radical radiotherapy who has been saved from cystectomy; the challenge is to improve on that figure. Little information has been published on the effect of chemotherapy on primary bladder tumours, particularly relating the UICC T stage to response.

Table 24.1
DISEASE STATUS AT LAST OBSERVATION*

Status	T1 N = 90	T2 N = 132	T3 N = 220	T4 N = 262
Alive:	48%	23%	29%	4%
(% disease-free)	(71)	(87)	(79)	(55)
Dead: local disease	21%	25%	23%	40%
Dead: local disease +				
metastases	10%	18%	15%	31%
Dead: metastasis	2%	5%	5%	8%
Dead: other causes	16%	25%	23%	14%

* Data from Hope-Stone (Chapter 15)

This paper reviews the results of three preliminary phase I/II studies designed to evaluate the problem of giving nephrotoxic drugs to patients with advanced pelvic disease. Two single agents, methotrexate and cis-platinum, and the three-drug combination of doxorubicin, cis-platinum and cyclophosphamide, have been assessed. Patients received methotrexate at a time when there were insufficient supplies of cis-platinum or if they were over 75 years old. *Table 24.2* shows the characteristics of the patients treated, indicating that the majority of patients had T4 tumours, and the patients receiving methotrexate were, on average, slightly older.

Table 24.2
PATIENT CHARACTERISTICS

Drug	N	Median Age (years)
Methotrexate 100 mg/m² /2-weekly + folinic acid	13 (7)*	69 (37–79)†
Cis-platinum 50 mg/m² /3-weekly	6 (4)	65 (54–70)
Doxorubicin 40 mg/m² Cyclophosphamide 75 mg/m² } 3-weekly Cis-platinum 75 mg/m²	6 (3)	62 (42–68)

* Figures in parentheses indicate number of T4 patients treated
† Age range

Table 24.3 gives the response to treatment as assessed after two treatments with the platinum-containing protocols, or six treatments with methotrexate. The small numbers of patients preclude any definite analysis of the effectiveness of the particular treatments. Although responses were observed with all three treatments, there was no patient in whom unequivocal lysis of a bi-manually palpable mass occurred, as

Table 24.3
EFFECT OF CHEMOTHERAPY ON RECURRENT PRIMARY BLADDER TUMOURS IN
PATIENTS WITHOUT CLINICAL EVIDENCE OF METASTASIS

Chemotherapy	N	Cystoscopic evidence of response	Evidence of symptomatic response for > 3/12
Methotrexate 100 mg/m²/2-weekly and folinic acid	13	2	3
Cis-platinum 50 mg/m²/3-weekly	6	1	1
Doxorubicin 40 mg/m² + Cyclophosphamide 750 mg/m² + Cis-platinum 75 mg/m²/3-weekly	6	3	1

has been well documented using radiotherapy. Furthermore, the
patients judged to have responded would have been considered as
responders only on less rigorous criteria than those used to assess the
response of measurable metastases. Four patients were considered to
have responded, as biopsy in the area of the tumour changed from
positive to negative: all four patients had relatively small masses and
post-irradiation fibrosis, which made assessment of the tumour size
impossible. The other two patients showing cystoscopic evidence of
response were assessed to have reduction in size of a bi-manually
palpable mass, but by no means as much as 50%.

This response rate is extremely low and is approximately half that
reported for these drugs in the literature when they have been used to
treat patients with measurable metastases. Results from my own limited
experience of treating such patients with metastases (*Table 24.4*)
confirm the difference in response rate between primary and metastatic tumours, and demonstrate that our response rate treating metastatic disease is as good as that reported in the literature. There are two
possible explanations for this: either the clones of cells which produce
the metastases have different biological properties from primary

Table 24.4
COMPARISON OF PRIMARY AND METASTATIC BLADDER CANCER RESPONSE TO
CHEMOTHERAPY

Chemotherapy	Patients with primary tumour and no metastases		Patients with clinically measurable metastases		Response rate taken from a review of the literature	
	N	Cystoscopic evidence of response	N	PR	N	PR
Methotrexate	13	2 (15%)	6	2 (33%)	145	35%
Cis-platinum	6	1 (17%)	16	6 (38%)	114	37%

N = number of patients treated; PR = partial response

tumour cells, as Fidler (1978) has demonstrated by cloning cells from primary tumours and metastases of experimental animal tumours, or, alternatively, the methods for assessing response of the primary are not as sensitive as those used to assess response of metastases. I favour the latter hypothesis for two reasons, as follows.

First, it is established that present clinical staging techniques underestimate the degree of response to radiotherapy, as witnessed by the number of patients with a mass palpable in the bladder after treatment, in whom histology reveals necrotic tissue only (Werf-Messing, 1980).

Second, if the objective and subjective responses in this series are combined, the overall response rate (44% in this series) approximates to that seen after chemotherapy for measurable metastases. The symptomatic responses almost all involved reduction of pain and of urinary frequency for sustained periods (the longest for 12 months and the shortest for 4 months), although in one patient there was cessation of haematuria and reduction of bladder pain. The most convincing evidence that these minor responses indicate tumour response was the disappearance of malignant cells on serial urine cytology (*Table 24.5*).

Table 24.5
CHEMOTHERAPY AND URINARY CYTOLOGY

Cytology response	Responders*	Non-responders
Continuously positive	0	7
Change from positive to negative	4	1
Continuously negative	5	4
Not done	2	2

* Responders: patients showing measurable or symptomatic response

In addition, two patients with T4 tumour receiving methotrexate at two-weekly intervals had repeated, but temporary, response of symptoms after each injection. When the dose was doubled, one of them had sustained control of symptoms lasting 6 months, though at examination under anaesthetic and on CT scan at 3 and 6 months there was no change in the size of the tumour mass. Additional indirect evidence that these equivocal responses were due to effect of the drug on tumour comes from the observation that responders survived better than non-responders (*Table 24.6*), and patients showing subjective responses were those with the larger T4 tumours (*Table 24.7*). It is possible that the use of more refined techniques such as flow cytometry of exfoliated tumour cells in the urine (Tribukait *et al.*, 1979) might help in the accurate quantitation of this type of response.

Table 24.6
SURVIVAL OF CHEMOTHERAPY RESPONDERS VS. NON-RESPONDERS

Patients	N	Alive at 6 months
Responders*	11	9
Non-responders	14	5

* Responders: patients showing measurable response or symptomatic response.

Table 24.7
EFFECT OF CHEMOTHERAPY ON RECURRENT PRIMARY BLADDER TUMOURS IN PATIENTS WITHOUT CLINICAL EVIDENCE OF METASTASIS

Tumour stage	N	Cystoscopic evidence of response	Evidence of symptomatic response for > 3/12
≤T3	11	5	1
T4	14	1	4

N = number of patients treated

Although of some palliative use, the response demonstrated in this study is of limited clinical value for patients with advanced disease. However, if the effect proved to be additive to the effect of radiotherapy it might reduce the number of patients having to undergo cystectomy. Some evidence in support of this concept was seen in a pre-trial pilot study where seven of 10 patients, given three doses of methotrexate before pre-operative or radical radiotherapy, had complete disappearance of tumour by 6 months after combined treatment was completed (Oliver, unpublished observations). This compares with a complete response rate after radical radiotherapy of 42% seen in the study by Hope-Stone *et al.* (Chapter 15) and a 38% complete response achieved in the Institute of Urology trial (Wallace and Bloom, 1976). These early results, which were achieved without any increase in side-effects of treatment, have led to the setting up by the London and Oxford Cooperative Urological Cancer Group of a randomized trial comparing the combination of radiotherapy and methotrexate with radiotherapy alone (*see* Chapter 25) as either pre-cystectomy treatment for patients under 65 years old or as radical treatment for patients over 65 years.

REFERENCES

FIDLER, I.J. (1978). Tumour heterogeneity and the biology of cancer invasion and metastasis. *Cancer Research,* **38**, 2651–2660

TRIBUKAIT, B., GUSTAFSON, H. and ESPOSTI, P.L. (1979). Ploidy and proliferation in human bladder tumors as measured by flow-cytofluometric DNA-analysis and its relation to histopathology and cytology. *Cancer,* **43**, 1742–1751

WERF-MESSING, B. VAN DER. (1980). Carcinoma of the bladder category T3 NX, 0–4 MO treated by pre-operative irradiation followed by cystectomy at the Rotterdam Radiotherapy Institute. In *Bladder Tumours and Other Topics in Urological Oncology,* Ed. by P.H. Smith, pp. 281. New York: Plenum Publishing Company (in press).

WALLACE, D.M. and BLOOM, H.J.G. (1976). The management of deeply infiltrating (T3) bladder carcinoma: controlled trial of radical radiotherapy versus pre-operative radiotherapy and radical cystectomy (first report). *British Journal of Urology,* **48**, 587–594

IIIC

Treatment of invasive tumours: integration
of chemotherapy into early treatment

25

A Clinical Trial of Methotrexate Combined with Radiotherapy and Surgery in Deeply Infiltrating (T3) Carcinoma of Bladder

The London and Oxford Cooperative Urological Cancer Group*

The results of the Institute of Urology Trial of radical radiotherapy versus pre-operative radiotherapy and cystectomy showed that the combined treatment produced a slight, but not significant, improvement in overall results. The trend in favour of the combined treatment was more marked in the younger patients and especially in those showing a good response (downstaging) to the initial radiotherapy (*see* Chapter 17 and Wallace and Bloom, 1976). This impressive effect of downstaging encouraged us to include in the next trial an increased pre-operative dose of irradiation with the addition of systemic chemotherapy in the hope of further increasing the local antitumour effect. In addition, since the majority of deaths in the first 18 months following cystectomy were due to metastases, it was hoped that the early exposure to chemotherapy might control distant micrometastases.

Several drugs assessed as active single agents in patients with advanced bladder cancer have been studied by this group. Disappointing

*Grant Williams (Chairman), Prof. M. Alderson, H.J.G. Bloom, H.T. Ford, W.F. Hendry, R.J. Shearer, P.A. Trott (The Royal Marsden Hospital); J. Malpas, R. Sandland, H. Whitfield (St. Bartholomew's Hospital); N. Howard, E. Newlands, P.F. Philip (Charing Cross Hospital); J. Boyd (St Helier Hospital); M. Snell (St Mary's Hospital); K. Durrant, G. Fellows, J.C. Smith (Oxford); R.T.D. Oliver, P.R. Riddle (St Peter's Hospitals); G.F. Abercrombie, I. Cade and J. Vinnicombe (Portsmouth)

results were obtained with doxorubicin and bleomycin (Turner *et al.,* 1979), but methotrexate given for 2 weeks produced objective evidence of response in 56% of 22 outpatients, and in 50% of 16 inpatients when given in higher dosage with folinic acid rescue (*see* Chapter 23, Turner *et al.,* 1977). Methotrexate was well tolerated by elderly patients, and side-effects were few, provided that care was taken to adjust its dosage if renal function was impaired. This drug was therefore selected as adjuvant in a new prospective trial for T3 bladder carcinomas. For logistic reasons, the preliminary three doses of methotrexate were to be given in hospital with folinic acid rescue, before radiotherapy. After completion of radiotherapy (with or without surgery), therapy with methotrexate without folinic acid rescue was to be maintained on an outpatient basis for 9 months.

The original T3 trial showed that the benefits of the combined treatment (pre-operative radiotherapy and cystectomy) were seen only in patients aged less than 65 years, partly because of the increased morbidity and mortality associated with cystectomy over this age (*see* Chapter 17). Pre-operative radiotherapy and cystectomy were therefore included in the protocol only for patients aged less than 65 years, and radical radiotherapy was to be given to patients over this age (with possible salvage cystectomy if indicated). It was also recognized that, in some centres, there was a preference to undertake cystectomy only in those patients who had had previous radical radiotherapy, and whose tumours had failed to respond or had recurred (*see* Chapter 15 and Vinnicombe and Abercrombie, 1978). It was agreed that such a centre could continue a policy of radical radiotherapy and salvage cystectomy for all ages of patients, provided that this policy was consistently followed throughout the trial. Finally, it was recognized that certain patients might not be fit for elective cystectomy on medical or psychological grounds and they, too, would be treated by radical radiotherapy.

Table 25.1
THE LONDON AND OXFORD COOPERATIVE UROLOGICAL CANCER GROUP

Group A; (i)	Pre-radiation methotrexate		(ii)
	4400 rad in 4.5 weeks ↓	compared with	4400 rad in 4.5 weeks ↓
	Elective radical cystectomy ↓		Elective radical cystectomy
	Maintenance methotrexate ↓		
Group B: (ii)	Pre-radiation methotrexate ↓		(ii)
	6400 rad in 6.5 weeks ↓	compared with	6400 rad in 4.5 weeks
	Post-radiation methotrexate ↓		↓
	Salvage cystectomy		Salvage cystectomy

Patients with T3 bladder tumours who are to be entered into this new trial are investigated to exclude distant metastases. Treatment is either by pre-operative radiotherapy and elective cystectomy, or radical radiotherapy with or without salvage cystectomy, according to the patient's age and the defined policy of the centre at which he is treated. Treatment is randomized between those who will, or will not, receive additional adjuvant methotrexate (*Table 25.1*). The protocol is reproduced in detail below.

AIMS OF STUDY

To test in patients with T3 bladder tumour without systemic metastases whether adjuvant treatment with methotrexate increases local control, reduces the risk of distant metastases and improves survival.

REQUIREMENTS FOR ADMISSION TO STUDY

(1) Histologically confirmed carcinoma of the urinary bladder — tumours may be either transitional cell or squamous cell carcinomas.
(2) On bi-manual examination, induration or a nodular mobile mass is palpable in the bladder wall, which persists after transurethral resection of the exophytic portion of the lesion; and/or there is microscopic invasion of deep muscle or extension through the bladder wall (UICC category T3).
(3) Absence of metastases on chest X-ray $\left.\right\}$ mandatory.
                                bone scan

                            liver scan $\left.\right\}$ optional.
                            lymphography
(4) Normal blood count and liver function tests.
(5) A measured creatinine clearance.

PREVIOUS TREATMENT

Patients who have previously been treated by diathermy, local excision or by interstitial radiation implant, but whose tumours progressed to category T3, are still eligible for the trial, but the nature and the date of commencement of the previous treatment must be entered in the Notification Form.

TREATMENT PROTOCOL

Patients will be randomly allocated to treatment with or without methotrexate. All patients over 65 years old will receive radical radiotherapy with or without methotrexate. Patients aged less than 65 years will be treated by pre-operative radiotherapy and 'elective' radical cystectomy, with or without methotrexate.

It is recognized that certain centres prefer to reserve cystectomy for cases where recurrence is confined to the bladder after previous radical radiotherapy — so-called 'salvage' cystectomy. If a collaborating centre states *at the outset* that it prefers to do only salvage cystectomies, then that centre will treat all patients primarily with radical radiotherapy, with or without methotrexate.

Some patients will not be fit for surgery. Such patients under treatment by surgeons who normally are committed to elective cystectomy will be randomized separately.

TREATMENT DETAILS

Preliminary chemotherapy

Creatinine clearance > 80 ml/min

Methotrexate 100 mg/m² intravenously as straight i.v. push followed by folinic acid rescue (15 mg i.m. at 24 hours).

Creatinine clearance 50–80 ml/min

As above, but in addition, oral folinic acid 15 mg 6-hourly will be given for 48 hours after the initial intramuscular injection.

Creatinine clearance < 50 ml/min

Patients with creatinine clearance of less than 50 ml/min should be treated only if facilities for measurement of methotrexate levels exist. Folinic acid should be continued until plasma methotrexate level is less than 5×10^{-8} (μmol/ℓ). Follow-up therapy should also not be given until that level has been reached.

Great care must be taken to ensure that folinic acid is given precisely as prescribed. A detailed explanation should be given to the patient and nursing staff of the dangers of missing out dosage and a chart should be drawn for each dose given. The responsible doctor or nurse should append their signature and the exact time of administration. **Patients should be well hydrated and the urine should be alkaline when receiving methotrexate. At least 3 litres oral fluid should be given in 24 hours, and patients should be receiving sodium bicarbonate 1 g b.d.** This regime should be given on days 0, 7 and 14.

Before each course, biochemical estimations of haemoglobin, differential white cell count and platelets, the serum SGOT level, serum creatinine, urea and electrolytes, should be performed. If there is any evidence of toxicity from the previous injection, such as a reduction in the white cell count of $< 3.0 \times 10^9/\ell$; in platelets $< 100 \times 10^9/\ell$; an increase in creatinine >130 mmol or urea >7.5 mmol; or if mouth ulcers are seen, then **delay** injection for 1 week and then give the normal dose but **in addition** to intramuscular folinic acid 15 mg at 24 hours, give **oral** folinic acid 15 mg 6-hourly for 48 hours.

Rest

The patient should rest for 7 days.

Radiotherapy

All patients will receive 4400 rad in 4.5 weeks (tumour dose 200 rad $\times$ 22 fractions) to the whole pelvis starting on day 21. Patients having radical radiotherapy will receive an additional 2000 rad in 2 weeks to the bladder only, to a total dose of 6400 rad. The pre-operative irradiated volume is to extend from the lower border of L5, down to the inferior margin of the obturator foramen and laterally to 1.5–2 cm beyond the edge of the bony pelvis. The suggested technique is an anterior direct field, and two lateral wedged fields (extending posteriorly from the pubis to ensure full coverage of the bladder and perivesical tissue, but sparing the rectum as much as possible).

For those patients receiving radical radiotherapy without elective surgery, an additional 2000 rad is given to the bladder and perivesical tissue, using an anterior direct field (approximately 8 $\times$ 9 cm) and two posterior oblique fields (approximately 8 $\times$ 9 cm).

Rest period for patients proceeding to elective cystectomy

Three weeks at home.

Radical cystectomy

This includes excision of external iliac, internal iliac and obturator nodes, with ileal loop diversion.

Maintenance chemotherapy

Creatinine clearance should be re-measured before starting maintenance chemotherapy.

Creatinine clearance > 80 ml/min

Methotrexate 100 mg i.v. with no folinic acid rescue, starting 1 month after completion of surgery or radiotherapy, repeated every 2 weeks for 3 months, and then every month for a further 9 months.

Creatinine clearance 50–80 ml/min

As above, giving methotrexate 50 mg i.v.

Creatinine clearance < 50 ml/min

To be treated with methotrexate only if radiommunoassay of metho-trexate is available and hospital admission for 48 hours is possible. Before each course, biochemical estimations of haemoglobin, differential white count and platelets, serum SGOT level and serum creatinine, urea and electrolytes, should be performed. If there is any evidence of toxicity from the previous injection such as a reduction in the white cell count $< 3.0 \times 10^9/\ell$; platelets $< 100 \times 10^9/\ell$; increase in creatinine > 130 mmol or urea > 7.5 mmol; or the occurrence of mouth ulcers, then **delay** injection for 1 week and then give the normal dose, but **in addition** to intramuscular folinic acid 15 mg at 24 hours, give **oral** folinic acid 15 mg 6-hourly for 48 hours.

Follow-up

All patients will be reviewed at not more than 3-monthly intervals for up to 5 years. Patients who have not had cystectomy should have cystoscopy at these times. Salvage cystectomy will be done at the discretion of the urologist concerned, if there is biopsy confirmation of recurrence in the bladder at least 6 months after completion of radical radiotherapy, provided that there are no distant metastases and the patient is fit.

PROGRESS TO DATE

So far, (between 1 June 1978 and 1 December 1979), 56 patients have been entered into the trial, and their treatment allocation is shown in *Table 25.2*. At this stage, of course, there is no indication whether the addition of methotrexate will have any influence on survival. However,

Table 25.2
THE LONDON AND OXFORD COOPERATIVE UROLOGICAL CANCER GROUP

Age of patients	(1 June 1978–1 December 1979) Treatment	Number of patients
Over 65 years	6400 rad	17
	6400 rad + MTX	17
Under 65 years	4400 rad + radical cystectomy	11
	4400 rad + radical cystectomy + MTX	8
	6400 rad	2
	6400 rad + MTX	1

no serious complications have been encountered as a result of including methotrexate in these treatment regimens, although one patient developed severe stomatitis and mucositis after receiving only two preliminary doses of chemotherapy, and one other patient developed a rise in serum creatinine.

REFERENCES

TURNER, A.G., DURRANT, K.R. and MALPAS, J.S. (1979). A trial of bleomycin versus Adriamycin in advanced carcinoma of bladder. *British Journal of Urology*, **51**, 121–124

TURNER, A.G., HENDRY, W.F., WILLIAMS, G.B. and BLOOM, H.J.G. (1977). The treatment of advanced bladder cancer with methotrexate. *British Journal of Urology*, **49**, 673–678

VINNICOMBE, J. and ABERCROMBIE, G.F. (1978). Total cystectomy — a review. *British Journal of Urology*, **50**, 488–491

WALLACE, D.M. and BLOOM, H.J.G. (1976). The management of deeply infiltrating (T3) bladder carcinoma: controlled trial of radical radiotherapy and radical cystectomy (first report). *British Journal of Urology*, **48**, 587–594

26

The Combination of Chemotherapy and Radiotherapy in Invasive Carcinoma of the Bladder

B. Richards and the Yorkshire Urology Cooperative Research Group

The therapeutic attack on carcinoma of the bladder has been directed mainly towards eradication of the primary tumour. This approach has been reasonably rewarding as long as the disease is superficial. Nevertheless, the outlook for patients with infiltrating cancer remains unsatisfactory. While there are significant differences in the survival rates in series of patients treated with primary radiotherapy (Rider and Evans, 1976; Wallace and Bloom, 1976; Miller, 1977), primary surgery (Wajsman *et al.,* 1975), or with a combination (Wajsman *et al.,* 1975; Wallace and Bloom, 1976; Miller, 1977), these differences are relatively small compared with the proportion of patients who die of their disease whatever treatment is employed. Differences in survival at 5 years may be about 10%, but 70% die, irrespective of the primary treatment.

Many patients die of metastatic disease which was not evident at the time of primary therapy. Thirty-four per cent of 281 patients with T3 bladder tumours reported by Rider and Evans died of distant metastases after treatment with radiotherapy (Rider and Evans, 1976). In other series, the primary treatment failed as a result of development of metastases in 26% of 205 patients with all categories of transitional cell carcinoma (Whitmore *et al.,* 1977), in 39% of 28 patients with T2 and T3 tumours, and in 35% of 96 cases of all T categories after radiotherapy followed by cystectomy (Prout, 1977). It is possible that some of these distant metastases may have occurred as a result of failure of local control of the tumour, but there was only evidence of intrapelvic disease in 20% of the 205 cases reported by Whitmore *et al.* (1977), in 25% of the 96 cases reported by Prout (1977), and in 26% of the recurrences in a series of 183 patients reported by Rubin (1971). Control of the primary tumour was satisfactory in these patients, and their deaths are likely to have been due to micrometastases, present but undetected at the time of initial treatment — an incidence of failure which it would be hard to reduce by improving the treatment of the bladder lesion itself. The presence of these micrometastases is a great challenge to the clinician and has led to the advocacy of adjuvant chemotherapy (Wallace and Bloom, 1976; De Kernion, 1977; Prout, 1977; Whitmore *et al.*, 1977), which should be more effective in the treatment of micrometastases than would be expected from the response rates when the tumour loads are larger (Schabel, 1975), partly because the vascularization of small tumours is better, so that drug delivery is likely to be more efficient, and partly because a higher proportion of the cells are in a proliferative phase of cell division.

The question of timing of the different aspects of combination therapy is interesting and important. In general, the aim of combining chemotherapy with radiotherapy is either to increase the efficiency of local control of the primary tumour (by an additive radiopotentiating effect) or to control micrometastases outside the field of radiotherapy. Radiotherapy, like chemotherapy, is more effective when the tumour bulk is small. Each method of treatment would benefit from any bulk reduction achieved by the other. On the other hand, each depresses the immune response (Mathé, 1978), and reduces the body's tolerance to the other. Which should be used first?

The answer is not in doubt when one of the treatments is very effective. Seminoma of the testis, for example, is very sensitive to radiotherapy, which should therefore be used first. Teratocarcinoma is often very sensitive to chemotherapy and the chance of a complete remission is diminished by prior irradiation (Stoter *et al.*, 1979). Unfortunately, the chemotherapeutic agents which are available are not very active in bladder cancer: objective responses can be expected in not more than 50% of patients treated by single agents or combination chemotherapy (Merrin *et al.*, 1975; Cross *et al.*, 1976; Turner *et al.*, 1977; Yagoda *et al.*, 1978; Williams *et al.*, 1980). The response rates in other series are very much less than this (Merrin *et al.*, 1975; Yagoda *et al.*, 1977; Turner *et al.*, 1979), although a 90% response rate to CISCA (cis-platinum, doxorubicin and cyclophosphamide) has been reported in one small series of 10 cases (Sternberg *et al.*, 1977).

There is little information about the response rate to chemotherapy in previously untreated patients with bladder cancer. In one trial, doxorubicin and 5-fluorouracil were given as the first treatment to 12 patients with advanced bladder cancer, with three objective responses. The response rate was no lower in the seven patients in the same series who had been treated previously with radiotherapy (Cross *et al.*, 1976).

As part of a toxicity study on the combination of chemotherapy and radiotherapy in T3 bladder cancers, instituted by the Yorkshire Urological Cancer Research Group, eight patients were given doxorubicin and 5-fluorouracil for 3 months (four cycles) before radiotherapy. The results of the combination were disappointing and the study was abandoned.

Chemotherapeutic agents are more likely to be found effective when the tumour mass is small and, until more effective agents are found, they are best employed after some bulk reduction has been achieved by radiotherapy. It seems that chemotherapy should be used soon after irradiation, or concurrently. However, there is no doubt that thera-peutically effective adjuvant chemotherapy imposes an added burden of toxicity on these patients, most of whom are already suffering toxic effects as a result of radiotherapy. Indeed, extensive prior radiotherapy has been cited as one of the causes of a poor response to chemotherapy (Yagoda *et al.,* 1977).

In an attempt to see whether the combination of radiotherapy and chemotherapy was safe and tolerable to the patient, a toxicity study was carried out by the Yorkshire Urological Cancer Research Group (Glashan *et al.,* 1977). Eighteen patients with T3 bladder cancers were given 4–11 courses of doxorubicin 50 mg/m² and 5-fluorouracil 500 mg/m² at 21-day intervals starting shortly after completing a radical course of radiotherapy. Four patients declined further therapy after 4–8 cycles because of nausea and vomiting. Haematological toxicity was mild, but myocardial damage was recognized in five patients after doxorubicin 300–500 mg/m², and contributed to the death of three (*Table 26.1*). This high incidence of cardiac toxicity is

Table 26.1

THE TOXICITY OF DOXORUBICIN AND 5-FLUOROURACIL ADJUVANT TO IRRA–
DIATION (18 PATIENTS)

Effect	*Number of patients*	*Comments*
Haematological Haemoglobin	1	Transfused
White count < 4800/mm³ at 21 days	2	Dose modified
Platelets	0	
Cardiac	5	
Gastrointestinal	4	Refused further treatment
Alopecia	18	

surprising, for it is rarely that the dose of doxorubicin is less than 500 mg/m² (Cortes *et al.,* 1975). The toxic effect might have been less if patients had been given prophylactic digoxin (Guthrie and Gibson, 1977), or if the dose had been given slowly over a period of 30 minutes.

Neither gastrointestinal nor cardiac toxicity was a problem until four courses of chemotherapy had been given, and it was concluded that the risk of toxicity was acceptable for an adjuvant study provided that chemotherapy was limited to four courses.

The initial results of this study, which was designed to test toxicity not tumour response, were better than expected. Fifteen of 18 patients (83%) survived for 1 year, as opposed to approximately 60% in other radical radiotherapy series (Rider and Evans, 1976; Wallace and Bloom, 1976). They have now been followed-up for 3 years and the survival still appears to be better than that in a group of patients fit for cystectomy but randomly allocated to radical radiotherapy in the series reported from the Marsden Hospital and the Institute of Urology (*Figure 26.1*) (Wallace and Bloom, 1976). It is comparable with that after radiotherapy and cystectomy in the same series.

The numbers in this study are too small to allow any definite conclusions about tumour response. However, the results suggest that adjuvant chemotherapy is unlikely to reduce survival, at least in the short term, and that a prospective randomized study is needed.

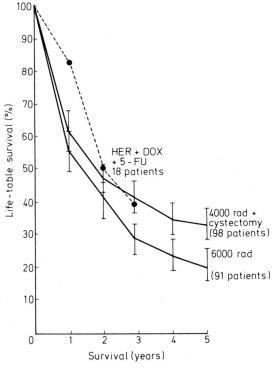

Figure 26.1 Comparison of survival of 18 patients treated in the YUCRG adjuvant chemotherapy toxicity study (Glashan et al., 1977) with survival in the Institute of Urology and Royal Marsden Hospital trial of pre-operative radiotherapy plus cystectomy versus radical radiotherapy plus salvage cystectomy (Wallace and Bloom, 1976)

Accordingly, such a study has been set up under the auspices of the Yorkshire Urological Cancer Research Group. Patients under 76 years of age, with a life expectancy of 3 months and having category T3 (UICC) transitional cell cancers of the bladder, are being randomly allocated to treatment with radiotherapy or to radiotherapy plus 4–11 courses, given at 3-weekly intervals, of doxorubicin 50 mg/m² and 5-fluorouracil 500 mg/m². Randomization is being carried out at diagnosis, and this has resulted in the loss of a number of patients who died of rapidly progressive disease without having adequate treatment (in five cases without having any treatment at all).

This study is not sufficiently advanced as yet to allow adequate follow-up — one-third of the patients entered within the last 6 months, and only six patients have been studied for more than a year and a half. Because, on theoretical grounds, it is expected that the main effect of added chemotherapy will be to influence the rate of development of overt metastases as a result of an effect on micrometastases which may have been present, although undetected, at the time of primary treatment, any influence it has on these micrometastases will not become apparent until patients have been followed-up for a considerable time, and it is inappropriate to report the results at this stage.

It is relatively unlikely that adjuvant chemotherapy will have a great impact on the number of patients who die as a result of rapid progression of the tumour before adequate treatment can be given. It remains to be seen whether the number of patients whose primary tumour is completely eliminated by radical radiotherapy will be influenced by chemotherapy. Currently, approximately 50% of the series as a whole has been rendered tumour-free within 6 months. This compares with the 30% of patients who are found to be tumour-free at cystectomy shortly after subradical pre-operative radiotherapy (Prout *et al.*, 1970; Wallace and Bloom, 1976; Miller, 1977; Slack *et al.*, 1977), and is comparable with the 38% of subjects rendered tumour-free by radical radiotherapy in the study reported from the Marsden Hospital and the Institute of Urology (Wallace and Bloom, 1976), with the 55% in a series from the M.D. Anderson Hospital (Miller, 1977) and with 55% having a reduction to T0 or T1 in a Leeds series (Smith *et al.*, 1980).

This YUCRG study is the first large prospective investigation of adjuvant chemotherapy following radical radiotherapy for transitional cell carcinoma of the bladder. At the present rate of accrual, it is expected that sufficient cases will be recruited within 18 months to establish whether there is at least 20% difference between these two treatments.

REFERENCES

CORTES, E.P., LUTMAN, G., WANKA, J., WANG, J.J., PICKREN, J., WALLACE, J. and HOLLAND, J.F.(1975). Adriamycin (NSC-123127) cardiotoxicity: a clinico-pathologic correlation. *Cancer Chemotherapy Reports*, **6**, 215–225

CROSS, R.J., GLASHAN, R.W., HUMPHREY, C.S., ROBINSON, M.R.G., SMITH, P.H. and wil
WILLIAMS, R.E. (1976). Treatment of advanced bladder cancer with adriamycin and 5-fluorouracil. *British Journal of Urology,* **48**, 609–615

DE KERNION, J.B. (1977). The chemotherapy of advanced bladder carcinoma. *Cancer Research,* **37**, 2771–2774

GLASHAN, R.W., HOUGHTON, A.L. and ROBINSON, M.R.G. (1977). A toxicity study of the treatment of T3 bladder tumours with a combination of radiotherapy and chemotherapy. *British Journal of Urology,* **49**, 669–672

GUTHRIE, D. and GIBSON, A.L. (1977). Doxorubicin cardiotoxicity: possible role of digoxin in its prevention. *British Medical Journal,* **2**, 1447–1449

MATHÉ, G. (1978). Chemotherapy, a double agent in respect of immune functions. *Cancer Chemotherapy and Pharmacology,* **1**, 65–68

MERRIN, C., CARTAGENA, R., WAJSMAN, Z., BAUMGARTNER, G. and MURPHY, G.P. (1975). Chemotherapy of bladder carcinoma with cyclpphosphamide and (1975). Chemotherapy of bladder carcinoma with cyclophosphamide and adriamycin. *Journal of Urology,* **114**, 884–887

MILLER, L.S. (1977). Bladder cancer: superiority of pre-operative irradiation and cystectomy in stages B2 and C. *Cancer,* **39**, 973–980

PROUT, G.R. (1977). The role of surgery in the potentially curative treatment of bladder carcinoma. *Cancer Research,* **37**, 2764–2770

PROUT, G.R., SLACK, H.N. and BROSS, I.D.J. (1970). Irradiation and 5-fluorouracil as adjuvants in the management of invasive bladder carcinoma. A co-operative group report after five years. *Journal of Urology,* **104**, 116–129

RIDER, W.D. and EVANS, D.H. (1976). Radiotherapy in the treatment of recurrent bladder cancer. *British Journal of Urology,* **48**, 595–601

RUBIN, P. (1971). Current concepts in genito-urinary oncology: a multidisciplinary approach. *Journal of Urology,* **106**, 315–338

SCHABEL, F.M. (1975). Concepts for systemic treatment of micrometastases. *Cancer,* **35**, 15–24

SLACK, H.N., BROSS, I.D.J. and PROUT, G.R. (1977). Five year follow-up results of collaborative study of therapy for carcinoma of the bladder. *Journal of Surgical Oncology,* **9**, 393–405

SMITH, P.H., AKDAS, A., CAMPBELL-ROBSON, L., FRANK, H.G. and WILLIAMS, R.E. (1980). Radiotherapy and chemotherapy in the management of invasive bladder cancer. *In preparation.*

STERNBERG, J.J., BRACKEN, R.B., HANDEL, P.B. and JOHNSON, D.E. (1977). Combination chemotherapy (CISCA) for advanced urinary tract carcinoma. A preliminary report. *Journal of the American Medical Association,* **238**, 2282–2287

STOTER, G., VENDRIK, C.P.J., STRUYUENBERG, A., BROUWERS, Th.M., SLEIJFER, D. Th., KOOPS, H.S., van OOSTEROM, A.T. and PINEDO, H.M. (1979). Combination therapy with cis-diammine-dichloro-platinum, vinblastine, and bleomucin in advanced testicular non-seminoma. *Lancet,* **1**, 941–945

TURNER, A.G., DURRANT, K.R. and MALPAS, J.S. (1979). A trial of bleomycin versus adriamycin in advanced carcinoma of the bladder. *British Journal of Urology,* **51**, 121–124

TURNER, A.G., HENDRY, W.F., WILLIAMS, G.B. and BLOOM, H.J.G. (1977). The treatment of advanced bladder cancer with methotrexate. *British Journal of Urology,* **49**, 673–678

WAJSMAN, Z., MERRIN, C., MOORE, R. and MURPHY, G.P. (1975). Current results from treatment of bladder tumors with total cystectomy at Roswell Park Memorial Institute. *Journal of Urology,* **113**, 806–810

WALLACE, D.M. and BLOOM, H.J.G. (1976). The management of deeply infiltrating (T3) bladder carcinoma: controlled trial of radical radiotherapy versus pre-operative radiotherapy and radical cystectomy (first report). *British Journal of Urology,* **48**, 587–594

WHITMORE, W.F. Jr., BATATA, M.A., HILDRIS, B.S., REDDY, G.M., UNAL, A., GHONEIM, M.A., GRABSTALD, H. and CHU, F. (1977). A comparative study of two pre-operative radiation regimes with cystectomy for bladder cancer. *Cancer,* **40**, 1077–1086

WILLIAMS, S.D., DONOGHUE, J.P. and EINHORN, L.H. (1980). Advanced bladder cancer: therapy with cis-platinum, adriamycin and five-fluorouracil. *In press.*

YAGODA, A., WATSON, R.C., WHITMORE, W.F., GRABSTALD, H., MIDDLEMAN, M.P. and KRAKOFF, I.H. (1977). Adriamycin in advanced urinary tract cancer: experience in 42 patients and review of the literature. *Cancer,* **39**, 279–285

YAGODA, A., WATSON, R.C., KEMENY, N., BARZELL, W.E., GRABSTALD, H. and WHITMORE, W.F. Jr. (1978). Diamminedichloride platinum II and cyclophosphamide in the treatment of advanced urothelial cancer. *Cancer,* **41**, 2121–2130

27

Adjuvant Post-Surgical Chemotherapy with Cyclophosphamide, Doxorubicin Hydrochloride and Cis-diamminedichloroplatinum in Patients with Bladder Cancer

C. Merrin

INTRODUCTION

Treatment of bladder cancer is effective when the tumour is localized to the mucosa or when superficial invasion of the muscle only is present (Whitmore *et al.*, 1977). Patients with more deeply infiltrating tumours have a high incidence of occult dissemination and their survival is limited. To improve these results, it is rational to explore the early use of systemic chemotherapy with drugs which have shown activity against metastatic bladder cancer (Merrin *et al.*, 1975; Yagoda *et al.*, 1976; Merrin, 1978), in combination with surgery in patients at risk of tumour dissemination. This chapter reviews the results from pilot studies where radical cystectomy has been combined with chemotherapy, using doxorubicin hydrochloride and cyclophosphamide in one group of patients, and cis-platinum in another group.

MATERIALS AND METHODS

Forty-six patients were entered in this study at Roswell Park Memorial Institute between September 1973 and February 1979. All the patients had transitional cell carcinoma of the bladder, confirmed histologically. The patients ranged in age from 49 to 75 years, with an average of 62 years. All cases were staged according to the classification of Jewett and Strong (1946), modified by Marshall (1952). The patients were evaluated by physical examination, excretory urography, bilateral pedal lymphography, hypogastric arteriography, chest X-ray, metastatic radiological survey, endoscopy, cytology, bi-manual palpation under anaesthesia, and routine biochemical and haematological tests. Two patients had stage A (T1) disease, five patients had stage B (T2 or T3a NO MO), two patients had stage C (T3b NO MO) and 37 patients had stage D1 (T3b N2 MO). There were 40 male and six female patients, All patients were submitted to radical cystectomy and ileal loop diversion. As soon as they recovered and before leaving the hospital, they were started on adjuvant chemotherapy.

Twenty-five patients (two stage A (T1 NO MO), five stage B (T3a NO MO), two stage C (T3b NO MO) and 16 stage D1 (T3b N2 MO)) received 40 mg/m² of doxorubicin hydrochloride intravenously every 3 weeks up to a total of 500 mg/m², and 200 mg/m² of cyclophosphamide per day for 4 days every 3 weeks for 3 years, or until progression of the disease.

Twenty-one patients (all stage D1 (T3b N2 MO)) received cis-diamminedichloroplatinum 50 mg/m² once weekly for 6 weeks and every 3 weeks thereafter. Cis-platinum was mixed with 37.5 g of manni-tol in 2000 ml of 5% dextrose in 0.5N saline and 40 mmol of potassium chloride. It was administered in a slow intravenous infusion lasting 6—8 hours once weekly for 6 weeks and every 3 weeks thereafter. Before each chemotherapy treatment the patients were evaluated by complete blood count, routine blood chemistries, serum creatinine, chest X-ray and, when indicated, metastatic radiological survey and bone and liver scans. Patients receiving doxorubicin underwent a complete cardiac evaluation, including electrocardiographic studies.

RESULTS

Doxorubicin and cyclophosphamide

In the group treated with the combination doxorubicin hydrochloride and cyclophosphamide, the two patients with stage A (T1 NO MO) tumours have remained free of disease for 36 and 49 months respectively. Of the five patients with stage B (T3a NO MO), three have remained free of disease for 51, 57 and 42 months respectively. The two other stage B (T3a NO MO) patients developed metastases after remaining free of disease for 25 and 26 months respectively. Of the two patients with stage C (T3b NO MO), one died from the progression of his tumour after 7 months' treatment and the other has remained alive and free of disease for 52 months.

Of the 16 patients with stage D1 (T3b N2 MO), seven (43.75%) have remained free of disease for 29–47 months (average 33 months). Two (12.5%) survived for 26 and 28 months respectively before developing metastases and dying from their disease. Three (18.5%) survived for 1 year or more (average 12.3 months) and four (25%) died from the progression of their tumour in less than 1 year (average 4.5 months).

Cis-platinum

Of the 21 patients with stage D1 (T3b N2 MO) treated with cis-platinum, 11 (52%) have remained clinically free of disease for 6–24 months (average 13.5 months). One patient who developed metastases after a 9-month disease-free period is still alive. Nine patients had recurrences and died from the progression of their disease within 2–10 months (average 5.6 months).

TOXICITY

In the group of patients receiving the combination of doxorubicin hydrochloride and cyclophosphamide (*Table 27.1*), mild to moderate nausea was observed in some patients, whilst alopecia occurred in all

Table 27.1
TOXICITY OF 25 PATIENTS ON POST-SURGICAL ADJUVANT CHEMOTHERAPY FOR BLADDER CANCER TREATED WITH DOXORUBICIN AND CYCLOPHOSPHAMIDE

Toxicity	*Number of patients*
Nausea	8
Vomiting	3
Cardiac effects	0
Mucositis	6 (Mild)
Alopecia	25
Leucopoenia	25 (Mild)
Thrombocytopoenia	0

patients. Mild to moderate leucopoenia was seen in all patients, 10–14 days after administration of the drug, though most returned to normal in time for the next scheduled doses. No thrombocytopoenia and/or cardiotoxicity was seen but some patients developed mild to moderate mucositis. In general, the drug combination was well tolerated and did not incapacitate any of the patients.

Table 27.2
TOXICITY OF 21 PATIENTS ON POST-SURGICAL ADJUVANT
CHEMOTHERAPY TREATED WITH CIS-PLATINUM

Toxicity	*Number of patients*
Renal effects	0
Leucopoenia	6 (Mild)
Hearing loss (high frequency)	3
Hearing loss (speech range)	0
Peripheral neuropathy	1
Nausea	21
Vomiting	21
Allergy	0

In the group treated with cis-platinum, (*Table 27.2*) no nephro-toxicity was observed. Six patients developed mild leucopoenia (3000–4000 WBC), three showed high-frequency hearing loss and one developed peripheral neuropathy. Different degrees of nausea and vomiting were present during the cis-platinum administration. The intensity of these symptoms varied greatly with time and some of the patients tolerated the cis-platinum infusion without any major dis-comfort.

DISCUSSION

The results of the treatment of locally invasive and/or occultly disseminated bladder cancer by surgery and/or radiotherapy have been disappointing (Whitmore *et al.*, 1977). The experience of Whitmore and Marshall (1962) and of Prout (1976) has shown that most of the patients with lymph node metastases treated by cystectomy alone will have a recurrence or die from their disease within 1 year and only 4% will survive 5 years (Whitmore and Marshall, 1962).

The combination of pre-operative radiation and cystectomy has improved survival in patients with locally invasive tumours, but did not alter prognosis in patients with occult or clinically evident tumour dissemination at the time of the treatment (Whitmore *et al.*, 1977)*. Therapeutic failure in these patients is not surprising, because they had systemic disease and received local treatment only. Consequently, this high-risk group of patients is in need of a more complete type of treatment combining local tumour reduction by surgery with systemic treatment by drug therapy. Our results in this limited study seem to demonstrate the possible value of such an approach. The number of

Editors' footnote: In the Institute of Urology trial survival of node positive cases after pre-operative radiotherapy and surgery was 24% at 3 years.

stage D1 (T3b N2 MO) patients in the first group who have remained free of disease for an average of 33 months is surprisingly high. In the second group, our follow-up is not as long, but the fact that more than half of the patients with advanced disease stage D1 (T3b N2 MO) are still clinically in remission for an average of 13 months is very encouraging, when we compare the survival of the same type of patients treated with surgery alone, or in combination with radiotherapy.

The question now arises whether pre-operative radiation is necessary when chemotherapy is used post-surgically. Radiotherapy has the advantage of producing local sterilization of the tumour, but it has the disadvantage of destroying some of the bone marrow reserve which is so necessary for an effective chemotherapy. This is of even more importance in the group of patients with the highest incidence of bladder cancer, who are in their sixth and seventh decades, a time when the bone marrow may be less capable of recovering after chemotherapy.

In this series most patients died from systemic disease and there were very few local recurrences, suggesting that the local sterilizing benefits of pre-operative radiotherapy may not be necessary when using post-surgical chemotherapy. This suggestion is based on a small number of patients, and needs confirmation by randomized studies, with large numbers of patients, comparing pre-operative radiotherapy, surgery and adjuvant chemotherapy on the one hand to surgery and adjuvant chemotherapy on the other.

REFERENCES

JEWETT, H.J. and STRONG, G.H. (1946). Infiltrating carcinoma of the bladder: relation of depth of penetration of the bladder wall to incidence of local extension and metastases. *Journal of Urology,* **55,** 336–372

MARSHALL, V.F. (1952). The relation of preoperative estimate to the pathologic demonstration of the extent of vesical neoplasms. *Journal of Urology,* **68,** 714–723

MERRIN, C. (1978). Treatment of advanced bladder cancer with cisdiammine-dichloroplatinum (II NSC 119 875): A pilot study. *Journal of Urology,* **119,** 493–495

MERRIN, C., CARTAGENA, R., WAJSMAN, Z., BAUMGARTNER, G. and MURPHY, G.P. (1975). Chemotherapy of bladder carcinoma with cyclophosphamide and adriamycin. *Journal of Urology,* **114,** 884–887

PROUT, G. (1976). In *Minutes of the Cooperative Studies Discussion Group on Bladder Cancer, National Cancer Institute, Bethesda, Maryland, October 26, 1976*

WHITMORE, W.F., JR., BATATA, M.A., GHONEIM, M.A., GRABSTALD, H. and UNAL, A. (1977). Radical cystectomy with or without prior irradiation in the treatment of bladder cancer. *Transactions of the American Association of Genito-Urinary Surgeons,* **69,** 100–103

WHITMORE, W.F. and MARSHALL, V.F.   (1962). Radical total cystectomy for cancer of the bladder: 230 consecutive cases five years later. *Journal of Urology,* **87**, 853–868

YAGODA, A., WATSON, R.C., GONZALEZ-VITALE, J.C., GRABSTALD, H. and WHITMORE, W.F. (1976). Cis-dichlorodiammineplatinum (II) in advanced bladder cancer. *Cancer Treatment Reports,* **60**, 917–923

IV

Immunotherapy

28

Immunity in Malignant Disease

R.T.D. Oliver

The idea of immunization of patients against their tumours has been with us since the end of the nineteenth century, when the first successes of immunization against infectious diseases were being reported (for review *see* Currie, 1972). As yet, despite considerable research effort, there is no demonstration in any clinical situation that an immunological manipulation has altered the patient's immunological response to his tumour in relation to long-term cure of that tumour, although there is some evidence for prolongation of survival of patients after treatments which are known to affect non-specifically the capacity for immune response.

This Chapter will review the evidence for immunosurveillance against neoplastic cell growth in experimental animals, and will consider the evidence in man for immunological reactivity of patients against their tumours and ways in which it may be possible to improve on this.

IMMUNOSURVEILLANCE AGAINST TUMOURS

The concept that host response was important in suppressing growth of tumours in man originated from a discussion initiated by Thomas at a Ciba Symposium in 1959. Subsequent to this meeting Burnett (1965) wrote at length on the concept of immunosurveillance against tumours being an important raison d'être for the complexities of the immune system and a logical complement to his theory of clonal selection, which he proposed for generating the diversity of the immune system.

Today it must be accepted that the totality of this theory is no longer acceptable, particularly as regards the idea that the immune response by T lymphocytes is continuously aborting growth of spon-taneous malignant transformation which threatens to overgrow the normal tissue. There are three pieces of information which argue against this simplistic interpretation:

(1) congenitally athymic mice develop no more tumours than mice with the same genetic background and normal thymic function (Rygaard and Poulsen, 1976);
(2) mice treated with antilymphocyte serum from birth to death, developed no more tumours than controls (Simpson and Nehlsen, 1971);
(3) studies of tumour occurrence in humans on immunosuppressive drugs after renal transplantation or because of autoimmune disease (Hoover and Fraumeni, 1973). Although these patients do have an increased incidence of some types of tumours, those tumours (such as lymphomas) that occur, are rare in normal populations, and there is no increase in the incidence of common tumours such as carcinoma of the lung or breast (*Table 28.1*).

Table 28.1
RELATIVE RISK OF VARIOUS TYPES OF CANCER IN
PATIENTS ON IMMUNOSUPPRESSIVE DRUGS

Type of cancer	Risk
Lymphoma	× 90
Cervical cancer	× 47
Liver cancer	× 30
Bladder cancer	× 10
Lung cancer	× 2.4

It is clear that the data argue against the original theory that malignant change was occurring all the time and that it was only the occasional mutation which managed to evade the host surveillance and developed into a malignant tumour. However, it is important to remember that none of this data proves conclusively that host response cannot suppress growth of tumours, as all that has been shown is that T-cell deficiency does not lead to the host being overwhelmed by spontaneous tumours. There are at least four separate interactive host-surveillance systems – T cells (Gorczynski and Norbury, 1974), B cells and antibodies (Farham *et al.,* 1978), macrophages (Evans and Alexander, 1970; Alexander, 1976) and NK (natural killer cells – possible immature T cells (Haller, 1979)) – which have been demonstrated to react against tumour cells in experimental animals and so far there are no reports on the effect of B-cell, macrophage or NK deficiency on tumour growth. Furthermore, if the occurrence of immunogenic malignant transformation was a rare event and usually led to tumour formation, rather than was common and often rejected, as envisaged in the original Burnett hypothesis, one might not expect the incidence of tumours to be different in immunosuppressed animals. If host response were important in suppressing tumour growth, this would be demonstrated only by study of survival from the first symptom until death. Most investigations of immunosurveillance have not focussed on this problem: there are no reports which compare survival and response to treatment in patients developing tumours on immuno-suppressive drugs with similar tumours arising spontaneously.

The clearest experimental evidence that would support this inter-pretation of the immunosurveillance hypothesis is the fulminating rate at which T-cell deficient mice die from tumour after infection with Polyoma virus (Allison and Law, 1968).

Additional information on the influence of anti-T lymphocyte immunosuppression on tumour growth comes from the study of renal graft recipients, who received a transplant from a cadaver donor who was subsequently found to have occult malignant disease at autopsy. Under these circumstances a foreign or allogeneic tumour can be trans-planted with the kidney. Although it is not invariably the case that a tumour will develop in the patient receiving the graft, when it does occur the tumours usually disseminate quite extensively. However, in the majority of patients, once the immunosuppressive drugs are stopped the kidney will be rejected and, at the same time, the tumour metastases will regress and disappear. It is unlikely that this type of immune response is a reaction developed to a specific tumour antigen, but dependent on an immune response to the foreign transplantation antigens on the tumour cells which were grafted with the kidney. None the less, it does provide evidence that tumour cells living in an environ-ment where the immune response is diminished, will grow quite freely, but when immunosuppression is stopped they are readily rejected. It is not clear, in the minority of patients who die, whether it is lack of anti-genicity of the graft tumour cells or failure of response of the patient which enables the graft to survive when immunosuppression is stopped.

EVIDENCE FOR HOST RESPONSE AGAINST HUMAN TUMOURS

In man, the evidence for specific host anti-tumour immune response suppressing growth of tumours is much less substantial than in experi-mental animals.

The most conclusive clinical evidence that the host is able to mount a response against its own tumour is the carefully documented series of 176 cases that Everson and Cole (1966) were able to collect, comprising patients whose tumour had undergone spontaneous regression of histo-logically documented tumours (*Table 28.2*). Of interest to the urologist was the high frequency of hypernephroma and bladder tumour regres-sion, (the latter mostly seen after urinary diversion). From looking at the list of tumour types it is clear that those tumours where regression

Table 28.2
COLLECTED CASES OF SPONTANEOUS REGRESSION OF
CANCER (EVERSON AND COLE, 1966)

Type of tumour	Number of cases
Hypernephroma	31
Neuroblastoma	29
Malignant melanoma	19
Choriocarcinoma	19
Bladder	13
Others	65
Total	176

has been reported are not the most frequently observed in the normal
population, suggesting that involvement of host response in anti-tumour
surveillance may be of importance for certain tumours only. Although
these regressions are exceptionally rare, the fact that minor fluctuation
in the size of metastases in patients with tumours of the type where
complete regressions have been documented, suggests that these
responses represent the tip of an iceberg of host tumour interactions.
Typical of the minor fluctuations are the changing pattern of cutaneous
tumour deposits seen in patients with melanoma where regressing and
growing deposits coexist in the same area of skin (Bodenham, 1968)
and the fluctuation in size of lung metastases seen in patients with
hypernephroma (Werf-Messing and Van Gilse, 1971). If these observations
are extreme examples of host—tumour interactions, it is possible that
the wide spectrum of behaviour seen with tumours of similar histological type may be an indication of a variable degree of host-induced
slowing of tumour growth.

Two tumours which show rather well this extreme spectrum of
behaviour are carcinoma of the breast and bladder. It has been well
documented that 15% of untreated patients with carcinoma of the
breast survive for 10 years (Bloom, 1964) and a similar percentage of
patients with untreated advanced bladder tumours have been reported
to survive for 5 years (Prout and Marshall, 1956). These patients often
have large locally invasive tumours without metastases. The difference
between this type of disease and the patient who dies rapidly with
multiple metastases is similar to the extremes seen in tuberculosis, one
individual surviving many years with chronic fibroid phthisis and
another dying in months, from miliary tuberculosis. Undoubtedly, the
degree of differentiation induced by the initial carcinogenic stimulus is
important in determining behaviour of the tumour. However, evidence
that immune response can influence occurrence of metastases comes
from the study of individual animal tumours that are primarily non-
metastatic but will produce lung metastases in animals which have been
immunosuppressed (*Table 28.3*; data from Eccles and Alexander, 1975).

Such a mechanism might explain the explosive development occasionally seen in patients after major surgery, of metastases to a primary which has been growing slowly for several years.

Most of the evidence that immune response can influence behaviour of experimental animals is from direct experiments monitoring the effect of various *in vivo* and *in vitro* immunological manipulations. In contrast, because of the difficulty of direct experimentation in man,

Table 28.3
CHEMICALLY INDUCED SARCOMA (ECCLES AND
ALEXANDER, 1975)

Procedure	Animals with pulmonary metastases
Thoracic duct drainage	5/8
Sham operation	0/3
Controls	0/5

most of the information from human tumours is indirect, as exemplified by the studies of normal host-cell infiltration in tumours and correlation of this with patients' survival. Results of this type of study of breast tumours show that there is a direct relationship between the number of long-term survivors at 15 years and the degree of mononuclear cell infiltration in tumours as shown in *Table 28.4* (data from Hamlin, 1968). Similar results have been reported from studies of

Table 28.4
HISTOLOGICAL GRADES AND SURVIVAL IN CARCINOMA OF
BREAST (HAMLIN, 1968)

| | | Degree of tumour cell differentiation | |
		++	+
Degree of lymphoid cell infiltration	−	18/34[a]	3/68
	+	12/27	29/88
	++		29/55

[a] Figures indicate number of patients alive for more than 15 years

carcinoma of the bladder (Pomerance, 1972). Evidence that not only lymphocytes may be involved in patients' reactivity against the tumours comes from several studies on macrophages in tumours. In experimental animals it is found that the higher the macrophage content, the less systemic metastases occur and, indeed, in one human tumour, Currie (1976) has found, as shown in *Figure 28.1,* that one of the enzymes produced by macrophages (lysozyme) is synthesized in much higher levels in tissue culture of biopsies from Stage I melanomas than

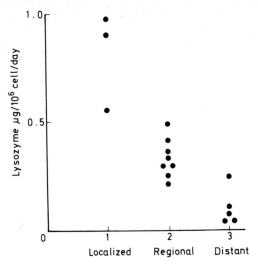

Figure 28.1 In vitro *lysozyme release from cultured malignant melanoma biopsies (reproduced from Currie 1976, by permission of the author)*

from similar biopsies of tumours which have already disseminated, such as Stage II and Stage III.

This type of information is indirect, in that there is no definite information that these cells which are found in tumours are, in fact, preventing growth of the malignant cell. However, in Burkitt's lymphoma there is now evidence to suggest that normal lymphocytes found in the tumour are able actually to kill the tumour cell *in vitro*.

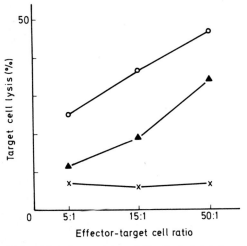

Figure 28.2 Cytotoxicity of T cells isolated from Burkitt lymphoma biopsy (modified from Jondal et al. (1975). Targets: o—o, purified tumour cells from same tumour; ▲—▲, EB virus transformed normal lymphocytes; x—x, EB virus negative tumour cell line

Burkitt's lymphoma is one tumour where it is very common to see an extremely rapid response to a very minimal dose of chemotherapy (Burkitt *et al.,* 1965). Although it is possible that it is simply a direct effect of the treatment, a more likely explanation is that, just by giving this single dose of drug, the balance between the host and the tumour is altered in favour of the host, and the tumour begins to undergo regression because of the activity of the host response against the tumour. In support of this, Klein and his colleagues (Jondal *et al.* 1975) in Stockholm have been able to separate the contaminating lymphocytes from the tumour cells of a biopsy from a patient with Burkitt's lymphoma, and then to show that these separated T-lymphocytes were able actually to kill chromium-labelled tumour cells, as shown in *Figure 28.2.* That this may also occur in other tumours is suggested by the results of studies on urological tumours undertaken in my own department (*Figure 28.3*) which have shown that the majority

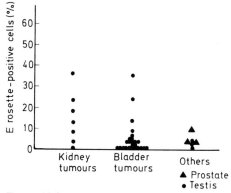

Figure 28.3 Frequency of E rosette-positive lymphocytes in tumour cell suspensions (as percentage of viable nucleated cells)

of tumour-infiltrating lymphocytes are T cells, which may constitute as much as 25% of nucleated cells in cell suspension prepared from tumours of the kidney and testis.

These observations demonstrate that there are now several human tumours investigated in depth, where there is evidence for a seemingly inadequate host response against their own tumour cells. In experimental animals there are several theories to explain how tumours escape immunological control, such as 'sneaking through' (Klein, 1969) or rapid shedding of tumour antigens so that immunological paralysis is induced by excess soluble antigen (Currie and Alexander, 1974). A third possibility is that there may be relative differences in response of individuals to a specific tumour antigen. In mice, for example, there is a suggestion that immune response associated with the H-2 transplantation antigens influence survival of animals with lymphomas (Lilly and Pincus, 1973). A similar phenomenon has been suggested as an explanation for the difference in HLA-antigen frequency between long-term survivors and patients who die early with a variety of tumours, such as carcinoma of the lung, Hodgkin's disease and acute leukaemia (for review *see* Oliver, 1977) and the indication from follow-up studies that certain HLA phenotypes may be of significance in predicting long-term survival (*Figure 28.4* from Oliver *et al.*, 1977).

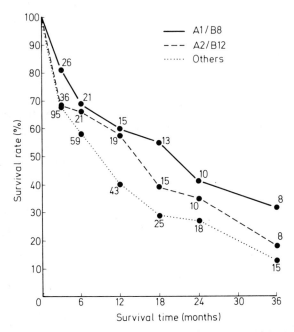

Figure 28.4 HLA phenotype and survival of patients with AML

Despite the clear suggestion, from these indirect approaches, for host response against autologous human tumours, there has been no entirely satisfactory quantitative *in vitro* assay established, although there have been many attempts to do so (Hellstrom *et al.*, 1971; O'Toole *et al.*, 1972; Takasugi *et al.*, 1974). This is because most *in vitro* assays have depended on cell lines established from primary tumours. These have been shown to change genetically after several generations *in vitro*, or to become contaminated with cells from other cell lines or other non-lytic microorganisms.

IMMUNOTHERAPY IN HUMAN TUMOURS

Just as for the immunological manipulations that have been used to counteract infectious disease, the approaches to immunotherapy of cancer are broadly divided into two categories — active immunotherapy and passive immunotherapy. Passive immunotherapy involves the transfer into a tumour-bearing individual either of serum immune against that specific tumour or of immune cells with reactivity directed against the tumour. Active specific immunotherapy, on the other hand, as when used in infectious disease, is of value as a prophylactic only after the majority of the tumour load has already been removed by other therapy such as surgery, radiotherapy or chemotherapy to eliminate the minimum residual tumour load or prevent recurrence of a tumour.

These two principal types of immunotherapy are subdivided on the basis of whether they are specific, in that the immunological reactivity is directed to a tumour antigen that is the specific target of the immunological attack, or non-specific — a general boost of immunological reactivity of the patient in the hope that it will also encompass a response of the patient to his own tumour. BCG (bacille Calmette-Guérin) has been the most widely used non-specific immunotherapeutic agent. This has been most successful when used as a local injection at a site where there are tumour cells, intrapleural as an adjunct to pneumonectomy in carcinoma of the lung, (McKneally *et al.*, 1976), intratumoural in treatment of cutaneous deposits of melanoma (Nathanson *et al.*, 1979) or carcinoma of the breast, or intravesical to treat recurrent carcinoma of the bladder (*see* Chapters 30,31). Passive non-specific immunotherapy is exemplified by the use of reagents such as thymosin, a soluble mediator involved in maturation of T cells in treatment of carcinoma of the lung (Cohen *et al.*, 1978) or interferon, which has been shown to improve survival of patients with osteogenic sarcoma (Strander, 1975).

So far, very little use has been made of the principle of passive specific immunotherapy in human tumours, predominantly because of the lack of well-documented human tumour-specific antigens, and the logistic difficulties of producing a specific reagent for each patient, although this was one of the most frequently attempted approaches to immunotherapy before 1970. Pairs of patients in the late stage of their disease were cross-immunized with cells prepared from biopsies performed on their tumour. Leucocytes taken from the patient after a 2-week interval would then be injected into the patient from whom the tumour originated. Approximately 150 such experiments have been reported in the literature. The logistical problems and the fact that response was even less frequent than that seen with chemotherapy (15% of patients showed partial and 5% complete regression of tumour) and the death of a mother after injection with her daughter's melanoma cells, has led to the abandoning of such experiments (for review *see* Hersh *et al.*, 1973). The recent development of techniques to produce large quantities of immune T cells by cloning experiments after *in vitro* immunization has opened up the possibility of re-exploring this approach, as have the results from Feneley *et al.*, 1981 (*see* Chapter 32) who injected immune pig lymphocytes into the vesical artery of patients with bladder cancer.

Active specific immunotherapy was first attempted in the first years of the twentieth century. In the period from 1930 to 1950 there was a considerable loss of interest in this approach because it was found that most of the effects observed were, in fact, due to immunization against transplantation antigens present on the tumour of other individuals, and not against tumour-specific antigens. With the demonstration in highly inbred strains of mice that tumour-specific antigens did exist, and the development of *in vitro* assays of tumour immunity in man, in the late 1960s there was a resurgence of interest. Animal experiments showed that a combination of non-specific immunotherapy with BCG plus specific immunotherapy with irradiated autologous tumour cells gave a more pronounced prolongation of survival in experimental animals than the use of either irradiated leukaemic cells or BCG on their own. Mathé in 1967 reported on a series of 18 patients with acute leukaemia, treated with combined active specific and non-specific immunotherapy, using BCG plus irradiated allogeneic blast cells (for review, *see* Mathé, 1977). Although Mathé's pioneering studies have been criticized in that they were not strictly randomized and the numbers were extremely small, there have subsequently been several studies of this type of approach in patients with acute myeloid leukaemia, four of which are summarized in *Table 28.5*, and show a similar trend to the results reported by Mathé.

Although there was a trend for better survival of patients receiving immunotherapy in all of these trials, this was so even when BCG was used alone (Oliver, 1977), bringing into question the need for the use of specific immunotherapy with irradiated leukaemia cells. There is, however, one study which has suggested that leukaemia cell antigen alone, without BCG, can improve first remission lengths and overall patient survival. Patients with acute leukaemia in remission were

Table 28.5
MEDIAN SURVIVAL IN AML IMMUNOTHERAPY TRIALS

Series	Chemotherapy	Immunotherapy + chemotherapy
Powles *et al.*, 1977	270 days (22)	510 days [c] (28)
MCR, 1978	330 days (24)	450 days [d] (47)
South-eastern Cancer Study Group (USA), 1977	336 days (17)	707 days [b] (18)
Whittaker and Slater (Cardiff), 1977	329 days (19)	455 days [a] (18)

Number of patients in parentheses
[a] $P < 0.02$; [b] $P < 0.05$; [c] $P = 0.03$; [d] $P = $ NS

injected with leukaemic blast cells after they had been treated with neuraminidase, an enzyme that removes sialic acid from the cell membrane. In animal experiments this procedure has been shown to increase the immunogenicity of tumour cells (Currie and Bagshawe, 1969). Comparison of the influence of treatment with BCG plus irradiated cells on length of remission as seen in the St Bartholomew's study, with the results that the American Group (Bekesi and Holland, 1977) were able to achieve using neuraminidase-treated cells without BCG, is shown in *Figure 28.5*. It is clear that neuraminidase-treated cells are having a more pronounced effect, although confirmation of this promising observation in other series of patients with acute myelogenous leukaemia is clearly necessary.

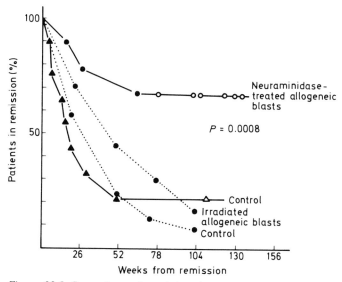

Figure 28.5 Comparison of remission duration in AML immunotherapy trials (data from Powles et al. (1977) and Bekesi and Holland (1977))

Recently, studies in our own laboratory (Lee and Oliver, 1978) have shown a possible explanation why, in humans, the evidence for patient-specific anti-leukaemia immune response has been so sparse. These studies were performed using an *in vitro* cell-mediated cytotoxicity assay, with patient's lymphocytes stimulated by their own specific leukaemic blast cells in the presence of normal allogeneic lymphocytes inactivated by mitomycin C used as an additional nonspecific stimulus. *Table 28.6* shows that, only when the patient's remission lymphocytes are cultured with the specific patient's leukaemia cells plus allogeneic lymphocytes, is significant cytotoxicity generated against that specific leukaemia cell. Culture with specific

Table 28.6
CYTOTOXICITY OF REMISSION LYMPHOCYTES AGAINT PATIENTS' OWN AML BLAST
CELLS (DATE FROM LEE AND OLIVER, 1978)

In vitro *immunization with:*	N	*Cytotoxicity (%)*
Autologous blast cell	34	3.7
Allogeneic blast cell	20	5.4
Autologous blast + allogeneic lymphocyte	36	19.0

leukaemia cells alone, or with allogeneic blast cells or allogeneic lympocytes alone, generates no cytotoxicity whatsoever against the patient's own specific leukaemia cells. In addition, it has been possible to demonstrate by absorption studies that the cytotoxicity against the specific blast cell cannot be removed by absorption with allogeneic blasts.

The conclusion from these studies must be that there is an antigenic determinant on the leukaemia cell which, although on its own was non-immunogenic, could induce an immune response under the right conditions of antigen help. This leukaemia antigen was shown to be unique for each patient tested. Currently, attempts are being made to apply the principles learnt from these *in vitro* studies to develop a new vaccine for *in vivo* use.

CONCLUSIONS

There is evidence that some human tumour cells do invoke immunological reactions from the host, though so far only in acute myelogenous leukaemia is there any evidence that immunotherapeutic manipulations known to be effective in experimental animals will lead to prolongation of survival. At this stage there is no claim for a curative effect of this therapy which, at best, can be seen as an important adjuvant to other approaches in the management of cancer patients. This is particularly so, when one considers that the other major approaches to treatment, such as surgery, radiotherapy and drugs for variable periods of time, actually suppress immunological reactivity in patients, and to date there has only been one study combining BCG with radiotherapy, which prolonged survival (Pines, 1976). The important conclusion to draw from this is that, just as has always been accepted for antibiotic therapy and combination chemotherapy of malignancy, the best combination therapy that can be devised would include active agents, all of which have slightly different mechanisms of action and side-effects. For this reason alone, the opposing effects of chemotherapy (or radiotherapy) and immunotherapy on immune response make them ideal candidates for combination therapy as immunotherapy will not add to the burden of side-effects induced by chemotherapy, although it must be remembered that the place for immunotherapy will be predominantly in situations of minimal residual disease. The next three Chapters focus on attempts to apply these principles to patients with bladder cancer.

REFERENCES

ALEXANDER, P. (1976). Surveillance against neoplastic cells — is it mediated by macrophages? *British Journal of Cancer,* **33**, 344—345

ALLISON, A.C. and LAW, L.W. (1968). Effects of antilymphocyte serum on virus oncogenesis. *Proceedings of the Society for Experimental Biology and Medicine,* **127**, 207—212

BEKESI, J.G. and HOLLAND, J.F. (1977). Active immunotherapy in leukaemia with neuraminidase-modified leukemic cells. *Recent Results in Cancer Research,* **62**, 78—89

BLOOM, H.J.G. (1964). The natural history of untreated breast cancer. *Annals of the New York Academy of Science,* **114**, 747—754

BODENHAM, D.C. (1968). A study of 650 observed malignant melanomas in the South West Region. *Annals of the Royal College of Surgeons of England,* **43**, 218—239

BURKITT, D., HUTT, M.S.R. and WRIGHT, D.M. (1965). The African lymphoma: preliminary observations on response to therapy. *Cancer,* **18**, 399—410

BURNETT, F.M. (1965). Somatic mutation and chronic disease. *British Medical Journal,* **1**, 338—342

COHEN, M.H., CHRETIEN, P.B. and IHDE, D.C. (1978). Thymosia fraction V prolongs the survival of small cell lung cancer patients treated with intensive chemotherapy. *Proceedings of the American Association for Cancer Research,* **19**, 466

CURRIE, G.A. (1972). 80 years of immunotherapy. *British Journal of Cancer,* **26**, 141

CURRIE, G.A. (1976). Serum lysozyme as a marker of host resistance. II: Patients with malignant melanoma, hypernephroma or breast carcinoma. *British Journal of Cancer,* **33**, 593—599

CURRIE, G.A. and ALEXANDER, P. (1974). Spontaneous shedding of TSTA by viable sarcoma cells: its possible role in facilitating metastatic spread. *British Journal of Cancer,* **29**, 72—75

CURRIE, G.A. and BAGSHAWE, K.D. (1969). Tumour specific immunogenicity of methylcholanthrene-induced sarcoma cells after incubation in neuraminidase. *British Journal of Cancer,* **23**, 141—149

ECCLES, S.A. and ALEXANDER, P. (1975). Immunologically-mediated restraint of latent tumour metastases. *Nature (London),* **257**, 52—53

EVANS, R. and ALEXANDER, P. (1970). Cooperation of immune lymphoid cells with macrophages in tumour immunity. *Nature (London)* **228**, 620—622

EVERSON, T.C. and COLE, W.H. (1966). *Spontaneous Regression of Cancer.* Philadelphia; W.B. Saunders

FARHAM, E., FESTENSTEIN, H. and DI GIORGIO, L. (1978). The role of antibody in the inhibition of meth A tumour growth. *Clinical and Experimental Immunology*, **33**, 377–385

GORCZYNSKI, R.M. and NORBURY, C. (1974). Immunity to murine sarcoma virus induced tumours. *British Journal of Cancer*, **30**, 118–128

HALLER, O. (1979). Generation in vivo of mouse natural cytotoxic cells. In *Natural and Induced Cell Mediated Cytotoxicity*. Ed. by G. Ruethmuller, P. Wernet and G. Ludkovicy, pp. 7–18. New York; Academic Press

HAMLIN, I.M.E. (1968). Possible host resistance in carcinoma of the breast: a histological study. *British Journal of Cancer*, **22**, 383–401

HELLSTROM, I., HELLSTROM, K.E., SJÖGREN, H.O. and WARNER, G.A. (1971). Demonstration of cell-mediated immunity to human neoplasms of various histological types. *International Journal of Cancer*, **7**, 1–16

HERSH, E.M., GUTTERMAN, J.U. and MAVEIGIT, G. (1973). In *Immunotherapy of Cancer in Man*, pp. 96–102. Springfield, Illinois; C.C. Thomas

HOOVER, R. and FRAUMENI, J.F. (1973). Risk of cancer in renal transplant patients. *Lancet*, **2**, 55–57

JONDAL, M., SVEDMYR, E., KLEIN, E. and SINGH, S. (1975). Killer T cells in a Burkitt's lymphoma biopsy. *Nature*, **255**, 405–407

KLEIN, G. (1969). Experimental studies in tumor immunology. *Federation Proceedings*, **28**, 1739–1753

LEE, S.K. and OLIVER, R.T.D. (1978). Leukaemia specific T cell mediated lymphocytotoxicity. *Journal of Experimental Medicine*, **147**, 912–922

LILLY, F. and PINCUS, T. (1973). Genetic control of murine leukenogenesis. *Advances in Cancer Research*, **17**, 231–277

McKNEALLY, M.F., MAVER, C. and KAUSEL, H.W. (1976). Regional immunotherapy of lung cancer with intrapleural B.C.G. *Lancet*, **1**, 377–379

MATHÉ, G. (1977). Follow-up of the first (1962) pilot study of active immunotherapy of acute lymphoblastic leukaemia. *Biomedicine*, **26**, 29–35

MEDICAL RESEARCH COUNCIL REPORT (1978). Immunotherapy of acute myeloid leukaemia. *British Journal of Cancer*, **37**, 1–14

NATHANSON, L., SCHOENFELD, D., REGELSON, M.D., COLSKY, J. and MITTELMAN, A. (1979). Prospective comparison of intralesional and multipuncture BCG in recurrent intradermal melanoma. *Cancer*, **43**, 1630–1635

OLIVER, R.T.D. (1977). Active specific and non-specific immunotherapy for patients with AML. In *Progress in Immunology III: Proceedings of the Third International Congress of Immunology, Sydney, Australia, 3–8 July 1977*. Ed. by T.E. Mandel, C. Cheers, C.S. Hosking, I.F.C. McKenzie and G.J.V. Nossal, pp. 572–578. Oxford; North Holland Publishing Co.

OLIVER, R.T.D., PILLAI, A., KLOUDA, P.T. and LAWLER, S.D. (1977). HLA linked resistance factors and survival in acute myelogenous leukemia. *Cancer*, **39**, 2337–2341

O'TOOLE, C., PERLMANN, P., UNSGAARD, H., MOBERGER, G. and EDSMYR, F. (1972). Cellular immunity to human urinary bladder cancer. 1. Correlation to clinical stage and radiotherapy. *International Journal of Cancer*, **10**, 77–91

PINES, A. (1976). A 5-year controlled study of BCG and radiotherapy for inoperable lung cancer. *Lancet*, **1**, 380–381

POMERANCE, A. (1972). Pathology and prognosis following total cystectomy for carcinoma of bladder. *British Journal of Urology*, **44**, 451–458

POWLES, R.L., RUSSELL, J., LISTER, T.A., OLIVER, R.T.D., WHITEHOUSE, J.M.A., PETO, R., CAHPUIS, B., CROWTHER, D. and ALEXANDER, P. (1977). Immuno-therapy for AML. *British Journal of Cancer,* **35**, 265–272

PROUT, G.R. and MARSHALL, V.F. (1956). The prognosis with untreated bladder tumors. *Cancer,* **9**, 551–558

RYGAARD, J. and POVLSEN, C.O. (1976). The nude mouse vs. the hypothesis of immunological surveillance. *Transplantation Reviews,* **28**, 43–61

SIMPSON, E. and NEHLSEN, S.L. (1971). Prolonged administration of anti-thymocyte serum in mice. 1. Histopathological investigations. *Clinical and Experimental Immunology,* **9**, 79–98

SOUTH-EASTERN CANCER STUDY GROUP. (1977). A controlled clinical trial of chemotherapy vs. BCG immunotherapy vs. no further therapy in remission maintenance of acute myelogenous leukemia (AML). *ASCO Abstracts,* **18**, 272

STRANDER, H. (1975). In *Report of the International Workshop on Interferon in the Treatment of Cancer.* Ed. by M. Krim. New York, p. 39. Cosponsored by the Memorial Sloan-Kettering Cancer Center and the Division of Cancer Treatment of the National Cancer Institute

TAKASUGI, M., MICKEY, M.R. and TERASAKI, P.I. (1974). Studies on specificity of cell-mediated immunity to human tumors. *Journal of the National Cancer Institute,* **53**, 1527–1538

THOMAS, L. (1959). In discussion in *Cellular and Humoral Aspects of the Hyper-sensitive State.* Ed. by H.G. Lawrence, p. 529. New York; Hoeber

WERF-MESSING, B. VAN DER and VAN GILSE, H.A. (1971). Hormonal treatment of metastases of renal carcinoma. *British Journal of Cancer,* **25**, 423–427

WHITTAKER, J.A. and SLATER, A.J. (1977). The immunotherapy of acute myelo-genous leukaemia using intravenous BCG. *British Journal of Haematology,* **35** 263–273

29

'Natural Killer' Cells in Chronic Bacterial Cystitis: Possible Implications for Immunosurveillance against Bladder Cancer

Carol O'Toole

Studies on lymphocyte cytotoxicity responses in patients with transitional cell carcinoma (TCC) of the urinary bladder have suggested that some cell lines of TCC origin share common antigens (O'Toole *et al.*, 1973; O'Toole, 1977). Cell lines obtained from non-malignant urothelium, squamous cell carcinoma of bladder and metastatic TCC lacked such antigen(s). The lymphoid cells exerting cytotoxicity in this system were identified as having receptors for the Fc portion of immunoglobulin (FcR+) and were found predominantly in patients with localized disease. Lymphocytes with similar attributes have also been detected in healthy persons and termed natural killer or NK cells (Bolhuis *et al.*, 1978; Pape *et al.*, 1979). The levels of cytotoxicity observed with healthy persons' cells were generally lower than those in patients with localized TCC (O'Toole, 1977). While screening subjects with no history of TCC for NK activity towards urothelial cell lines, several patients with chronic cystitis were encountered who showed significantly increased NK activity compared with healthy individuals. The specificity and nature of the cells mediating this reaction were examined in detail in one such case. The results demonstrate that these effector cells shared a similar target specificity to those in TCC patients but appeared to differ in being FcR−. The demonstration that bacterial infection increases NK activity against TCC cells may be one explanation for the benefit of intravesical BCG treatment of superficial tumours reported by Morales (Chapter 31).

MATERIALS AND METHODS

Case history

MG, a 72-year-old female with a history of chronic cystitis, presented in March 1977 with haematuria. Bladder biopsy showed numerous plasma cell infiltrates in the submucosa. The transitional epithelium had small areas of ulceration but was otherwise normal. The urine contained 1.4×10^6 granulocytes/ml, many with ingested bacteria. Urine cultures gave counts $>10^5$ *Enterobacter cloacae*. The patient was followed for 12 months, during which time bacterial infection persisted.

Control subjects

Forty-seven hospital workers were included in this study. There were 30 females and 17 males, aged from 40–60 years.

Experimental methods (see Appendix, p. 284)

RESULTS

The levels of NK activity by lymphocytes from healthy donors against allogeneic urothelial cell lines are shown in *Table 29.1*. Lymphocytes from the patient MG showed elevated lysis of certain cell lines, compared

Table 29.1
LEVELS OF NK ACTIVITY AGAINST ALLOGENEIC CELL LINES BY LYMPHOCYTES FROM HEALTHY DONORS (N = 47)

Effector:target ratio	Mean ± SD% corrected isotope release					
	T24	RT4	J82	TCC SuP	SCaBER	HCV-29
100 : 1	10 ± 7	8 ± 6	5 ± 2.9	3.3 ± 2.8	3 ± 2.5	5.8 ± 4.3
50 : 1	6.5 ± 5.4	5 ± 5	2.6 ± 1.8	2.4 ± 1.4	2 ± 1.5	4.7 ± 3.7

with any of the 47 normal donors tested. *Figure 29.1* shows the results of two tests on three target cell lines. MG's effector cells showed higher cytotoxicity against T24 and RT4 targets, than two normal donors. No differences between MG and normal donors were evident in lytic activity towards HCV–29 non-malignant urothelial cells. As shown in *Figure 29.1*, incubation of effectors for up to 48 hours at 37^0C before testing

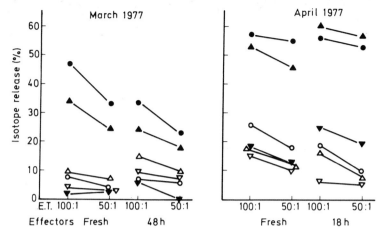

Figure 29.1 Serial tests on lymphocytes from patient (MG) with chronic cystitis for NK activity against allogeneic cell lines. Target cells: T24 •–•, RT4 ▲–▲ derived from TCC; HCV-29 ▼–▼ derived from non-malignant urothelium. Open symbols show results with lympho-cytes from two healthy donors. E:T = effector lymphocyte:target cell ratio. Patient's and control lymphocytes were tested immediately after isolation and after 48 hours or 18 hours pre-incubation at 37° C

did not change the patterns of reactivity. MG was tested for cytotoxicity on four occasions during 12 months with similar results.

To examine further the target specificity, MG's effector cells were pre-incubated on target cell monolayers before measuring NK activity. *Figure 29.2* shows an experiment in which cytotoxicity was detected

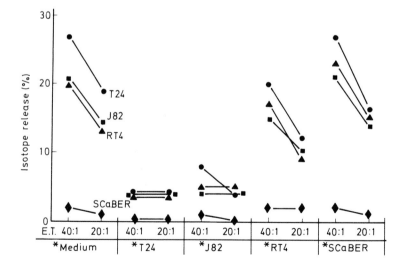

Figure 29.2 Specificity of target cell lysis shown by pre-absorbing MG lymphocytes on mono-layers for 8 hours before testing. ■–■ J82, derived from TCC; ♦–♦ SCaBER, derived from a squamous carcinoma of bladder. Other symbols as in text to Figure 29.1*

against three cell lines derived from TCC (T24, J82 and RT4), while no effect was found on SCaBER, a line derived from a squamous cell carcinoma of bladder. Effector cells pre-incubated on T24 and J82 monolayers showed greatly reduced lytic activity against T24, J82 and RT4 cells. RT4 cells were anomalous, in being susceptible to lysis but with a very poor capacity to absorb effector cells. SCaBER cells were without absorption capacity.

To determine whether the mechanism of cytolysis by MG effectors involved FcR+ cells, depletion experiments were performed. Monolayers of the cell line TCC SuP complexed with B85 antiserum were used as absorbant. TCC SuP was chosen as absorbant and target in these experiments as it was not lysed by MG effectors in the absence of added antibody. Lymphocytes from MG and control donors were compared in NK and ADCC activity before and after FcR+ depletion. *Figure 29.3* shows that removal of FcR+ cells had no effect on NK

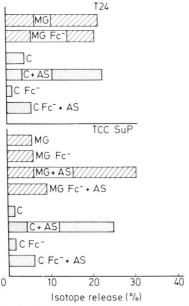

Figure 29.3 Differential effect of depletion of FcR+ lymphocytes on NK and ADCC by effector cells from MG and healthy control donor (C). AS: heterologous rabbit antisera (B85) to urothelial cells. Target cells T24 and TCC SuP derived from TCC. Effector lymphocyte: target cell ratio 20:1

activity of MG cells on T24 targets. However, ADCC by both MG and control donor cells was significantly reduced after FcR+ depletion. Further experiments showed that NK activity was not affected by inclusion of aggregated human IgG in concentrations up to 5 mg/ml in the assay. Under these conditions, ADCC was inhibited up to 80%. Specific depletion of NK effectors from MG on monolayers of T24 and J82 had no effect on ADCC capacity.

DISCUSSION

The data presented suggest, but do not prove, that chronic bacterial cystitis caused increased NK cell activity against allogeneic TCC targets. In this case, the increase in NK activity was restricted to three cell lines derived from TCC and was reproduced in four separate tests during a 12-month period. Three other urothelial cell lines of malignant and non-malignant origin were not preferentially lysed by the patients' lymphocytes when compared with those from healthy donors. Bacteria have previously been shown to influence cellular and humoral responses to neoplastic and normal tissues. An increase in NK activity has been described after injection of BCG (Wolfe *et al.*, 1976). Immunization of some mouse strains with group A streptococci induced specific cyto-toxicity to cardiac cells (Senitzer *et al.*, 1977). BCG injection has also been reported to cause development of antibodies cross-reactive with certain neoplastic cells (Bucana and Hanna; 1974; Minden *et al.*, 1974). Cross-reacting antibodies have been described between the common antigen of Enterobacteriaceae and human kidney and colon cells (Holmgren *et al.*, 1972). The results shown here indicate that cross-reactive antigens to some TCC may also exist within this group of bacteria.

The NK activity detected in this patient was functionally distinct from ADCC. Effector cells were specifically adsorbed on to target cell monolayers without affecting ADCC, while depletion of FcR+ cells had no effect on NK but reduced ADCC capacity in the same effector-cell preparations. These results, showing cell-mediated cytotoxicity to be independent of ADCC, are similar to those of De Landazuri *et al.* (1974) in a rat lymphoma. Several other observations indicate that NK activity against TCC cells was an immunoglobulin-independent function in this donor: pre-incubation of effector cells at 37°C for as long as 48 hours did not lead to a loss of cytotoxicity. Cytophilic antibody is known to be shed under such conditions (Kumagai *et al.*, 1975). NK function was not diminished in the presence of aggregated IgG, while ADCC was significantly reduced. These features of NK cells are similar to those reported in healthy donors by Bolhuis *et al.* (1978) and Kay *et al.* (1979). These authors found that NK was a predominantly immunoglobulin-independent phenomenon. Using the target cell T24, Pape *et al.* (1979) suggested that NK activity in healthy donors could follow both IgG-dependent and independent pathways. It remains to be determined what role previous bacterial exposure has in the generation and specificity of NK cell activity in humans.

In view of the wide variety of antigens present on different bacteria, it is unlikely that the phenomena demonstrated in this report will be produced by all bacteria causing urinary infection. However, if BCG could be shown to induce similar responses, it might provide an explanation for the benefit of intravesical BCG in the treatment of superficial bladder tumours reported by Morales (*see* Chapter 31). Use of this assay to study patients receiving such treatment will be of considerable interest. In addition, in view of the known incidence of bacterial colonization of tumours in the bladder, it will be important to correlate this observation with NK cell levels before drawing any firm conclusion on the role of these cells in surveillance.

APPENDIX: Details of the experimental method

Defibrinated blood was mixed with a 3% gelatin solution in a 3:1 v/v ratio, and incubated for 1 hour at 37°C to sediment erythrocytes. The leucocyte-plasma layer was removed and centrifuged at 700 *g* for 10 minutes. Pelleted cells were resuspended in Tris-buffered Hanks' solution (TH) containing 10% heat-inactivated (56°C for 1 hour) foetal calf serum (FCS). The cell suspension was layered over Ficoll-Paque and centrifuged at 400 *g* for 40 minutes at 20°C. Lymphocytes were collected from the interface and washed three times in TH. Mononuclear cells were counted in Turk's stain. Lymphocytes were maintained at a density of 2×10^6/ml in tissue culture medium (199 with Hanks' salts containing 10% FCS, 100 IU penicillin, 100 μg streptomycin and 0.3 mg glutamine/ml) at 37°C in air + 5% CO_2 before testing.

Target cells

Six cell lines of urothelial origin were tested: T24, RT4, J82 and TCC SuP derived from TCC, and SCaBER derived from a pure squamous cell carcinoma of bladder (O'Toole, 1977). HCV−29, a culture of non-malignant urothelium, was obtained from Dr J. Fogh (Sloan-Kettering Cancer Institute, New York). The lines were grown in monolayers and were free of mycoplasma contamination.

Cellular absorbants

Confluent target monolayers at densities of $1-2 \times 10^6$ cells in 25 cm² flasks were used 2 days after plating. Four million lymphocytes in 4 ml tissue culture medium were incubated on the monolayers for 8 hours at 37°C in air + 5% CO_2. Non-adherent cells were collected and washed three times in TH solution before testing.

Depletion of FcR+ lymphocytes

Confluent target monolayers in 75 cm² flasks were treated with 10 ml 0.25% glutaraldehyde in Hanks' solution for 5 minutes at 4°C, 10 ml of a 1/200 dilution of hyperimmune rabbit serum to urothelial cells

(B85) were added for 30 minutes at 22°C. B85 was heat-inactivated (56°C, 30 minutes) before use. The monolayers were then washed three times with Hanks' solution. Five million lymphocytes in 10 ml Hanks' solution were added per flask and left for 30 minutes at 22°C. Non-adherent cells were collected and washed three times in TH solution.

Tests for lymphocyte function

Chromium–51 isotope release assay for NK activity

Target cells at confluency in 25 cm² flasks were labelled with 50 μCi Na$_2$ ^{51}CrO$_4$ (specific activity 200–500 Ci/g Cr) for 18 hours at 37°C in air + 5% CO_2. Cells were collected by treatment with a solution containing 0.02% EDTA and 0.05% trypsin at 37°C for 5–10 minutes. Cells were washed three times in tissue culture medium. Viability estimated by trypan blue dye exclusion was $\geqslant$ 95%. Cytotoxicity assays were done in 10 × 75 mm borosilicate culture tubes each containing 5 × 10^3 target cells. Lymphocytes were added at the ratios indicated. The incubation medium was 199 containing 5% FCS, antibiotics and glutamine with a total volume of 1 ml/tube. Each parameter was tested in duplicate tubes. The tubes were centrifuged at 200 g for 5 minutes, then incubated at 37°C in air + 5% CO_2 for 18–20 hours. The results are presented as mean percentage isotope release, corrected for spontaneous isotope release by targets incubated without effector cells. Spontaneous isotope release from all targets averaged $\leqslant$ 1% per hour. Maximum variation in percentage release between duplicates was ± 2.5%.

Antibody-dependent cytotoxicity (ADCC)

Heat-inactivated rabbit antiserum B85, prepared against the T24 cell line, was added at a final dilution of 1:2000 to the assay described above. This serum before absorption induced cytotoxicity by K cells against all urothelial cell lines tested. At the dilution used, the serum was not toxic to any target in the absence of effector cells.

ACKNOWLEDGEMENTS

This work was supported by Grant Ca20216 from the National Cancer Institute. I wish to thank Drs W.M. Murphy and L.G. Koss for reviewing the pathology, and A. Balows and D. Brenner, Center for Disease Control in Atlanta, Georgia, USA for identification of the bacteria.

REFERENCES

BOLHUIS, R.J.H., SCHUIT, H.R.E., NOOYEN, A.M. and RONTELTAP, C.P.M. (1978). Characterisation of natural killer (NK) and killer (K) cells in human blood: discrimination between NK and K cell activities. *European Journal of Immunology*, **8**, 731–740

BUCANA, C. and HANNA, M.G. JR. (1974). Immunoelectronmicroscopic analysis of surface antigens common to *Mycobacterium bovis* (BCG) and tumor cells. *Journal of the National Cancer Institute*, **53**, 1313–1323

DE LANDAZURI, M.O., KEDAR, E. and FAHEY, J.L. (1974). Simultaneous expression of cell-mediated cytotoxicity and antibody-dependent cellular cytotoxicity to a syngeneic rat lymphoma: separation and partial characterisation of two types of cytotoxic cells. *Cellular Immunology*, **14**, 193–205

HOLMGREN, J., HAMMARSTRÖM, S., HOLM, S.E., AHLEN, J., ATTMAN, P.O. and JODAL, U. (1972). An antigenic relationship between human kidney, colon and the common antigen of Enterobacteriaceae. *International Archives of Allergy and Applied Immunology*, **43**, 89–97

KAY, H.D., BONNARD, G.D. and HERBERMAN, R.B. (1979). Evaluation of the role of IgG antibodies in human natural cell-mediated cytotoxicity against the myeloid cell line K562. *Journal of Immunology*, **122**, 675–685

KUMAGAI, K., ABO, T., SEKIZAWA, T. and SASAKI, M. (1975). Studies of surface immunoglobulins on human B lymphocytes. I. Dissociation of cell-bound immunoglobulins with acid pH or at 37°C. *Journal of Immunology*, **115**, 982–987

MINDEN, P., McCLATCHY, J.K., WAINBERG, M. and WEISS, D.W. (1974). Shared antigens between *Mycobacterium bovis* (BCG) and neoplastic cells. *Journal of the National Cancer Institute*, **53**, 1325–1331

O'TOOLE, C., UNSGAARD, B., ALMGÅRD, L.E. and JOHANSSON, B. (1973). The cellular immune response to carcinoma of the urinary bladder. Correlation to clinical stage and therapy. *British Journal of Cancer*, **28**, 266–275

O'TOOLE, C. (1977). A [51] chromium isotope release assay for detecting cytotoxicity to human bladder cancer. *International Journal of Cancer*, **19**, 324–331

PAPE, G.R., TROYE, M., AXELSSON, B. and PERLMANN, P. (1979). Simultaneous occurrence of immunoglobulin-dependent and immunoglobulin-independent mechanisms in natural cytotoxicity of human lymphocytes. *Journal of Immunology*, **122**, 2251–2260

SENITZER, D., CAFRUNY, W., PANSKY, B. and FREIMER, E.H. (1977). Spontaneous and induced cell-mediated reactivity to syngeneic cells. *Nature (London)*, **268**, 158–159

WOLFE, S.A., TRACEY, D.E. and HENNEY, C.S. (1976). Introduction of 'natural killer' cells by BCG. *Nature (London)*, **262**, 584–586

30

Intravesical BCG Therapy for Ta and T1 Bladder Tumours: Histopathology and Toxicity

M.R.G. Robinson and C.C. Rigby

The majority of Ta and T1 category transitional cell carcinomas of the bladder (UICC, 1978) are easily and effectively controlled by endoscopic diathermy or resection. Some, however, require alternative therapy because they progress to more invasive disease and others because they recur too rapidly for endoscopic treatment to be effective.

The tumours which recur rapidly, but remain in the Ta and T1 category because they do not invade beyond the lamina propria, pose a particular problem for the urologist. If their sites of recurrence are confined to the epithelium of the bladder, they can be cured by total cystectomy. This, however, is a drastic treatment for the patient, with a high morbidity and mortality for what is essentially non-invasive malignant disease. Many alternatives, such as external and intravesical radiotherapy, hydrostatic pressure, hyperthermia, and intravesical chemotherapy, have been suggested for these recurrent tumours. None are entirely satisfactory and, recently, interest has grown in immunotherapy for these patients.

As a clinical discipline, active non-specific tumour immunotherapy with BCG (bacille Calmette-Guérin) has been practised for more than a decade. BCG increases reticulo-endothelial system function, augments the antibody response and increases delayed hypersensitivity responses to a variety of antigens. It may also cross-react with antigen on the surface of some tumour cells (Hersh et al., 1977). Morales et al. (1976) have observed that the antigenicity of bladder tumours has been well documented by Bubenik et al. (1970) and by Catalona and Chretien

(1973), and this suggests that BCG immunotherapy may be useful in the eradication of non-invasive bladder neoplasms. For effective immunotherapy, direct BCG tumour contact may be essential (Baldwin *et al.*, 1974). The bladder is a suitable organ for bringing BCG into contact with tumour by intravesical instillation, or by direct endo-scopic injection into the malignant lesion. Observation by cystoscopy and biopsy during the follow-up of the tumours is easily performed at regular intervals.

Several workers have now reported studies of BCG immunotherapy in the management of recurrent non-invasive transitional cell bladder neoplasms. Morales (1976) reported the results for 15 patients with transitional cell tumours and one with squamous cell tumour, who completed a course of treatment. He administered 120 mg of lyophilized BCG (Institut Armand Frappier, Montreal) in 50 ml normal saline instilled into the bladder via a urethral catheter, and 5 mg of the same BCG administered intradermally by Heaf gun into the thigh, weekly for 6 consecutive weeks. Before BCG therapy, the 16 patients had a total of 53 recurrent tumours during an interval of 162 patient-months. Following BCG therapy, these patients yielded seven recurrences during the follow-up of 222 patient-months. Six weeks after completion of treatment, biopsy of the location of the previous tumours, which had been resected or diathermized before BCG treat-ment, showed granulomatous inflammation with multinucleated giant cells, lymphocytes and plasma cells. Toxicity of BCG therapy in this series was slight. Three patients had low-grade fever for less than 24 hours and three had urinary frequency and urgency.

Douville *et al.* (1978) have reported six patients with recurrent bladder papillomata, who were treated both by BCG abdominal scari-fication and BCG intravesical instillations without resection. The scarification dose was, as in Morales' series, 5 mg, and the intravesical dose of 120 mg in normal saline was repeated weekly for 6 weeks. Four of their six patients were completely cleared of tumour without pre-treatment resection. All four responders had systemic toxic reactions to BCG, and two of these were severe, requiring hospitalization and anti-tubercular drugs.

Toxicity of BCG cancer immunotherapy has been well documented. Rosenberg *et al.* (1978) reported eight patients with disseminated BCG infection following a single injection of living BCG directly into malig-nant melanomas. Clinical features of this toxicity were persistent fever commencing 9–20 days after BCG injection, and severe liver function abnormalities peaking approximately 20 days after injection. All their patients had raised serum transaminase and alkaline phosphatase levels. Serum bilirubin was raised in only one patient. Fever, chills, malaise and arthralgia lasted for 7–22 days before subsiding. Liver function abnormalities sometimes took 6 months to return to normal. Biopsies of the liver and bone marrow revealed the presence of disseminated BCG granulomas in these organs. The clinical course of this toxicity was not influenced by treatment with isoniazid. Robinson *et al.* (1976) reported widespread interstitial granulomas at post-mortem examination in patients who received intratumour freeze-dried Glaxo BCG immunotherapy for carcinoma of the prostate. The organs affected were the lungs, bone marrow, kidney, liver, spleen and heart (*Figure 30.1*). These lesions often persisted for months after immunotherapy and were not associated with clinical symptoms other than pyrexia, lasting for approximately 48 hours after BCG injection. From these observations it must be concluded that, in planning BCG immunotherapy for non-invasive bladder cancer, the risks of disseminated BCG toxicity must be considered against the possible benefits of this treatment.

Martinez-Pineiro (1978) reported that intravesical BCG alone may be as effective in the treatment of superficial bladder tumours as the combination of intravesical and intradermal immunotherapy or direct injection into the tumours. In addition, in 1978 the Yorkshire Urological Cancer Research Group and the Institute of Urology, London,[a] began a study of intravesical BCG only in the treatment of non-invasive bladder neoplasms. This trial has two objectives. The first is to determine histological changes produced in the bladder epithelium and the tumour cells, and the second is to determine the local and systemic toxicity produced by this treatment. The preliminary results of this trial have been reported recently (Richards *et al.,* 1979). Twenty-seven patients have been entered in this study. They all have transitional cell tumours clinically staged as T1 NX MX (UICC). Patients have been excluded if they have other neoplasms, are unfit for repeated cystoscopy and biopsy under general anaesthesia, or are not expected to live for more than 3 years. They have all been Mantoux tested before entry to the trial and after 6 months' treatment. All have received weekly instillations of one ampoule freeze-dried Glaxo BCG, diluted in 50 ml normal saline, instilled via a urethral catheter into the bladder and retained for at least 2 hours, weekly for 4 weeks and then monthly for 11 months. Twenty-one patients have had cystoscopy and biopsy only before the first four instillations of BCG, the tumours not being resected until the first cystoscopy at 1 month. Six patients had their tumours resected before commencing therapy. Cystoscopies have been repeated 1 month after initial treatment (at which any residual tumour was resected) and then at 3-monthly intervals thereafter. At each cystoscopy, a biopsy has been taken of the tumour surface, the tumour base, normal bladder epithelium and any epithelium which appeared to

[a]B. Richards, York; R.S. Adib, Wakefield; M.R.G. Robinson, Pontefract; C.C. Rigby, London; R.C.B. Pugh, London.

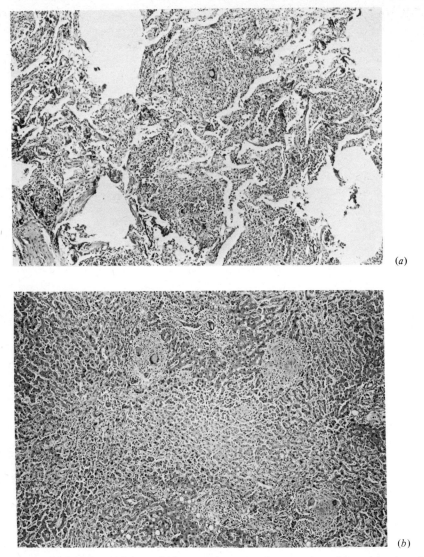

(a)

(b)

Figure 30.1 Widespread interstitial macrophage granulomas, some with multinucleated giant cells, showing associated lymphocyte and plasma cell infiltration. Found post-mortem in a patient who died 3 months after immunotherapeutic injection of BCG into his prostatic tumour. (a) Lung (H.E. × 16. Magnification × 3); (b) Liver (H.E. × 16. Magnification × 3); (c) Heart (H.E. × 40. Magnification × 3); (d) Bone marrow (H.E. × 40. Magnification × 3)

be abnormal. As this is a histological and toxicity study, the protocol does not demand delayed cutaneous hypersensitivity tests other than the Mantoux test, or quantitative lymphocyte studies.

Histologically granulomatous lesions have been observed in biopsies from 10 of the 27 patients, similar to those described by Morales

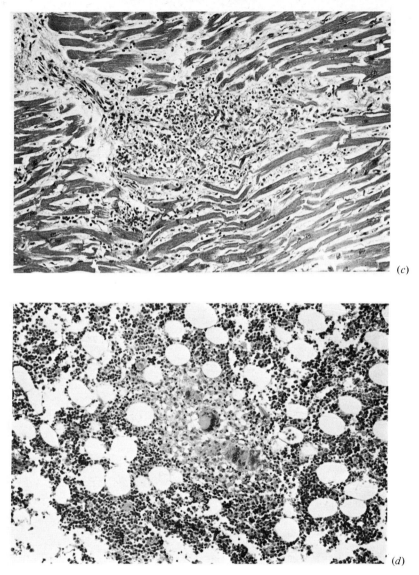

(c)

(d)

(1976). They feature multinucleated giant cells and macrophages with infiltration of the surrounding tissues by lymphocytes and plasma cells (*Figures 30.2, 30.3*). They are similar to the reactions produced by the direct injection of BCG into prostatic carcinoma (Robinson *et al.,* 1976). These granulomata are found only in the subepithelium and not usually in close proximity to the malignant epithelial cells. Tumour necrosis in association with granulomata has not been demonstrated histologically.

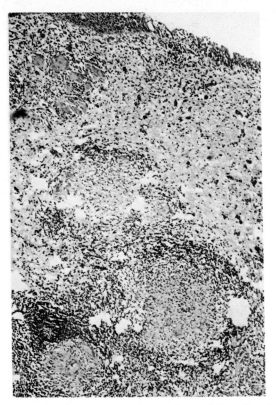

Figure 30.2 Cystoscopic biopsy obtained 7 weeks after the commencement of intravesical BCG immunotherapy. Scattered granulomatous lesions are visible in the lamina propria. (H.E. × 16, Magnification × 4)

Systemic toxicity has been observed in two of 27 patients. Both had persistent fever and abnormal liver function tests. One of them had complete remission of seven of her eight tumours, but they rapidly recurred when therapy was suspended because of toxicity, and she was admitted to hospital. The toxicity did not respond to isoniazid, but she recovered when subsequently treated with ethambutol and rifampicin. The other patient recovered without anti-tuberculous drugs, but his tumour category rapidly progressed to T4 and it is possible that, in this case, there was tumour enhancement induced by BCG. Before treatment however, his T1 category tumour was poorly differentiated (G3 category, UICC).

Seven of the 21 patients had an erythrocyte sedimentation rate which, during therapy, became raised to above 30 mm in the first hour. Transient abnormal liver function tests have been observed in three other patients.

Local toxicity characterized by frequency and dysuria has been reported in 25% of these patients. Usually this has been transient, but

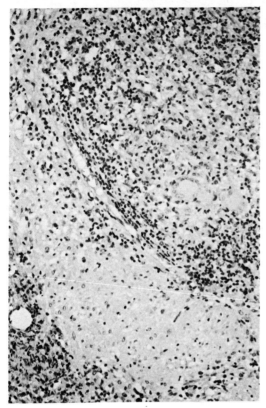

Figure 30.3 Extensive macrophage granuloma found in a bladder biopsy taken 7 weeks after commencement of immunotherapy, in a second patient. There is an intense lymphocyte infiltration; some plasma cells, eosinophils and polymorphonuclear leucocytes are also present. (H.E. × 40, Magnification × 4)

it caused temporary incontinence in one patient and required treatment to be interrupted in two more.

Preliminary tumour response has not been impressive in this study. The tumours of the 21 patients who were not initially resected have regressed in four, not changed in 10 and progressed in seven. In three of the four which regressed, the tumour was solitary and the effect of biopsy must be taken into account. In the fourth, complete regression of all but one of eight tumours was noted. The frequency with which endoscopic surgery was required was not influenced in 19 of the 21 recurrent cases. An apparent reduction in tumour recurrence has been noted in only two cases. The Mantoux reaction became more marked in four patients during treatment. One of these had no further recurrences over a period of 10 months. The recurrence rate was unchanged in the other three patients.

DISCUSSION

There is no doubt that systemic toxicity of intravesical BCG therapy can be severe, requiring hospitalization and anti-tuberculous drugs. This may be associated with widespread multiple granulomata in many organs and, as in our cases, may not respond to therapy with isoniazid alone. Such systemic toxicity may result from depression of the patient's immune competence and may be associated with tumour enhancement, as possibly occurred in the patient with a poorly differentiated tumour which progressed to T4 category. The Yorkshire study has demontrated that this toxicity can occur, even if the drug is administered by the intravesical route only.

The results of intravesical BCG therapy alone, as used in this study, have not been as effective in producing tumour regression and reducing recurrence as those reported in earlier studies of combined intradermal and intravesical therapy, even though several patients developed typical BCG granulomata in the sub-epithelium of the bladder mucosa. Bloomberg *et al.* (1975) in a series of experiments on dogs reported that, while both saline injections and BCG instillations produced only mild congestion in the normal bladder mucosa, whether or not they had been previously sensitized by BCG inoculation, direct injection of BCG into the bladder epithelium produced a marked inflammatory action in some non-sensitized dogs and in all dogs which had been inoculated with BCG. They concluded that it was possible to produce BCG reactions in the bladder by BCG instillations, only after the epithelium had been traumatized by resection or biopsy. This may be the mechanism by which the BCG granulomata were produced in the Yorkshire patients. The lower incidence of local granulomatous reaction in unsensitized individuals is possibly an explanation for the higher incidence of systemic toxicity, as there is no barrier to the spread of the organism.

The precise role of BCG immunotherapy for superficial bladder tumours still has to be established. Further attention should also be paid to the source of BCG used, and to the mode and frequency of its administration. In future trials, particular emphasis should be placed on the assessment of patients' initial and subsequent immune status, using such assays as that reported by O'Toole (*see* Chapter 29).

REFERENCES

BALDWIN, R.W., BOWEN, J.G., EMBLETON, M.J., PRICE, M.R. and ROBINS, R.A. (1974) Cellular and humoral responses to neoantigens associated with chemically-induced tumours. In *Progress in Immunology, II. vol. 3: Biological Aspects II,* Ed. by L. Brent and J. Holborow, pp 239–248 Amsterdam; North Holland

BLOOMBERG, S.D., BROSMAN, S.A., HAUSMAN, M.S., COHEN, A. and BATTENBERG, J.D. (1975). The effects of BCG on the dog bladder *Investigative Urology*, **12**, 423–427

BUBENIK, J., PERLMANN, P., HELMSTEIN, K. and MOBERGER, G. (1970). Cellular and humoral immune responses to human urinary bladder carcinomas. *International Journal of Cancer*, **5**, 310–319

CATALONA, W.J. and CHRETIEN, P.B. (1973). Correlation among host immuno-competence and tumor stage, tumor grade and vascular permeation in trans-itional carcinoma. *Journal of Urology*, **110**, 526–528

DOUVILLE, Y., PELOUZE, G., ROY, R., CHARROIS, R., KIBRITÉ, A., MARTIN, M., DIONNE, L., COULONVAL, L. and ROBINSON, J. (1978). Recurrent bladder papil-lomata treated with bacillus Calmette-Guérin : a preliminary report (Phase I Trial). *Cancer Treatment Reports*, **62**, 551–552

HERSH, E.M., GUTTERMAN, J.U. and MAVLIGIT, G.M. (1977). BCG as adjuvant immunotherapy for neoplasia. *Annual Review of Medicine*, **28**, 489–515

MARTINEZ-PINEIRO, J.A. (1978). Introduction of immunology and immuno-therapy of bladder tumours. *Paper read at the Second International Conference on Bladder Tumours, Eriche, Sicily, 1978*, To be published in *Bladder Tumours and Their Topics in Urological Oncology*. Ed. M. Paveone-Macaluso, P.H. Smith and M.R.G. Robinson. New York: Plenum Publishing Co Ltd

MORALES, A., EIDINGER, D. and BRUCE, A.W. (1976). Intracavitary bacillus Cal-mette-Guérin in the treatment of superficial bladder tumours. *Journal of Urology*, **116**, 180–183

MORALES, A. (1976). Adjuvant immunotherapy in superficial bladder cancer. *Workshop on Genito-Urinary Cancer Immunology. NCI Monograph 49*. Ed. by J.C. Bailor and E.H. Weisberg, pp. 315–319. Washington DC: US Department of Health, Education & Welfare

RICHARDS, B., ROBINSON, M.R.G., ADIB, R.S., RIGBY, C.C. and PUGH, R.C.B. (1981). Intravesical BCG in non-invasive carcinomas of the bladder. *Proceedings of the XVIII Congress of the International Urological Society, Parish, 1979.* In press

ROBINSON, M.R.G., RIGBY, C.C., PUGH, R.C.B. and DUMMONDE, D.C. (1976). Pro-static carcinoma: intratumour BCG immunotherapy. *Workshop on Genito-Urinary Cancer Immunology. NCI Monograph 49*. Ed. by J.C. Bailor and E.H. Weisberg, pp. 351–353. Washington DC: US Department of Health, Education & Welfare

ROSENBERG, S.A., SEIPP, C. and SEARS, H.F. (1978). Clinical and immunologic studies of disseminated BCG infection. *Cancer*, **41**, 1771–1780

UICC (1978). *TNM Classification of Malignant Tumours*. 3rd ed. Geneva; UICC

31

Intravesical and Systemic BCG Treatment for Superficial Bladder Cancer: Results and Method of Evaluation

Alvaro Morales

Though control of superficial bladder cancer is readily achieved by endoscopic surgical procedures when the tumours are small and few in number, this treatment needs to be repeated frequently in the majority of patients (Greene *et al.*, 1973). In addition, tumour recurrences are so widespread and frequent that they cannot be controlled by endoscopic means alone. These considerations have prompted the search for additional approaches to the prophylaxis and treatment of non-invasive bladder cancer. Vesical instillation of antineoplastic agents has been used for many years in the prevention and eradication of these tumours. Recent results on the effectiveness of thiotepa and ethoglucid have already been discussed elsewhere (*see* Chapters 7 and 8).

The antigenicity of bladder cancer has been repeatedly demonstrated (Bubenik *et al.*, 1970; O'Toole *et al.*, 1972; Bean, 1977). This would suggest that an immunological approach may have a part to play in the management of these neoplasms. Experimental studies have shown the efficacy of bacillus Calmette-Guérin (BCG) in inducing tumour regression and, in the clinical situation, the intratumoural administration of the vaccine has been noted to produce favourable responses in patients with several types of tumour (DeKernion *et al.*, 1975; McKneally *et al.*, 1978). The most relevant factors contributing to the success of BCG therapy have been defined by Bast *et al.*, (1974). Evidently, no other tumour, with the possible general exception of cutaneous malignancies, fulfills the requirements of small tumour burden, adequate dose and close intimate contact between BCG and tumour as does the superficial vesical neoplasm.

In this Chapter, experience of the use of regional BCG for prophylaxis of recurrent bladder cancer is summarized.

PATIENTS AND METHODS

Twenty-three patients with histologically diagnosed transitional cell carcinoma of the bladder were treated. To qualify for entry to the study, a patient must have had no less than two documented recurrences, in separate endoscopic examinations, within 2 years before the onset of treatment. In every case the tumours were superficial and were completely resected, thus leaving no endoscopic evidence of residual tumour. There were 16 men and seven women, ranging in age from 43 to 88 years (mean 72 years).

BCG

Throughout the trial the vaccine from the Institut Armand Frappier, Montreal, was used. One hundred and twenty milligrams of the lyophilized vaccine were re-suspended in 50 ml of sterile normal saline for use as a bladder instillation. Five milligrams of reconstituted BCG were employed for intradermal immunization.

The treatment protocol established that every patient should receive weekly intradermal and intravesical immunizations with BCG, starting within one week of transurethral resection. For the intradermal route, the anterior aspect of a thigh was cleaned with alcohol and allowed to dry. Utilizing a multiple puncture apparatus (Heaf gun) with a six-pronged head, ten impacts were administered to an area of approximately 5 × 5 cm. A small amount of the BCG suspension was spread over the area of skin punctures and allowed to dry. The procedure was repeated until all the vaccine was used. The area was covered with a dry dressing and the patient was instructed to leave it undisturbed for 24 hours. For the intravesical administration, the patient was suitably prepared for routine bladder catheterization under sterile conditions. A number 8F catheter was interted into the bladder, all urine was removed and a sample sent for routine culture. The BCG suspension was instilled into the bladder and the catheter removed immediately afterwards. The patient was instructed to retain the medication for not less than 2 hours at which time he was allowed to void. Both the intradermal and intravesical administration of the vaccine were repeated at weekly intervals for 6 weeks. For the intradermal applications, alternate thighs were used.

In all patients, follow-up cystoscopic examinations were performed at 3 to 6-month intervals from the onset of treatment. At endoscopy, any obvious tumour or areas suggestive of recurrence were biopsied utilizing cold-cup forceps. In the absence of mucosal changes suggestive of tumour, samples from pre-selected areas (usually four) were obtained. Urinary cytological examinations were performed on fresh voided specimens and on samples obtained at the time of cystoscopy.

RESULTS

The duration of the follow-up periods differs among patients. The pre-BCG period ranges from 7 to 43 months, the post-BCG from 14 to 52 months. The follow-up interval before treatment does not equal the corresponding duration after treatment, for each subject. Thus, for comparison of the effects of therapy, equal periods before and after treatment were used. Data on the entire set of patients, and the statistical analysis using the Wilcoxon test, are summarized in *Table 31.1*.

The least square method was used to estimate the slopes of the pre- and post-BCG linear regression lines. The Cochrane Q (*Table 31.2*) test (Sokal and Rohlf, 1969) was applied to determine trend. In this test the patients were scored for the presence or absence of a tumour during four equal intervals before and after BCG therapy. *Table 31.2* gives

Table 31.1
WILCOXON SIGNED-RANK TEST

Patient number	Number of tumours pre-BCG	Number of tumours post-BCG	d_i	Rank of absolute value of d_i
1	9	0	9	20.5
2	6	0	6	14.5
3	9	1	8	18.5
4	6	0	6	14.5
5	4	2	2	1.0
6	9	0	9	20.5
7	6	2	4	8.5
8	5	2	3	3.5
9	16	2	14	23.0
10	4	0	4	8.5
11	6	0	6	14.5
12	8	3	5	12.0
13	3	0	3	3.5
14	8	4	4	8.5
15	4	0	4	8.5
16	8	0	8	18.5
17	7	0	7	17.0
18	3	0	3	3.5
19	4	0	4	8.5
20	3	0	3	3.5
21	6	0	6	14.5
22	4	0	4	8.5
23	11	1	10	22.0

$\Sigma(\text{ranks } d_i < 0) = 0$
$\Sigma(\text{ranks } d_i > 0) = 276$
$T = \min (\Sigma(\text{ranks } d_i < 0), \Sigma(\text{ranks } d_i > 0))$
$= 0$

$\mu = n(n + 1)/4 \quad \sigma^2 = (2n + 1)\,\mu/6$
$= 23 \times 24/4 \qquad = 47 \times 138/6$
$= 138 \qquad\qquad = 1081$
$\qquad\qquad\qquad \sigma = \sqrt{1081} \cong 32.88$

$$Z = \frac{|T - \mu|}{\sigma}$$
$= 4.20$
$P = {} < 10^{-3}$

Table 31.2
THE COCHRANE'S Q TEST

Patient number	Pre-BCG intervals*					Post-BCG intervals				
	1	2	3	4	Σ	1	2	3	4	Σ
1	1	0	1	1	3	0	0	0	0	0
2	0	1	0	1	2	0	0	0	0	0
3	0	1	1	1	3	0	0	0	1	1
4	0	1	0	1	2	0	0	0	0	0
5	1	1	0	1	3	0	0	1	0	1
6	0	1	0	1	2	0	0	0	0	0
7	0	1	0	1	2	0	1	0	0	1
8	0	1	1	1	3	0	0	0	1	1
9	0	1	1	1	3	1	0	0	0	1
10	0	1	0	1	2	0	0	0	0	0
11	0	0	1	1	2	0	0	0	0	0
12	1	1	0	1	3	0	1	1	0	2
13	0	1	0	1	2	0	0	0	0	0
14	1	1	1	1	4	1	1	0	0	2
15	0	0	0	1	1	0	0	0	0	0
16	1	0	0	1	2	0	0	0	0	0
17	1	0	0	1	2	0	0	0	0	0
18	0	0	0	1	1	0	0	0	0	0
19	1	0	1	1	3	0	0	0	0	0
20	1	0	0	1	2	0	0	0	0	0
21	0	1	0	1	2	0	0	0	0	0
22	0	1	0	1	2	0	0	0	0	0
23	1	1	0	1	3	0	0	0	1	1
Totals	9	15	7	23	54	2	3	2	3	10

*0 denotes the absence of a recurrence during interval, 1 denotes the presence of recurrence(s)

$Q \sim x$

$$Q = (a-1)\,(a \, \Sigma\,(\Sigma Y) - (\Sigma\Sigma Y)\,) / (a\Sigma\Sigma Y - \Sigma(\Sigma Y)\,)$$

$a = 4$ $b = 23$

Pre-BCG: $Q = 23.85$
          $x^2\ 0.001;3 = 16.27$
          $\therefore P < 10^{-3}$

Post-BCG: $Q = 0.46$
          $x^2\ 0.05;3 = 7.82$
          $\therefore P > 0.05$

some details of the analysis. For the 23 patients in the trial, a statistically significant ($P < 10^{-3}$) positive (upward) trend in recurrence was detected for the pre-BCG period. No trend ($P > 0.05$) following BCG therapy is evident. This analysis indicates that BCG administration reduces the number of recurrent tumours, disrupting an upward trend in the recurrence pattern.

Further examination of the follow-up data reveals that it was feasible to classify the patients into three groups on the basis of their response to treatment. Class A consists of 12 of the 23 patients (52%) who remained entirely tumour-free during the post-BCG follow-up. Class B, which accounts for 30% of the group, is composed of seven patients (Cases 1, 3, 4, 8, 9, 17 and 23) in whom improvement is evident following BCG administration. In this group there was an average reduction of 83% in the number of tumours. Class C, the remaining 17%, is made up of the four patients (Cases 5, 7, 12 and 14) whose pattern of recurrence did not appear to be altered by the therapy under study.

The three groups were analyzed for factors which could account for the differences in response. A one-way analysis of variance (Ott, 1977) showed that the differences in ages among groups were significant, both

Table 31.3
AGE COMPARISONS BETWEEN GROUPS

Variable	Class A	Class B	Class C	Classes A & B	Classes B & C
Number of patients	12	7	4	19	11
Mean age at diagnosis	73.83	70.86	56.50	72.74	65.64
Mean age at treatment	76.08	73.29	58.50	75.05	67.91

A = patients who remained tumour-free; B = patients who improved; C = patients showing no evidence of benefit

at diagnosis ($F = 5.74$; df = 2,20; $P < 0.05$) and treatment ($F = 5.30$; df = 2,20; $P < 0.05$). Employing Fischer's test for multiple comparisons (Ott, 1977), it appears that mean ages at diagnosis and treatment in group C were significantly ($P < 0.05$) lower than the mean ages of groups A or B. Mean age comparisons between groups are summarized in *Table 31.3*

SIDE-EFFECTS

Untoward reactions to the vaccine were generally mild and self-limiting. In the majority of cases they consisted of malaise, low-grade fever and bladder irritability (dysuria and urinary frequency) lasting for a few days and not requiring specific treatment. In five subjects, however (Cases 8, 12, 15, 20 and 23), symptoms of bladder irritability were severe enough to require the use of urinary analgesics (phenazopyridine) and anticholinergic medication. Cases 15 and 20 responded promptly to the medication. Case 23 developed chills and high fever (40°C) after the fourth treatment but the symptoms subsided promptly after administration of isoniazid and streptomycin which were continued during the remaining two immunizations. Cessation of BCG administration after five treatment sessions was necessary for cases 8 and 12. Case 12 developed severe cystitis and secondary bilateral ureteric obstruction. The most severe generalized reactions were observed in patient 8 in whom migratory polyarthritis and cutaneous erythema of the palms occurred. In three other patients, a lower urinary tract, probably iatrogenic, infection with *Escherichia coli* was documented during treatment. In all three cases, a rapid response to antibiotics was obtained.

DISCUSSION

The results of this study indicate that the simultaneous intradermal and intravesical administration of BCG favourably alters the pattern of recurrence of superficial bladder cancer. Fifty-two per cent of the patients with a previous history of multiple recurrences have remained tumour-free for periods ranging from 15 to 52 months. As observed with other solid tumours (Eilber *et al.*, 1976) the response to therapy with BCG is not an all-or-nothing phenomenon. In 30% of the patients, although one or more recurrences were observed in the post-treatment period, its frequency was reduced by 83%, which corresponded to an extended mean disease-free interval increasing from 4 months before treatment to 20 months after treatment. It is conceivable that a longer period of immunization could have improved the outcome in these patients; such a possibility, however, has not as yet been studied. Our recent findings of tumour recurrence after 2 years of urothelial stability clearly suggest that periodic boosting of immunity may be necessary to maintain the effect of the vaccine.

Following our initial publications (Morales *et al.*, 1976; 1978) on the effect of BCG in superficial bladder cancer, confirmatory evidence has appeared in the literature (Martinez-Piñiero and Muntañola, 1977; Douville *et al.*, 1978; Lamm *et al.*, 1980). The recent studies of Lamm *et al.* (1980) are particularly relevant because they constitute the first properly controlled and randomized trial to assess the effect of BCG in superficial vesical neoplasms.

Undesirable side-effects directly attributable to the regimen of immunizations were tolerable. For the majority of patients they were minor and self-limiting and, except for the lower-tract manifestations, have been common findings during BCG therapy (Sparks *et al.*, 1973). Our present experience with administration of BCG suggests that the routine use of prophylactic isoniazid or an alternative antitubercular medication is not necessary but becomes mandatory in the presence of severe reactions.

The endoscopic appearance of the bladder epithelium may be deceptive following BCG therapy. A reddened, velvety mucosa may simply represent a residual inflammatory reaction or, alternatively, the ominous presence of carcinoma in situ. On the other hand, we have observed raised mucosal lesions highly suggestive of tumour recurrence which, on histological examination, proved to be granulomatous inflammation (*Figure 31.1*), a hallmark of effective BCG immunization.

In this trial, age appeared to be a possible determinant of treatment success. The subjects who showed complete or partial response were

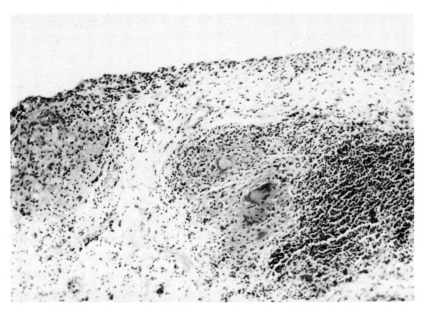

Figure 31.1 Microphotograph of a biopsy specimen from the bladder 12 weeks after onset of treatment. The mucosa is denuded and there is a marked granulomatous inflammatory reaction

significantly older on average ($P < 0.05$) than the four patients in whom the vaccine proved ineffective. Definitive answers on the role of age as a prognostic variable will require a larger population. No other factors emerged as a predictor of therapeutic success.

This study was designed to investigate the role of BCG as an adjuvant to surgery in the prevention of tumour recurrences; the effect of the vaccine alone in the destruction of superficial tumours is being investigated in a trial soon to be completed. The results presented here, essentially a Phase II investigation, have provided a reasonable judgement on the degree of efficacy and the nature of adverse effects of BCG at a particular dose and form of administration. A larger Phase III trial has independently confirmed the validity of our results (Lamm *et al.* 1980). Modifications to the present protocol and addition of other therapeutic modalities may enhance these gratifying results.

Editor's footnote. The discordant results presented in Chapter 30 and 31 are a reflection of the current uncertainty on the role of immunotherapy in cancer today. The significance of the relatively higher toxicity and lower antitumour activity in patients receiving intravesical treatment without systemic treatment requires further investigation.

REFERENCES

BAST, R.C., ZBAR, B., BORSOS, T. and RAPP, J.H. (1974). BCG and Cancer. *New England Journal of Medicine,* **290**, 1413–1420

BEAN, M.A. (1977). Some immunological considerations relevant to the study of human bladder cancer. *Cancer Research,* **37**, 2879–2884

BUBENIK, J., PERLMANN, P., HELMSTEIN, K. and MOBERGER, G. (1970). Immune response to urinary bladder tumours in man. *International Journal of Cancer,* **5**, 39–46

DeKERNION, J.B., GOLUB, S.H., GUPTA, R.K., SILVERSTEIN, M. and MORTON, D.L. (1975). Successful transurethral intralesional BCG therapy of a bladder melanoma. *Cancer,* **36**, 1662–1667

DOUVILLE, Y., PELOUZE, G., ROY, R., CHARROIS, R., KIBRITÉ, A., MARTIN, M., DIONNE, L., COULONVAL, L. and ROBINSON, J. (1978). Recurrent bladder papillomata treated with bacillus Calmette-Guérin: A preliminary report, (phase I trial). *Cancer Treatment Reports,* **62**, 551–552

EILBER, F.R., MORTON, D.F., HOLMES, E.C., SPARKS, F.C. and RAMMING, K.P. (1976). Adjuvant immunotherapy with BCG in the treatment of lymph node metastases from malignant melanoma. *New England Journal of Medicine,* **294**, 237–240

GREENE, L.F., HANASH, K.A. and FARROW, G.M. (1973). Benign papilloma or papillary carcinoma of the bladder? *Journal of Urology,* **110**, 205–207

LAMM, D.L., THOR, D.E., HARRIS, S.C., REYNA, J.A., STOGDILL, V.D. and RADWIN, H.M. (1980). BCG immunotherapy of superficial bladder cancer. *Journal of Urology* (in press)

McKNEALLY, M.F., MAUER, C.M. and KAUSEL, H.W. (1978). Regional immunotherapy of lung cancer using post-operative intrapleural BCG. *Progress in Cancer Research and Therapy,* **6**, 161–171

MARTÍNEZ-PIÑIERO, J.A. and MUNTAÑOLA, P. (1977). Non-specific immunotherapy with BCG vaccine in bladder tumours. *European Urology,* **3**, 11–22

MORALES, A., EIDINGER, D., and BRUCE, A.W. (1976). Intracavitary bacillus Calmette-Guérin in the treatment of superficial bladder tumors. *Journal of Urology,* **116**, 180–183

MORALES, A., EIDINGER, D. and BRUCE, A.W. (1978). Adjuvant BCG immunotherapy in recurrent superficial bladder cancer. *Progress in Cancer Research and Therapy,* **6**, 225–243

O'TOOLE, C., PERLMANN, P., UNSGAARD, B., MOBERGER, G. and EDSMYR, R. (1972). Cellular immunity to human urinary bladder carcinoma I. Correlation to clinical stage and radiotherapy. *International Journal of Cancer,* **10**, 77–91

OTT, L. (1977). In *An Introduction to Statistical Methods and Data analysis,* pp. 384–388. Boston, Duxbury Press

SOKAL, R.R. and ROHLF, F.J. (1969). In *Biometry. The Principles and Practice in Biological Research,* pp. 613–616. San Francisco; W.H. Freeman & Co

SPARKS, F.C., SILVERSTEIN, M.J., HUNT, J.S., HASKELL, C.M., PILCH, Y.H. and MORTON, D.L. (1973). Complications of BCG immunotherapy in patients with cancer. *New England Journal of Medicine,* **289**, 827–830

32

The Logistics of Adoptive Immunotherapy for Cancer using Pig Lymph Node Cells

R.C.L. Feneley, V.C. Harral and M.O. Symes

INTRODUCTION

The clinical management of patients with advanced invasive bladder carcinoma presents a major problem when cystectomy or radiotherapy are contraindicated. In such circumstances the possibility of adoptive immunotherapy was initially explored. Since April 1971, 108 patients with a variety of advanced malignant neoplasms have received a single infusion of tumour-immune pig mesenteric lymph node cells into the blood supply of their tumour. The principal tumours treated have been carcinoma of the urinary bladder and carcinoma of the ovary.

Experimental studies in tumour-bearing mice (Prichard-Thomas and Symes, 1978a, b; Lai and Prichard-Thomas, 1979) have indicated that, for an antitumour effect to be observed, the pig lymph node cells must be immunized against the relevant species antigens (tumour or skin) and make contact with the tumour, i.e. be injected i.v. to treat pulmonary tumours or i.p. to treat intraperitoneal tumours.

Thirty-one patients with invasive transitional cell carcinoma of the urinary bladder were treated, either by infusion of tumour-immune pig mesenteric lymph node cells into the tumour blood supply, followed 6 weeks later by 5500 rad, or by radiotherapy alone. The patients were paired before treatment using four criteria : age (nearest decade), sex, clinical stage (T3 or T4) and histological grade (average or high). The first patient in each pair then received combined treatment and the second, radiotherapy alone. Administration of pig cells before radio-therapy offered no advantage to the patient in terms of the incidence of remission or the length of survival after treatment (Symes *et al.*,

1978a). The patients in these two groups were compared retrospectively with a third group of six patients matched for clinical and pathological characteristics, and who had received pig cells followed by palliative radiotherapy (4000 rad) (Symes and Riddell, 1973). This last group of patients showed a significantly higher incidence of remissions (5/6) and lived longer than either of the other two groups. One explanation put forward for this difference was that radical (or high-dose) radio-therapy (5500 rad) interfered with a host antitumour immune response initiated by lymphokines released as a result of the initial pig cell antitumour reaction (Feneley *et al.*, 1974).

As a result of this potential effect of radical radiotherapy on the host response, the antitumour action of pig cells given alone in treatment was studied. Twenty-four patients with invasive transitional cell carcinoma of the bladder, that had failed to respond to a course of radical radiotherapy (5500–6000 rad) received a single infusion of pig cells as their sole treatment (Symes *et al.*, 1978b). In 23 of the patients the recurrent tumour was seen at endoscopy, and in 20 there was extra-vesical spread, detected by bi-manual examination under anaesthesia. In 15 of the patients the presence of recurrent tumour was confirmed histologically. Following treatment, six patients showed complete disappearance of their tumour at endoscopy and in five patients the extra-vesical tumour mass completely resolved. A further three patients showed a partial remission (i.e. > 50% reduction in tumour size seen at endoscopy). One patient is alive and tumour-free 5 years and 8 months after treatment, and a second at 1 year and 3 months, while a third patient, although alive 3 years after treatment, showed endoscopic evidence of recurrent tumour after 2 years and 8 months.

Finally, five patients with T3 or T4 carcinoma of the ovary, who had previously received the maximum possible surgery ± radiotherapy, received a single injection of tumour-immune pig lymph node cells (Turner and Symes, 1979). In four patients, the pig cells were injected into the tumour blood supply and two of these patients received, in addition, an intraperitoneal injection of cells. One patient died 12 days after treatment. At autopsy the tumours in the abdominal cavity and liver showed massive recent haemorrhagic necrosis. A second patient, who was known to have extensive intraperitoneal tumour deposits at the time of pig cell therapy, died 2 months later from progressive cachexia. However, at autopsy there was no evidence of tumour present in the peritoneal cavity. Two further patients had objective evidence of tumour remission, the first for a period of 2 months during which there was no evidence of previously persistent ascites, and the second for 4 months, during which time she lived a normal life and gained weight. However, both these patients eventually died from progressive disease. The fifth patient was 27 years of age and presented with a pleural effusion due to metastatic deposits from a carcinoma of the ovary. The primary lesion which was used to immunize the pig was the sole evidence of intra-abdominal tumour. She received pig cells by a combination of the intrapleural and intravenous routes. One to 2 weeks thereafter, she developed painful enlargement of the ipsilateral cervical and axillary nodes, following which, her effusion resolved. She is alive and well, 4 years and 8 months after treatment.

It may therefore be pertinent to review the logistic problems associated with the administration of this treatment.

LOGISTICS OF PIG LYMPH NODE CELL TREATMENT

Supply of pigs

The pig was originally chosen as a lymph node cell donor as it is readily available and relatively inexpensive. An approximately 20 kg female animal, costing £20 is normally used.

The pig possesses a long confluent chain of mesenteric lymph nodes, which can be immunized by implantation of tumour fragments into pockets made between the leaves of the mesentery. A cell suspension

Table 32.1
THE RESULTS OF CULTURE FOR MICRORGANISMS OF 2 ml ALIQUOTS OF PIG LYMPH NODE CELL SUSPENSIONS IN MEDIUM 199. BOTH AEROBIC AND ANAEROBIC CULTURES WERE MADE IN NUTRIENT BROTH

Outcome of culture	Number	Contaminating microorganisms
Sterile	73	Nil
Growth of microorganisms	26	23 coliforms*
		3 *Streptococcus faecalis**
		1 *Staphylococcus albus*

*One culture yielded a mixed growth of coliforms and *Strep. faecalis*

can readily be prepared from the nodes, seven days after immunization. Two millilitres of this suspension are cultured, both aerobically and anaerobically, in nutrient broth. The suspension in 73% of cases failed to yield any growth of microorganisms (*Table 32.1*).

Personnel and equipment

The urological team undertakes the clinical management of the patients receiving adoptive immunotherapy but close collaboration with the consultant immunologist is necessary to coordinate the preparation and administration of the lymph node cells. The patient is admitted to

hospital for cystoscopy, and a biopsy of 2–3 g of the tumour is undertaken by transurethral resection at a routine operating session. The
biopsy is transported to the Medical School in a fresh solution of
normal saline. One week later, the pig lymph node cell infusion is
performed under general anaesthesia, via a catheter introduced into the
femoral artery and passed up to the internal iliac artery on the side of
the bladder tumour, or to the abdominal aorta in cases where both
sides of the bladder are involved. Pneumatic cuffs are placed on both
thighs to occlude the arterial blood flow to the lower limbs during the
infusion. The patient normally leaves hospital 3–5 days later.

The pig surgery is conducted in a purpose-built animal operating
suite, and this is available in the University of Bristol Medical School.
One operator and, preferably, an assistant are required. As anaesthesia, O_2/N_2O and fluothane are administered to the pig from a
Boyles' apparatus via a nose cone.

The preparation of the pig lymph node cell suspensions has to be
performed quickly, in order to minimize cell death; two workers are
therefore essential. The procedure is carried out in a sterile vertical
lamina air-flow tissue culture cabinet in the Medical School. Thereafter, the cell suspension (100 ml) is transported to the patient in a
standard MRC blood transfusion bottle, placed in an ice bucket.

Cost of treatment

The cost of treatment with pig lymph node cells compares favourably
with other methods of managing advanced carcinoma of the bladder.

Table 32.2
A COMPARISON OF THE DEMAND FOR NATIONAL HEALTH SERVICE FACILITIES
AS BETWEEN AN INFUSION OF TUMOUR-IMMUNE PIG LYMPH NODE CELLS AND
TOTAL CYSTECTOMY, IN THE TREATMENT OF PATIENTS WITH RESIDUAL CARCI–
NOMA OF URINARY BLADDER FOLLOWING RADICAL RADIOTHERAPY (1977/78
COSTS)*

Variable	Infusion of pig lymph node cells	Cost of item (£)	Total cystectomy	Cost of item (£)
Length of stay in hospital	3 days	550	21 days (including some time in ITU	5000
Time spent in operating theatre	1 hour	450	3 hours	1400
Drugs given	Nil	–	I.V. fluids) for Blood) major Antibiotics) surgery	100
Extras	7 pigs	350	Time of stoma therapist	900
General Services			Stoma apparatus	
Inpatient costs		450	for rest of life	3200
Total costs		1800		10 600

* For seven patients treated in 1977

The comparison between immunotherapy and total cystectomy for recurrent lesions following radical radiotherapy is detailed in *Table 32.2.* The total cost* of immunotherapy has been estimated at £1800, and of surgery at £10600 in an NHS hospital. A note of caution should, however, be sounded. A series of 24 such patients treated by immunotherapy, is not adequate for comparison with the results of cystectomy. However, in a number of such patients, cystectomy is not possible and it is in any case associated with a high morbidity. In contrast, there do not seem to be any contraindications to the administration of immunotherapy, beyond suitability of the patient for a short general anaesthetic. In addition, we have observed no post-treatment complications.

FUTURE PROSPECTS

It is suggested that the logistic problems associated with this form of immunotherapy can conveniently be accommodated within existing National Health Service resources, provided that a University Medical School or similar facility is associated with the hospital concerned.

It is, however, of the greatest importance that any future studies should be in the form of prospective controlled trials.

Future trials of adoptive immunotherapy planned in Bristol, for stage T3 or T4 invasive transitional cell carcinoma of the bladder, will study the effect of tumour-immune pig lymph node cells, followed after 6 weeks by 4000 rad in 15 fractions compared with 5500 rad in 25 fractions alone.

ACKNOWLEDGEMENTS

We thank Mrs M. Stephens and Mr D. Loban for performing bacteriological culture of the pig lymph node cell suspensions. We are indebted to Mr G.W. Sweetnam, Animal Superintendent, University Medical School, for his continued advice concerning animal welfare. The clinical studies described were in part supported by the Cancer Research Campaign.

REFERENCES

FENELEY, R.C.L., ECKERT, H., RIDDELL, A.G., SYMES, M.O. and TRIBE, C.R. (1974). The treatment of advanced bladder cancer with sensitised pig lymphocytes. *British Journal of Surgery,* **61**, 825–827

*For 7 patients treated in 1977

LAI, T. and PRICHARD-THOMAS, S. (1979). The effect of immunisation and route of administration on the anti-tumour action of pig mononuclear cells. *British Journal of Surgery,* **66**, 367

PRICHARD-THOMAS, S. and SYMES, M.O. (1978a). The use of immunologically competent cells from pig mesenteric lymph nodes to treat pulmonary tumours in mice. *Cancer Immunology and Immunotherapy,* **5**, 129–134

PRICHARD-THOMAS, S. and SYMES, M.O. (1978b). Observations on the effect of radiotherapy, followed by injection of pig lymph node cells, in reducing the number of pulmonary tumours induced by intravenous injection of tumour cells into isogenic mice. *Cancer Immunology and Immunotherapy,* **5**, 135–139

SYMES, M.O., ECKERT, H., FENELEY, R.C.L., LAI, T., MITCHELL, J.P., ROBERTS, J.B.M. and TRIBE, C.R. (1978a). Adoptive immunotherapy and radiotherapy in the treatment of urinary bladder cancer. *British Journal of Urology,* **50**, 328–331

SYMES, M.O., ECKERT, H., FENELEY, R.C.L., LAI, T., MITCHELL, J.P., ROBERTS, J.B.M. and TRIBE, C.R. (1978b). Transfer of adoptive immunity by intra-arterial injection of tumor-immune pig lymph node cells: treatment of recurrent urinary bladder carcinoma after radical radiotherapy. *Urology,* **12**, 398–401

SYMES, M.O. and RIDDELL, A.G. (1973). The use of immunised pig lymph-node cells in the treatment of patients with advanced malignant disease. *British Journal of Surgery,* **60**, 176–180

TURNER, G.M. and SYMES, M.O. (1979). The use of sensitised pig lymph node cells in the treatment of carcinoma of the ovary. *British Journal of Cancer,* **40**, 823

Overview and Conclusions

H.J.G. Bloom, R.T.D. Oliver and W.F. Hendry

Bladder cancer is a disease with increasing incidence where there has been no further major improvement in survival since that which followed the introduction of megavoltage radiotherapy and modern techniques of surgery and anaesthesia in the 1950s. This book has provided an assessment of many of the controversial aspects of the current management of this disease and defines avenues for future progress.

Little controversy remains concerning the diagnosis and importance of clinical staging and histological grading of bladder tumours, although debate continues on the malignant potential of the papillary non-invasive tumour (loosely called 'papilloma' by some) which the new UICC classification has now set apart from other T1 tumours and designated as 'Ta'. The chapter on pathological staging by Dr Pugh re-emphasizes the importance of an accurate assessment of the precise extent of submucosal invasion in T1 tumours. In addition, he draws attention to a deficiency in the application of the UICC TNM classification by calling for the continuous reassessment of tumour staging on the basis of serial biopsy specimens rather than on the once-and-for-all category based on the first histological assessment.

Cytology in carcinoma of the bladder, although less well established than in carcinoma of the cervix, is generally under-used in the UK. Its potential as a screening test and in assessing response to treatment is emphasized in the chapter by Dr Esposti. This author also demonstrates the potential use of quantitative DNA histograms as measured in the cytofluorograph for a more precise measurement of response to treatment. It is hoped that this approach may provide additional information to that which may be obtained by drug screening techniques using cell culture and human tumour xenograft models to predict treatment response, thereby permitting a more selective treatment for the individual patient.

So far, there are few clinical situations where the role of CT scanning has clearly been established. Although the data for bladder cancer are only preliminary and larger studies correlating CT stages with the pathological stage found in the surgical specimen are urgently required, it seems that computerized tomography may reduce the considerable error rate of 25–30 per cent currently accepted in clinical staging techniques. Errors in staging may explain the discrepancy in the London Hospital results (Chapter 15) where patients with T3 tumours had a greater survival than those with T2 lesions.

The generally long natural history of patients with non-invasive malignant disease of the bladder often makes evaluation of treatment difficult. Recognition of high risk groups in this category is an important step in rationalizing treatment. Mr Riddle and also Mr England and his colleagues emphasize the possibility of classifying patients with papillary tumours on the basis of their response to chemotherapy to help in early selection of resistant cases for radical surgical treatment.

Only recently has flat carcinoma in situ been recognized as having an importance far beyond that warranted by its incidence as a purely primary condition. A study of its histopathology and natural history has provided information regarding steps in the development of bladder malignancy. Its early recognition and treatment may prevent neoplastic progression to the invasive stage. The demonstration of its high responsiveness to chemotherapy and lack of responsiveness to irradiation has important implications for its future management, since at the present time the only locally curative procedure is cystourethrectomy.

More controversy surrounds the treatment of invasive tumours than any other aspect discussed in this book. The problem is trying to balance the threat to life of the disease against the disturbance to function imposed by its treatment. Interstitial radiotherapy, as reported by Mr Grant Williams and his colleagues, is less used today than previously. It is an attractive technique compared with external beam therapy or cystectomy because it provides intensive local treatment, spares normal surrounding tissues and preserves bladder function. However, its scope is strictly limited, the technique being suitable only for highly selected tumours of limited size and depth of invasion. For the larger more extensive and more undifferentiated tumours, there is no place for this technique alone, although it may have a role as part of a combined approach with external beam therapy and/or systemic chemotherapy: this approach could reduce the need for cystectomy.

The controversies regarding external beam megavoltage radiotherapy techniques, particularly with regard to dose, fractionation and field size are to be found in the chapters by Dr Hope-Stone, Professor Edsmyr, Dr Bloom and Dr Whitmore. Although some data reported seem to favour inclusion of the regional lymph nodes in the irradiated volume, the conflicting data from Dr Hope-Stone, whose policy is to treat the bladder alone, merely serve to highlight the absence of controlled studies in this field. However, assessment of the relative merit of treating the bladder alone as opposed to the bladder and regional lymph nodes by external beam therapy is difficult, since, even with treatment portals of restricted size, the nodes must receive a substantial percentage of the tumour dose from the crossfiring beams. A further problem in comparing results with those in the London Hospital series arises from the discrepancy in prognosis between stages T2 and T3 cases: survival is greater for patients with tumours in the more advanced category.

Attempts to achieve a greater response of tumours to radiotherapy have been made by increasing the dose of irradiation and by changing treatment fractionation schedules. There is of course a limit to the maximum tumour dose which can be given. This is imposed by the risk of serious injury to normal tissues but, even with doses which approach or, in some cases, exceed the tolerance of adjacent organs, not more than about 50 per cent of bladder cancers will be eradicated. With pre-operative irradiation, a reduced dose of 2000 rad given over 1 week immediately followed by surgery, although producing less tumour downstaging in the available time to cystectomy, is currently achieving comparable survival rates to those following 4000 rad in 4 weeks with surgery after an interval of 1 month. Professor Edsmyr has investigated a new fractionation technique of radical radiotherapy using three fractions of irradiation per 24 hours and has reported encouraging early results: further follow-up is awaited with interest.

It is generally believed that tumour radiosensitivity is related to local tissue oxygenation at the time of treatment and that tumour resistance is largely due to hypoxic conditions resulting from progressive tumour growth outstripping its blood supply. The use of hyperbaric oxygen during irradiation to overcome tumour-cell hypoxia in patients with bladder cancer has been disappointing. The administration of chemical radiosensitizers, chiefly the electron-affinic nitroimidazole drugs, to obtain a greater selective tumour response has produced promising results in laboratory studies, but has yet to be evaluated clinically.

Compared with X-ray or gamma-ray irradiation, particle beam therapy with, for example, fast neutrons, is less dependent on oxygen and has a greater biological effect on tissues. Treatment with such beams may achieve greater local and regional control of relatively radio-resistant tumours of which bladder cancer is a good example.

The place for cystectomy in the treatment of deeply invasive tumours continues to be debated. The main controversy centres around the optimum timing for surgery: should it be carried out as a routine elective procedure following planned pre-operative irradiation or held in reserve as a 'salvage' procedure for failure after radical radiotherapy?

One factor which has become clear in recent years and is relevant to this debate, is the prognostic significance of a reduction in tumour stage ('downstaging') by radiotherapy. Such treatment-induced down-staging is important following radical radiotherapy and also after pre-operative irradiation: the former being assessed by follow-up cysto-scopies and bi-manual examinations, and the latter by examination of the surgical specimen (*see* Chapters 15, 17 and 18). The good survival of patients without tumour in their bladder after radical radiotherapy was used by Dr Hope-Stone and his colleagues to justify radical radio-therapy as routine treatment for deeply invasive tumours and to postpone the discussion about cystectomy until it was clear that the tumour had not been eradicated. However, in the Institute of Urology controlled trial of radical radiotherapy versus pre-operative radiotherapy and elective cystectomy (Chapter 17), survival of downstaged patients after pre-operative radiotherapy and elective cystectomy was better than that of downstaged patients after radical radiotherapy, although the difference was not statistically significant.

As far as non-downstage cases, i.e. non-responders to radiotherapy are concerned, there is little debate about the need for cystectomy as early as possible after the patient has been defined as a 'non-responder'. In the Institute of Urology trial, non-downstaged patients proceding to elective cystectomy did better than non-responders following radical radiotherapy who did not undergo salvage cystectomy. Although the higher survival rate in this study was seen in patients after salvage cystectomy, it should be remembered that such cases represent, in effect, a highly selected group since, in spite of local failure, their tumours must remain operable without detectable metastases.

The Institute of Urology study also demonstrated the importance of age — there was no benefit for elective cystectomy in patients over the age of 65 years and limited benefit for those in the 60—65 year age group: the greatest benefit for the combined treatment was seen in patients under the age of 60 years.

Metastatic disease from carcinoma of the bladder can undoubtedly respond to certain cytotoxic agents. In terms of response to single drugs, this tumour is more responsive than carcinoma of the kidney and colon, and seems to be as responsive as carcinoma of the breast and squamous-cell carcinoma of the head and neck. In none of the studies of chemotherapy for metastatic bladder cancer has there been a sub-stantially greater benefit for drug combinations compared with single agents. At present it appears that the most effective agents against transitional-cell carcinoma of the bladder are methotrexate, cis-platinum and doxorubicin, of which methotrexate is the best tolerated.

The use of chemotherapy as an adjuvant in the primary treatment of malignant disease is being widely explored in patients with breast and head-and-neck cancer. Since these tumours appear to have a response rate similar to that of single agent chemotherapy for transitional-cell carcinoma of the bladder, it is surprising that so little has been done to explore the role of chemotherapy in the primary treatment of bladder cancer. Preliminary results from three pilot trials of adjuvant chemotherapy in patients with carcinoma of the bladder are reported (*see* Chapters 25–27). It is clear that, with special attention to dose and timing, drugs can be given early in combination with other treatment without a serious increase in side-effects. It will require another 2–3 years before survival information will emerge from these strictly randomized trials which have been set up in the UK by the London/-Oxford and also the Yorkshire Urology Groups.

Although immunotherapy is not established as a therapeutic modality for any form of cancer, the responses reported of superficial tumours treated by intravesical BCG (*see* Chapter 31) and of invasive tumours treated by intra-arterial tumour-immune pig lymphocytes (*see* Chapter 32) does suggest that the immunological aspects of bladder cancer are worth further investigation.

We hope that this book has demonstrated the important interrelationships and the need for cooperation between the urologist, radiotherapist, medical oncologist and pathologist to obtain the best management for patients with bladder cancer and prospects for improved survival and function.

Index